Global Health and Critical Care Medicine

Editors

KRISTINA E. RUDD
WANGARI WAWERU-SIIKA

CRITICAL CARE CLINICS

www.criticalcare.theclinics.com

Consulting Editor
GREGORY S. MARTIN

October 2022 • Volume 38 • Number 4

ELSEVIER

1600 John F. Kennedy Boulevard • Suite 1800 • Philadelphia, Pennsylvania, 19103-2899

http://www.theclinics.com

CRITICAL CARE CLINICS Volume 38, Number 4
October 2022 ISSN 0749-0704, ISBN-13: 978-0-323-96181-3

Editor: Joanna Collett
Developmental Editor: Hannah Almira Lopez

Critical Care Clinics (ISSN: 0749-0704) is published quarterly by Elsevier Inc., 360 Park Avenue South, New York, NY 10010-1710. Months of issue are January, April, July, and October. Business and Editorial Offices: 1600 John F. Kennedy Blvd., Suite 1800, Philadelphia, PA 19103-2899. Customer Service Office: 6277 Sea Harbor Drive, Orlando, FL 32887-4800. Periodicals postage paid at New York, NY and additional mailing offices. Subscription prices are $266.00 per year for US individuals, $735 per year for US institutions, $100.00 per year for US students and residents, $296.00 per year for Canadian individuals, $921.00 per year for Canadian institutions, $338.00 per year for international individuals, $921.00 per year for international institutions, $100.00 per year for Canadian students/residents, and $150.00 per year for foreign students/residents. To receive student/resident rate, orders must be accompanied by name of affiliated institution, date of term, and the signature of program/residency coordinator on institution letterhead. Orders will be billed at individual rate until proof of status is received. Foreign air speed delivery is included in all *Clinics* subscription prices. All prices are subject to change without notice. POSTMASTER: Send address changes to *Critical Care Clinics*, Elsevier Periodicals Customer Service, 11830 Westline Industrial Drive, St. Louis, MO 63146. **Customer Service: 1-800-654-2452 (US). From outside of the US, call 1-314-447-8871. Fax: 1-314-447-8029. E-mail: journalscustomerservice-usa@elsevier.com (for print support) or journalsonlinesupport-usa@elsevier.com (for online support).**

Reprints. For copies of 100 or more of articles in this publication, please contact the Commercial Reprints Department, Elsevier Inc., 360 Park Avenue South, New York, NY 10010-1710. Tel.: 212-633-3874; Fax: 212-633-3820; E-mail: reprints@elsevier.com.

Critical Care Clinics is also published in Spanish by Editorial Inter-Medica, Junin 917, 1er A, 1113, Buenos Aires, Argentina.

Critical Care Clinics is covered in *MEDLINE/PubMed (Index Medicus), EMBASE/Excerpta Medica, Current Concepts/ Clinical Medicine, ISI/BIOMED,* and *Chemical Abstracts.*

Contributors

CONSULTING EDITOR

GREGORY S. MARTIN, MD, MSC
Professor, Division of Pulmonary, Allergy, Critical Care and Sleep Medicine, Research Director, Emory Critical Care Center, Director, Emory/Georgia Tech Predictive Health Institute, Co-Director, Atlanta Center for Microsystems Engineered Point-of-Care Technologies (ACME POCT), President, Society of Critical Care Medicine, Atlanta, Georgia, USA

EDITORS

KRISTINA E. RUDD, MD, MPH
Assistant Professor, The Clinical Research, Investigation, and Systems Modeling of Acute Illness (CRISMA) Center, Department of Critical Care Medicine, University of Pittsburgh, Pittsburgh, Pennsylvania, USA

WANGARI WAWERU-SIIKA, MBChB, MMed, FRCA
Clinical Associate Professor, Department of Anaesthesia, Aga Khan University, Nairobi, Kenya; Department for Continuing Education, University of Oxford, Oxford, United Kingdom

AUTHORS

MARY B. ADAM, MD, MA, PhD
AIC Kijabe Hospital, Kijabe, Kenya; ACQUIRE Africa Mission Healthcare Corporate Offices, Nairobi, Kenya

ANNE ALENYO-NGABIRANO, MD
Emergency Physician and COVID Emergency Coordinator, Ministry of Health, Kampala, Uganda

AMELIE VON SAINT ANDRE-VON ARNIM, MD
Department of Pediatrics, Division of Pediatric Critical Care, Department of Global Health, University of Washington, Seattle Children's, Seattle, Washington, USA

ANDREW C. ARGENT, MB, BCh, MMed(Paeds), MD(Paeds), DCH(SA), FCPaeds(SA), FRCPCH(UK), Cert Crit Care (Paeds) (SA)
Professor Emeritus, Department of Paediatrics and Child Health, University of Cape Town, Red Cross War Memorial Children's Hospital, Rondebosch, Cape Town, South Africa

HARSHIT ARORA, MBBS
Dayanand Medical College and Hospital, Non-academic Junior Resident, Department of Surgery, Punjab Institute of Medical Sciences, Jalandhar, India

DIPTESH ARYAL, MD
National Coordinator, Nepal Intensive Care Research Foundation, Kathmandu, Nepal

AMADO ALEJANDRO BAEZ, MD, MPH, PhD, FACEP, FCCM
Professor of Emergency Medicine and Epidemiology, Vice-Chair, Department of
Emergency Medicine, Medical College of Georgia, Augusta, Georgia, USA; Universidad
Nacional Pedro Henriquez Ureña (UNPHU), Santo Domingo, Dominican

TIM BAKER, MBChB, PhD
Department of Global Public Health, Karolinska Institutet, Stockholm, Sweden;
Department of Emergency Medicine, Muhimbili University of Health and Allied Sciences,
Ifakara Health Institute, Dar es Salaam, United Republic of Tanzania; Department of
Clinical Research, London School of Hygiene & Tropical Medicine, London, United
Kingdom

VARUN BANSAL, MBBS
Department of General Surgery, Seth Gordhandas Sundersas Medical College and King
Edward Memorial Hospital, Mumbai, India

LIA M. BARROS, DNP, AGACNP-BC
Division of Pulmonary, Critical Care, and Sleep Medicine, University of Washington
Medical Center, Seattle, Washington, USA

BRIAN JASON BROTHERTON, MD, MS
Department of Critical Care, AIC Kijabe Hospital, Kijabe, Kenya; Department of Critical
Care Medicine, University of Pittsburgh School of Medicine, Pittsburgh, Pennsylvania,
USA

DABOTA YVONNE BUOWARI, MBBS, DA
Department of Accident and Emergency, University of Port Harcourt Teaching Hospital,
Port Harcourt, Rivers State, Nigeria

BEVERLY CHESEREM, BM
Department of Neurosurgery, Aga Khan University Hospital, Nairobi, Kenya

Md JOBAYER CHISTI, MD, PhD
ARI Ward, Dhaka Hospital, Nutrition and Clinical Services Division, ICDDRB, Dhaka,
Bangladesh

MARTIN W. DÜNSER, MD
Department of Anesthesiology and Intensive Care Medicine, Kepler University Hospital
and Johannes Kepler University Linz, Linz, Austria

EUGENE WESLEY ELY, MD, MPH
Division of Allergy, Pulmonary, and Critical Care Medicine, Department of Medicine,
Critical Illness, Brain Dysfunction, and Survivorship (CIBS) Center, Vanderbilt University
Medical Center, Geriatric Research, Education, and Clinical Center (GRECC), Tennessee
Valley Healthcare System, Nashville, Tennessee, USA

ISABELLA FARIA, MD
Visiting Graduate Student, Program in Global Surgery and Social Change, Boston,
Massachusetts, USA; Faculdade de Medicina da Universidade Federal de Minas Gerais,
Belo Horizonte, Brazil

KRISHNAN GANAPATHY, M Ch (Neurosurgery), FICS, FACS, FAMS, PhD
Distinguished Professor, Tamilnadu Dr MGR Medical University, Director Apollo
Telemedicine Networking Foundation, Chennai, India

LALIT GUPTA, MBBS DA, DNB, MNAMS
Department of Anaesthesia and Critical Care, Maulana Azad Medical College, New Delhi, India

SAI PRAVEEN HARANATH, MBBS, MPH, FCCP
Medical Director, Apollo eACCESS TeleICU, Apollo Health City, Jubilee Hills, Hyderabad, Telangana, India

CARL HENEGHAN, MA, MRCGP, DPhil
Nuffield Department of Primary Care Health Sciences, University of Oxford, Oxford, United Kingdom

ROBERTO JABORNISKY, MD
Universidad Nacional Del Nordeste, Argentina, Pediatric Intensive Care Unit (Hospital Juan Pablo II and Hospital Olga Stuky) Argentina, Sociedad Latinoamericana de Cuidados Intensivos Pediátricos, LARed Network

YEWANDE KAMUNTU, PharmD
Program Manager, Expanding Access to Diagnosis and Treatment of Hypoxemia, Clinton Health Access Initiative, Kampala, Uganda

IMMACULATE KARIUKI-BARASA, MB, ChB, MMed
AIC Kijabe Hospital, Kijabe, Kenya

PAULINE KIMEU, MBCHB, DipPEC (SA)
Emergency Medicine Kenya Foundation, Nairobi, Kenya

GATEBE KIRONJI, MD, MPH
Vituity Emergency Medicine, Saint Agnes Hospital, Baltimore, USA

NIRANJAN KISSOON, MB, BS, FRCP(C), FAAP, MCCM, FACPE
British Columbia Children's Hospital and The University of British Columbia, Vancouver, British Columbia, Canada

ARTHUR KWIZERA, MD
Associate Professor and Staff Intensivist, Department of Anaesthesia and Critical Care, Makerere University, College of Health Sciences, Kampala, Uganda

HENRY KYOBE-BOSA, MD
Epidemiologist and Incident Commander COVID Task Force, Ministry of Health, Uganda Peoples Defense Forces, Uganda; Kellogg College, University of Oxford, United Kingdom

TSEGAZEAB LAEKE, MD
Division of Neurosurgery, Department of Surgery, College of Health Science, Addis Ababa University, Addis Ababa, Ethiopia; Department of Clinical Medicine, Faculty of Medicine, University of Bergen, Bergen, Norway; NIHR Global Health Research Group on Neurotrauma, University of Cambridge, Cambridge, United Kingdom

JENNIFER MAKIN, MD
Assistant Professor, Gynecological Specialties, Department of Obstetrics, Gynecology and Reproductive Science, The University of Pittsburgh Medical Center Magee-Womens Hospital, Pittsburgh, Pennsylvania, USA

MATTHEW F. MART, MD, MSc
Division of Allergy, Pulmonary, and Critical Care Medicine, Department of Medicine, Vanderbilt University Medical Center, Critical Illness, Brain Dysfunction, and Survivorship

(CIBS) Center, Vanderbilt University Medical Center, Geriatric Research, Education, and Clinical Center (GRECC), Tennessee Valley Healthcare System, Nashville, Tennessee, USA

PAUL MBUVI, MBCHB
Kenyatta National Hospital, Nairobi, Kenya

MERVYN MER, MD, MMed, PhD
Department of Medicine, Divisions of Critical Care and Pulmonology, Charlotte Maxeke Johannesburg Academic Hospital and Faculty of Health Sciences, University of the Witwatersrand, Johannesburg, South Africa

TRUFOSA MOCHACHE, MBCHB, DipPEC (SA)
Emergency Medicine Kenya Foundation, Nairobi, Kenya

GRACE MUKUNDI, BSc Nursing
Emergency Medicine Kenya Foundation, Nairobi, Kenya

NDIDIAMAKA L. MUSA, MD
Paediatric Critical Care, University of Washington, Seattle, Washington, USA

ADAN MUSTAFA, MBCHB, DipPEC (SA)
Emergency Medicine Kenya Foundation, Nairobi, Kenya

BENJAMIN MUTISO, MBChB
Department of Neurosurgery, University of Nairobi, Kenyatta National Hospital, Nairobi, Kenya

BENARD D. MUTWIRI, BSc
School of Nursing and Midwifery, Aga Khan University, Nairobi, Kenya

PATIENCE A. MUWANGUZI, PhD
Head, Department of Nursing, College of Health Sciences, Makerere University, Kampala, Uganda

JANE NAKIBUUKA, PhD
Senior Consultant and Head of ICU, Department of Medicine, Intensive Care Unit, Mulago National Referral Hospital, Kampala, Uganda

EUNICE NDIRANGU-MUGO, PhD, MScANP, BScN
School of Nursing and Midwifery, Aga Khan University, Nairobi, Kenya

ARY SERPA NETO, MD, MSc, PhD
Australian and New Zealand Intensive Care Research Centre (ANZIC-RC), School of Public Health and Preventive Medicine, Monash University, Melbourne, Victoria, Australia; Department of Critical Care, University of Melbourne, Parkville, Victoria, Australia; Department of Intensive Care, Austin Health, Heidelberg, Victoria, Australia; Department of Critical Care Medicine, Hospital Israelita Albert Einstein, Sao Paulo, Brazil

DAVID NGUGI, Diploma Nursing
Emergency Medicine Kenya Foundation, Nairobi, Kenya

NATHAN D. NIELSEN, MD, MSc
Division of Pulmonary, Critical Care, and Sleep Medicine, Section of Transfusion Medicine and Therapeutic Pathology, Departments of Medicine and Pathology, University of New Mexico School of Medicine, Albuquerque, New Mexico, USA

SALLY NJONJO, BSc Nursing
Emergency Medicine Kenya Foundation, Nairobi, Kenya

EMILY NYAGAKI, MSc Digital Business
Emergency Medicine Kenya Foundation, Nairobi, Kenya

NELSON NYAMU, MD, MRCEM
MMed Family Medicine, DipPEC (SA), Emergency Medicine Kenya Foundation, Nairobi, Kenya

CHARLES OLARO, MD
Director Clinical Services, Ministry of Health, Kampala, Uganda

CHRISTIAN OWOO, MBChB, DA, FGCS, MPH
Department of Anaesthesia, University of Ghana Medical School, College of Health Sciences, Department of Anaesthesia, Korle Bu Teaching Hospital, Accra, Ghana; Ghana Infectious Disease Centre, Kwabenya, Ga East, Accra, Ghana; University of Ghana Medical Centre, Legon, Accra, Ghana

MARK J. PETERS, MBChB, MRCP, FRCPCH, FFICM, PhD
University College London Great Ormond St Institute of Child Health, Paediatric Intensive Care Unit, Great Ormond St Hospital NHS Foundation Trust, London, United Kingdom

ANNETTE PLÜDDEMANN, PhD
Nuffield Department of Primary Care Health Sciences, University of Oxford, Oxford, United Kingdom

JUAN CARLOS PUYANA, MD
Professor of Surgery, Critical Care Medicine, and Clinical Translational Science, Director for Global Health-Surgery, University of Pittsburgh, UPMC Presbyterian, Pittsburgh, Pennsylvania, USA

MADIHA RAEES, MD
Division of Critical Care Medicine, Department of Anesthesia and Critical Care Medicine, Children's Hospital of Philadelphia, Philadelphia, Pennsylvania, USA

SUCHITRA RANJIT, MD, FCCM
Pediatric ICU, Apollo Children's Hospital, Chennai, India

NAKUL RAYKAR, MD, MPH
Faculty, Program in Global Surgery and Social Change, Harvard Medical School, Faculty, Division of Trauma and Emergency Surgery, Faculty, Center for Surgery and Public Health, Assistant Professor of Surgery, Brigham and Women's Hospital, Boston, Massachusetts, USA

ELISABETH D. RIVIELLO, MD, MPH
Division of Pulmonary, Critical Care, and Sleep Medicine, Beth Israel Deaconess Medical Center, Harvard Medical School, Boston, Massachusetts, USA

NOBHOJIT ROY, MD, MPH, PhD
WHO Collaborating Center for Research on Surgical Care Delivery in LMICs, Mumbai, India; The George Institute of Global Health, New Delhi, India

KRISTINA E. RUDD, MD, MPH
Assistant Professor, The Clinical Research, Investigation, and Systems Modeling of Acute Illness (CRISMA) Center, Department of Critical Care Medicine, University of Pittsburgh, Pittsburgh, Pennsylvania, USA

MEDDY RUTAYISIRE, MD
Case Management Committee, Department of Anaesthesia and Critical Care, Makerere University, College of Health Sciences, Kampala, Uganda

CARL OTTO SCHELL, MD
Department of Global Public Health, Karolinska Institutet, Stockholm, Sweden; Centre for Clinical Research Sörmland, Uppsala University, Eskilstuna, Sweden; Department of Medicine, Nyköping Hospital, Nyköping, Sweden

BENJAMIN K. SCOTT, MD
Associate Professor of Anesthesiology and Critical Care, University of Colorado School of Medicine, Aurora, Colorado, USA

CORNELIUS SENDAGIRE, MD, MBChB, MMed
Lecturer, Cardiac Anaesthesiologist and Intensivist, Department of Anaesthesia and Critical Care, Makerere University, College of Health Sciences, Kampala, Uganda

BHAVNA SETH, MD, MHS
Division of Pulmonary and Critical Care Medicine, Department of Medicine, Johns Hopkins School of Medicine, Baltimore, Maryland, USA

CONSTANCE S. SHUMBA, PhD, Msc, BSc
School of Nursing and Midwifery, Aga Khan University, Nairobi, Kenya

KAPIL DEV SONI, MD
Additional Professor, Critical and Intensive Care, Jai Prakash Narayan Apex Trauma Center, All India Institute of Medical Sciences, New Delhi, India

JANET SUGUT, MBCHB
Emergency Medicine Kenya Foundation, Nairobi, Kenya

NEIL THIVALAPILL, MS
Data Analyst, Institute for Public Health and Medicine, Northwestern University Feinberg School of Medicine, Chicago, Illinois, USA

THEOGENE TWAGIRUMUGABE, MD, PhD
Department of Anesthesiology, Kigali University Teaching Hospital, University of Rwanda, College of Medicine and Health Sciences, School of Medicine and Pharmacy, Kigali, Rwanda

SUKRITI VERMA, MBBS
Himalayan Institute of Medical Sciences, Non-academic Junior Resident, GTB Hospital, New Delhi, India; WHO Collaborating Center for Research on Surgical Care Delivery in LMICs, Mumbai, India

MARTIN GERDIN WÄRNBERG, MD, PhD
Department of Global Public Health, Karolinska Institutet, Stockholm, Sweden; Function Perioperative Medicine and Intensive Care, Karolinska University Hospital, Solna, Sweden

BENJAMIN WACHIRA, MBCHB, MD
Assistant Professor Emergency Medicine, Aga Khan University, Nairobi, Kenya

GRACE WANJIKU, MD, MPH
Assistant Professor Emergency Medicine, The Warren Alpert Medical School of Brown University, Providence, Rhode Island, USA

BETH WAWERU, BScN, MscN
School of Nursing and Midwifery, Aga Khan University, Nairobi, Kenya

WANGARI WAWERU-SIIKA, MBChB, MMed, FRCA
Clinical Associate Professor, Department of Anaesthesia, Aga Khan University, Nairobi, Kenya; Department for Continuing Education, University of Oxford, Oxford, United Kingdom

Contents

Critical illness is a state of ill health with vital organ dysfunction, a high risk of imminent death if care is not provided, and the potential for reversibility. An estimated 45 million adults become critically ill each year. While some are treated in emergency departments or intensive care units, most are cared for in general hospital wards. We outline a priority for health systems globally: the first-tier care that all critically ill patients should receive in all parts of all hospitals: Essential Emergency and Critical Care. We describe its relation to other specialties and care and opportunities for implementation.

This review provides insights on the current state of roles and responsibilities, on-the-job training, barriers, and facilitators of critical care nursing (CCN) practice. Some of the established roles and training of CCN were providing care for acutely ill patients, delivering expert and specialist care, working as a part of a multidisciplinary team, monitoring, and initiating timely treatment, and providing psychosocial support and advanced system treatment, especially in high-income countries. In low-resource settings, critical care nurses work as health care assistants, technical or ancillary staff, and clinical educators; manage medications; care for mechanically ventilated patients; and provide care to deteriorating patients.

Trauma is a leading cause of morbidity and mortality globally, with a significant burden attributable to the low- and middle-income countries (LMICs), where more than 90% of injury-related deaths occur. Road injuries contribute largely to the economic burden from trauma and are prevalent among adolescents and young adults. Trauma systems vary widely across the world in their capacity of providing basic and critical care to injured patients, with delays in treatment being present at multiple levels at LMICs. Strengthening existing systems by providing cost-effective and efficient solutions can help mitigate the injury burden in LMICs.

workers (HCWs). The recent COVID-19 pandemic has resulted in millions of severely ill patients, many of whom who have required hospital and intensive care unit (ICU) admission. The discipline of critical care is a vital and integral component of pandemic preparedness. Safe and effective critical care has the potential to improve outcomes, motivate individuals to seek timely medical attention, and attenuate the devastating sequelae of a severe pandemic. To achieve this, suitable critical care planning and preparation are essential.

CRITICAL CARE CLINICS

SERIES OF RELATED INTEREST

Emergency Medicine Clinics
https://www.emed.theclinics.com/
Clinics in Chest Medicine
https://www.chestmed.theclinics.com/

THE CLINICS ARE AVAILABLE ONLINE!
Access your subscription at:
www.theclinics.com

Preface

Global Critical Care: Innovation for the Sickest Patients Worldwide

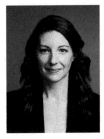
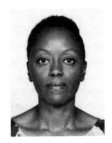

Kristina E. Rudd, MD, MPH   Wangari Waweru-Siika, MBChB, MMed, FRCA
Editors

Global critical care emphasizes and promotes the practice of critical care medicine worldwide, with consideration of the epidemiologic, resource, logistical, and health systems contexts in which different people live. This concept has been established for at least several decades. Although the first World Congress of Intensive Care Medicine held in 1973 drew delegates from only four countries, the group has grown to become the World Federation of Intensive and Critical Care, with membership from more than 85 critical care societies from across the globe.

While traditionally limited to a few highly resourced intensive care unit (ICU) environments, critical care as a discipline has moved beyond the walls of the ICU to other places where seriously ill patients need care, from emergency departments, to acute care wards, to operating theatres, and beyond. This growth of critical care as a philosophic approach and a system of care delivery, rather than care provided in a specific place, has been driven by the multidisciplinary nature of the field, particularly on a global level. This is beautifully exemplified by the diverse authorship in this unique collection, which includes nurses, trauma surgeons, pediatricians, obstetrician-gynecologists, medical ethicists, anesthesiologists, pulmonologists, epidemiologists, emergency medicine physicians, neurosurgeons, and others. Global critical care acknowledges and embraces the variation in human, material, economic, and other resources across diverse settings. This challenge of providing excellent, timely, appropriate, ethical care despite variable resources leads to tremendous innovation that benefits the entire discipline.

This collection features collaborative articles from a highly diverse group of authors who are thought leaders from a wide range of geographic and resource settings. The collection opens with an article focused on the current concept of essential emergency and critical care, outlining a global critical care approach and laying out strategies for

Crit Care Clin 38 (2022) xvii–xviii
https://doi.org/10.1016/j.ccc.2022.07.009
0749-0704/22/© 2022 Published by Elsevier Inc.   criticalcare.theclinics.com

implementing this essential care worldwide (Buowari et al). Ndirangu-Mugo et al focuses specifically on development of the global critical care nursing workforce, an important bedrock to the provision of critical care in any setting. This is followed by several articles that focus on the provision of critical care for special populations; those with trauma or other acute surgical needs (Dev Soni et al), children (Argent et al), and those with life-threatening neurologic conditions (Raees et al). Other articles focus on developing health systems' capacity to provide critical care, whether that is broadly in limited-resource settings, such as Uganda (Kwizera et al), or during public health emergencies, such as the COVID-19 pandemic (Mer et al), or focused more narrowly on the provision of essential resources, such as blood for transfusion (Faria et al) or supplemental oxygen (Mart et al). The next several articles present innovative approaches to the development of health systems' capacity to deliver important components of critical care, such as telemedicine services (Ganapathy et al) or cardiac ultrasound (Waweru-Siika et al), or focus on educational tools, such as simulation, to enhance provision of key critical care services (Nyamu et al). Finally, our closing article presents ethical challenges that arise in the care of critically ill patients in resource-limited settings, with lessons to be learned for the entire field of global critical care (Kariuki-Barasa and Adam). Together, these articles represent the innovation and diversity that are signature features of the field of global critical care and present potential solutions to guide our field as we strive to provide excellent, life-saving care to the sickest patients around the globe.

Kristina E. Rudd, MD, MPH
The Clinical Research, Investigation, and
Systems Modeling of Acute Illness (CRISMA) Center
Department of Critical Care Medicine
University of Pittsburgh
3520 Fifth Avenue, Suite 100
Pittsburgh, PA 15026, USA

Wangari Waweru-Siika, MBChB, MMed, FRCA
Department of Anaesthesia
Aga Khan University
3rd Parklands Avenue, PO Box 30270
Nairobi 00100, Kenya

E-mail addresses:
ruddk@pitt.edu (K.E. Rudd)
wangari.siika@aku.edu (W. Waweru-Siika)

Essential Emergency and Critical Care

A Priority for Health Systems Globally

Dabota Yvonne Buowari, MBBS, DA[a],
Christian Owoo, MBChB, DA, FGCS, MPH[b,c,d,e],
Lalit Gupta, MBBS, DA, DNB, MNAMS[f], Carl Otto Schell, MD[g,h,i],
Tim Baker, MBChB, PhD[g,j,k,l],*, The EECC Network Group

KEYWORDS

- Critical care • Emergency care • Global health • Essential health services
- Quality of care • Low- and middle-income countries

KEY POINTS

- Critical illness is common, and the majority of critically ill patients are cared for outside intensive care units in emergency departments and general hospital wards.
- The COVID-19 pandemic has led to surges of critical illness that have threatened to overwhelm health systems.
- Essential Emergency and Critical Care (EECC) has been defined as the care that all critically ill patients should receive in all wards and units in all hospitals in the world.

Continued

[a] Department of Accident and Emergency, University of Port Harcourt Teaching Hospital, Along East West Road, Alakahia, Port Harcourt, Rivers State 23401, Nigeria; [b] Department of Anaesthesia, University of Ghana Medical School, College of Health Sciences, Guggisberg Avenue, Korle Bu, GA-029-4296 Accra, Ghana; [c] Department of Anaesthesia, Korle Bu Teaching Hospital, Guggisberg Avenue, Korle Bu, GA-029-4296 Accra, Ghana; [d] Ghana Infectious Disease Centre, Kwabenya, Ga East, Municipal Hospital, GE-255-9501 (PQ47+FGV), Accra, Ghana; [e] University of Ghana Medical Centre, Indian Ocean Link, University of Ghana, GA-337-6980 (JRJ7+WJP) Accra, Ghana; [f] Department of Anaesthesia and Critical Care, Maulana Azad Medical College, 2 Bahadur Shah Zafar Marg, New Delhi 110002, India; [g] Department of Global Public Health, Karolinska Institutet, Solna Väg, Stockholm, 171 77, Sweden; [h] Centre for Clinical Research Sörmland, Uppsala University, Sveavägen entré 9 Mälarsjukhuset, Eskilstuna, 631 88 Sweden; [i] Department of Medicine, Nyköping Hospital, Nyköping 61185, Sweden; [j] Department of Emergency Medicine, Muhimbili University of Health and Allied Sciences, United Nations Road, Dar es Salaam, P.O. Box 65001, Tanzania; [k] Department of Clinical Research, London School of Hygiene & Tropical Medicine, Keppel Street, London, WC1E 7HT, UK; [l] Ifakara Health Institute, 5 Ifakara Street, Plot 463 Mikocheni, Dar es Salaam, P.O. Box 78 373, Tanzania
* Corresponding author. Department of Emergency Medicine, Muhimbili University of Health and Allied Sciences, Dar es Salaam, P.O. Box 65001, Tanzania
E-mail address: tim.baker@ki.se

Crit Care Clin 38 (2022) 639–656
https://doi.org/10.1016/j.ccc.2022.06.008
0749-0704/22/© 2022 Elsevier Inc. All rights reserved.

Continued

- The large unmet need for EECC across medical specialties in hospitals is likely to contribute to substantial numbers of preventable deaths.
- EECC is an essential component of Universal Health Coverage and can help health systems cope with pandemics and other public health emergencies.

Worldwide, an estimated 45 million people suffer from critical illness each year.[1] Critical illness is "a state of ill health with vital organ dysfunction, a high risk of imminent death if care is not provided, and the potential for reversibility."[2]. Patients of all ages and conditions can deteriorate and become critically ill at any point in the health care system. Although critical illness is often thought of as something mostly relevant to intensive care units (ICUs) or emergency departments (EDs), most critically ill patients are cared for in general hospital wards.[3–7] This article outlines a priority for health systems globally: the first-tier care that all critically ill patients should receive, described as essential emergency and critical care (EECC), its relation to other specialties, approaches and initiatives, and opportunities for implementation.

NEGLECTED CARE OF CRITICALLY ILL PATIENTS

The care of critically ill patients is often overlooked in hospitals, resulting in delayed and low-quality care.[8–10] Hospitals are largely organized by specialty, providing care focused on diagnosing and providing definitive treatments rather than illness severity, and there can be gaps in critical care provision. The gaps are largest in low-staffed and low-resourced settings, such as in general wards and hospitals in low-and middle-income countries (LMICs).[11] In studies from Malawi, only 10%–29% of hypoxic hospitalized patients received supplemental oxygen, and 75% of children who died from pneumonia never received oxygen.[4,12,13] Even in high-income countries, a substantial proportion of preventable deaths and ICU admissions have been seen to be preceded by a lack of clinical monitoring or basic organ support.[14,15] Health policies have little emphasis on critical care and health systems often lack structures and fail to ensure implementation and coverage of critical illness care.[8,16,17] The likely result is substantial preventable mortality.[18,19]

CARE OF CRITICALLY ILL PATIENTS AT DIFFERENT RESOURCE LEVELS

Treating critical illness can be done at different resource levels. The highest resource level is typically seen in ICUs, in advanced EDs, or in operating theaters. Such units, when available, can provide sophisticated, advanced critical care, including mechanical ventilation, cardiovascular support, and other advanced organ support through intensive human and material resources.[20] Many hospitals have high dependency units (HDUs), which commonly provide care for critically ill patients that is one step down from ICUs but of greater intensity than care in general wards. HDUs may provide vital organ support, up to but not including invasive mechanical ventilation. Critically ill patients are also often managed in general wards, cared for by nurses and doctors who may lack specialist training in the care of such patients. Available resources for care also depend greatly on the existing resources in the health system. In general, smaller health facilities and district hospitals have fewer resources than university or referral centers, hospitals in LMICs have fewer resources than those in high-income countries,[17] and there are fewer staff and services available in hospitals in the night-time and at weekends. Even when resources are low, critical care in the form of early identification of critical illness and the provision of first-tier care has the potential to stabilize vital organ functions and save lives.[18]

THE COVID-19 PANDEMIC

The COVID-19 pandemic has highlighted the need for critical care. Each wave of the pandemic has led to a surge of critically ill patients requiring hospital care and treatment for their life-threatening conditions.[21] Health systems have repeatedly become overstretched, with wards, HDUs, and ICUs becoming full or overwhelmed, and additional and off-service staff drafted in to work in areas of need. Critically ill patients suffering from other conditions have been unable to access care, and there have been acute shortages of vital treatments such as oxygen.[22] Huge global efforts have been made to scale-up intensive care in the pandemic, including designing new mechanical ventilators, shipping advanced ICU equipment around the world, and expanding ICU capacities.[23] However, it is clear that the fundamental barriers to effective provision of care to critically ill patients could not be overcome with only the procurement of equipment.[24,25] These barriers include a lack of staff trained in emergency and critical care; health systems and hospitals that were not prepared for the surge of critically ill patients; and a lack of established standards, guidelines, and protocols for managing critical illness in low-resource settings.[21]

THE OPTIMAL APPROACH TO THE CARE OF CRITICALLY ILL PATIENTS

Ideally, all critically ill patients should have the opportunity to receive all the care that they would benefit from. However, the realities of resource constraints mean that approaches need to be context-appropriate and balanced with competing priorities in the local health system. The highest priority care should be introduced before other care. Costs and cost-effectiveness considerations are vital to aid decisions about optimal approaches for maximum impact on population health, guided by ethical principles, such as autonomy, equity, beneficence, and justice.[26]

ESSENTIAL EMERGENCY AND CRITICAL CARE

EECC has been developed as the most simple, effective treatments and actions that can save the lives of patients with critical illness: the "first tier" of care for critical illness that is less complex than intermediate or advanced forms of emergency and critical care (**Fig. 1**).

EECC is defined as the care that all critically ill patients should receive in all hospitals in the world,[27] and is the care that supports vital organ functions; the universal care for all critical illnesses, irrespective of the patient's age, socio-economic status, underlying condition, or treating specialty. EECC is intended to be feasible in all wards and units in all hospitals, complementing specialty-based care and guidelines, and to be task-shared among doctors, nurses, and other health workers. EECC provides a means to bridge the commonly found quality gap between current practices in care for critical illness and best-practice guidelines. It does not aim to be comprehensive—in addition to EECC, patients should receive other care, such as nursing care, diagnostics, definitive and symptomatic care of their condition, end-of-life care if appropriate, and if needed and available, higher levels of emergency and critical care.

EECC is divided into two domains—the *identification* and the *treatment* of critical illness. Each domain requires resources (hospital readiness) to enable the processes of care (clinical practice) to ensure effective coverage of care (**Fig. 2**).

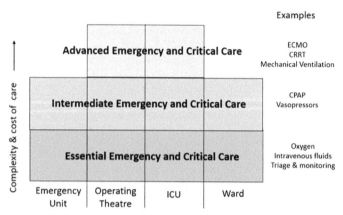

Fig. 1. The relationship between essential, intermediate, and advanced emergency and critical care. CPAP, continuous positive airway pressure; CRRT, continuous renal replacement therapy; ECMO, extracorporeal membrane oxygenation. (*Adapted from* Schell CO, Gerdin Wärnberg M, Hvarfner A, et al. The global need for essential emergency and critical care. Crit Care. 2018;22(1):284. Published 2018 Oct 29. https://doi.org/10.1186/s13054-018-2219-2.)

The content of EECC has recently been specified through a consensus of global experts.[28] EECC contains 40 processes—30 clinical processes and 10 general processes, including such items as triage and monitoring using vital signs, oxygen therapy, intravenous fluids, and patient positioning (**Table 1**). For the provision of these clinical processes, hospital readiness requirements have been specified, divided into the categories of equipment, consumables, drugs, human resources, training, routines, guidelines, and infrastructure.

RELATIONSHIP BETWEEN ESSENTIAL EMERGENCY AND CRITICAL CARE AND OTHER APPROACHES, INITIATIVES, AND DISCIPLINES

EECC is not a standalone specialty but is rather part of all acute disciplines and is complementary to specialty-based diagnostics and definitive therapies. There are

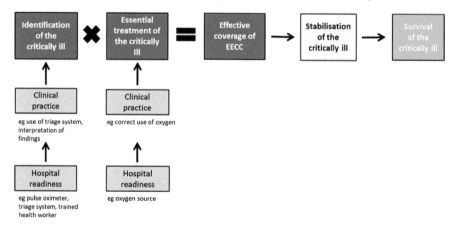

Fig. 2. EECC: a conceptual framework. (*Adapted from* Schell CO, Gerdin Wärnberg M, Hvarfner A, et al. The global need for essential emergency and critical care. Crit Care. 2018;22(1):284. Published 2018 Oct 29. https://doi.org/10.1186/s13054-018-2219-2.)

Table 1
The clinical processes in essential emergency and critical care

Identification of Critical Illness

Critical illness is identified as soon as possible so that timely care can be provided.

1. The hospital uses vital signs-based triage to identify critical illness
   1.1 Triage/identification of critical illness includes the use of these vital signs
       1.1.1 Pulse rate
       1.1.2 Blood pressure
       1.1.3 Respiratory rate
       1.1.4 Oxygen saturation
       1.1.5 Temperature
       1.1.6 Level of consciousness (eg, "alert, verbal, pain, unresponsive," "alert, confusion, voice, pain, unresponsive" or Glasgow Coma Scale)
       1.1.7 Presence of abnormal airway sounds heard from the bedside (eg, snoring, gurgling, stridor)
       1.1.8 The overall condition of the patient (health worker's concern that the patient is critically ill)
   1.2 Triage/identification of critical illness is conducted at these times
       1.2.1 When a patient arrives at hospital seeking acute care
       1.2.2 For hospital in-patients, at least every 24 h, unless otherwise prescribed, with increased frequency for patients who are at risk of becoming critically ill or who are critically ill, and then less frequently again when patients are stabilizing
       1.2.3 When a health worker, or the patient or guardian, is concerned that a patient may be critically ill
       1.2.4 During and after surgery or anesthesia
       1.2.5 During and after transport/transfer of a patient who is critically ill or at risk of becoming critically ill
       1.2.6 Following a treatment or action (re-evaluation)

Care of Critical Illness

Essential care of critical illness is initiated as soon as critical illness is identified and involves these clinical processes when appropriate:

Airway

Care for a blocked or threatened airway
   2. Placing the patient in the recovery position (lateral position)
   3. Age-appropriate airway positioning (eg, chin lift or jaw thrust in adults, neutral position in young children)
   4. Removal of any visible foreign body from the mouth or use of age-appropriate chest thrusts/abdominal thrusts/back blows in choking
   5. Suction for secretions that are obstructing the airway
   6. Insertion of an oro-pharyngeal (Guedel) airway

(continued on next page)

Table 1
(continued)

Breathing Care for hypoxia or respiratory distress	7. Optimizing the patient's position (eg, sitting-up or prone) 8. Oxygen therapy using nasal prongs, facemask, or mask with a reservoir bag (non-rebreathing mask) 9. Bag-valve-mask ventilation in threatened or manifest respiratory arrest
Circulation Care for a threatened circulation or shock	10. Optimizing the patient position (eg, lying flat, head-down, raised-legs, lateral tilt in pregnancy) 11. Compression and elevation to stop bleeding 12. Appropriate bolus of intravenous fluid 13. Oral rehydration solution or other appropriate oral fluids for dehydration without shock 14. Intramuscular adrenaline for anaphylaxis 15. Uterine massage and/or oxytocin when indicated
Reduced Conscious Level Care for a reduced level of consciousness	16. Treating an unconscious patient as having a threatened airway (eg, recovery position, etc.) 17. Dextrose (intravenous or buccal) in unconsciousness or seizures unless bedside blood glucose testing rules out hypoglycemia or there is a clear alternative cause 18. Protecting patients with a seizure from harm 19. Quick-acting antiseizure medication (eg, intravenous/rectal diazepam, or magnesium sulfate in pregnancy/post-partum) 20. Cooling in severe hyperthermia with a reduced level of consciousness
Other Care in essential emergency and critical care Other immediate or ongoing care of critical illness	21. Insertion of an intravenous cannula when critical illness is identified 22. Insertion of an intraosseous cannula, if indicated, if an intravenous cannula is not possible 23. Stabilizing the cervical spine in possible cervical spine injury 24. Appropriate antibiotics for sepsis 25. Treatment of pain and anxiety (eg, with needs-based psychological support, medication) 26. Keeping the patient warm using blankets and other means (including skin-to-skin care for babies) 27. Feeding (including breastfeeding for babies), naso-gastric feeding and dextrose for nutrition and to avoid hypoglycemia 28. Prevention of delirium (eg, sleep hygiene, provision of the patient's glasses or hearing aid) 29. Regular turning of immobilized patients 30. Mobilizing the patient as early as possible

General Processes

Care is provided according to these general processes:

1. Assistance from additional or senior staff is sought when a critically ill patient is identified
2. Essential emergency and critical care is respectful and patient-centered
3. EECC is provided without considering the patient's ability to pay
4. Critically ill patients are cared for in locations that facilitate observation and care (eg, designated beds, a bay, or a unit for critically ill patients)
5. Infection, prevention, and control measures are used including hand hygiene and separation of patients with a suspected or confirmed contagious disease from those without
6. Communication is clear, including:
   - Within the care team when a patient is identified as critically ill (eg, verbal communication, at staff handovers, visible color coding)
   - Within the care team about the planned essential emergency and critical care (eg, continue oxygen therapy, give intravenous fluids)
   - Documentation in the patient notes about the vital signs, when critical illness has been identified and the treatments and actions conducted
   - Effective and respectful communication with the patient and family
7. If there is poor response to treatment, or if the patient deteriorates, other indicated essential emergency and critical care clinical processes are used
8. Clinical processes are discontinued that are no longer indicated (eg, if a patient improves or if they are deemed to no longer be in the patient's best interest)
9. It is recognized when essential emergency and critical care alone is not sufficient to manage the critical illness
10. Essential emergency and critical care is integrated with care that is outside the scope of essential emergency and critical care (eg, the need for prompt investigations, definitive treatment of underlying conditions, including following disease-specific best-practice guidelines, end-of-life care, referral)

Addendum: Extended identification of critical illness

To maintain feasibility of the essential emergency and critical care package, only a limited number of signs for the identification of critical illness are included. However, if time and expertise allow, there are additional signs that are not part of essential emergency and critical care that aid the identification of critical illness:

- Presence of respiratory distress (eg, unable to complete sentences; accessory muscle use; chest recessions; grunting or head nodding)
- Cyanosis
- Capillary refill time
- Cold or warm extremities
- Presence of severe dehydration (eg, decreased skin turgor; dry mucous membranes; sunken fontanelle)
- Confused, agitated, or disoriented mental state
- Presence of prostration or lethargy
- Presence of a generalized seizure
- Inability to stand or walk without help
- Inability to breastfeed or feed in a young child
- Presence of severe acute malnutrition

Modified from Schell CO, Gerdin Wärnberg M, Hvarfner A, et al. The global need for essential emergency and critical care. Crit Care. 2018;22(1):284. Published 2018 Oct 29. https://doi.org/10.1186/s13054-018-2219-2.

considerable specialty-based initiatives and approaches to improving the care and outcomes of sick patients. Some that include simple elements have had a significant impact. Introducing oxygen systems for child pneumonia in Papua New Guinea reduced mortality by 35%.[29] A surgical safety checklist reduced mortality and surgical complications by more than 40%.[30] Strategies should be adopted for the implementation of EECC within existing initiatives with the goal of increasing their positive impact and reducing the unmet need for life-saving basic care for critically ill patients.

Essential Emergency and Critical Care and Basic Emergency Care

The World Health Organization (WHO)/International Committee of the Red Cross Basic Emergency Care (BEC), developed in collaboration with the International Federation of Emergency Medicine, is a training course designed for frontline physicians and nurses embedded within the emergency care systems framework.[31,32] It focuses on the initial management of patients suffering trauma, difficulty in breathing, shock, and altered mental states; "treatment of individuals with acute life- or limb-threatening conditions,"[33] "the care given in the first few hours after the onset of an acute medical or obstetric problem or the occurrence of an injury."[34] EECC has its primary focus on severity—critical illness anywhere in the hospital at any point of the patient's illness. EECC includes only the first-tier, life-saving, supportive care of patients' vital functions, whereas BEC extends beyond this to the provision of diagnostics and definitive therapies. The initiatives have extensive overlap and complement each other to ensure that basic life-saving care is provided in all settings.

Essential Emergency and Critical Care and Early Critical Care Services

Early critical care services are the initial care provided to critically ill patients when they become critically ill, often at arrival to the hospital. It has been defined as "the early interventions that support vital organ function during the initial care provided to the critically ill patient,"[11] and stresses the importance of ensuring continuity of care in the transition from the arrival unit to inpatient care. EECC and early critical care have substantial overlap, with EECC focusing on the most essential, low-cost, feasible care, and the provision of care throughout critical illness. EECC is the first tier of early critical care services, not limited by specialty, geographical location in the hospital, or by the different time points in the in-patient journey.

Essential Emergency and Critical Care, Levels of Critical Care, and Intensive Care Units

Critical care has been described in several levels, from the more basic up to the more advanced.[35] In these terms, EECC is the most basic level of critical care—the foundation that should be provided in all hospital settings. Although EECC is enough to stabilize and save the lives of many patients, some will require more advanced care to survive. For those for whom EECC is sufficient, transfer to resource-intensive ICUs can be avoided, thereby conserving such a highly rationed resource for those for whom it is necessary. Although ICUs comprise only a small percentage of acute hospital beds, they are an expensive resource[36] and can consume 20% of hospital resources.[37] When more advanced levels of care are available, such as HDUs and ICUs, clear referral and selection policies are required to ensure the optimal selection of patients. EECC could reduce the burden of low ICU bed space capacities, especially in LMICs, by averting the progression to organ failure and even death from preventable causes.

Essential Emergency and Critical Care, Primary Health Care, and Universal Health Coverage

As the WHO acknowledges, primary health care, including care in first-line district hospitals, is fundamental for the equitable delivery of health care to populations.[38,39] Primary health care is a core part of universal health coverage—the equity-based goal that all people should receive the health services they need without financial hardship. EECC, by its definition, can be regarded as the emergency and critical care component of primary health care and universal health coverage, providing an approach for the equitable provision of care to critically ill patients everywhere in the world. EECC should be seen as integral to primary health care and universal health coverage—strengthening basic health care services through an integrated equity-based approach that will lead to optimal population health.

Trauma care

Trauma is a leading cause of premature death and disability globally.[40,41] Trauma can cause critical illness through direct damage to vital organs, the systemic effects of trauma and inflammation, or complications such as hemorrhage, infection, and renal damage. Recent work has focused on improving trauma care within health systems globally. This has included the initial care of trauma patients through approaches, such as advanced trauma life support (ATLS) and referral systems for transferring the critically injured patient from basic health centers to designated trauma centers.[42] EECC has a vital role to play in the initial and ongoing care of critically ill trauma patients, including preventing and managing a blocked airway, supplementary oxygen, the control of hemorrhage, and fluid resuscitation.[43] EECC should be integrated into trauma systems and be a prioritized focus in trauma care. ATLS and similar programs revolve around many of the principles of EECC, allowing for integration of these approaches.

Surgery and Anesthesia

The World Health Assembly in 2015 unanimously adopted a resolution to strengthen emergency and essential surgical and anesthesia services.[44] Although surgical interventions have been shown to be efficacious and cost-effective, 5 billion people lack access to safe surgery.[45,46] Many surgical patients become critically ill, either due to their underlying surgical condition and comorbidities, to the stress of the surgery and anesthesia, or complications in the perioperative period. EECC has a crucial role in the care of perioperative critical illness, including preoperative stabilization, safe anesthesia, identification of the deteriorating surgical patient, and the provision of the low-cost, effective resuscitative measures that can reduce the risk of "failure to rescue" and the high postoperative mortality rates that have been identified in LMICs.[47,48] EECC should be an integral part of perioperative care and included as a necessary component in the scale-up of surgical services, such as the National Surgery, Obstetric, and Anesthesia Plans implemented in many countries.[49]

Emergency Obstetric Care

Preventing maternal and neonatal critical illnesses and deaths is the goal of emergency obstetric care. Common obstetric conditions leading to critical illness include hemorrhage, eclampsia, and sepsis.[50,51] Much work has been done to improve acute obstetric care, including the approaches of basic emergency obstetric and neonatal care (BEmONC) and comprehensive emergency obstetric and neonatal care.[52,53] BEmONC includes many EECC elements, such as the resuscitation of the critically ill mother and newborn. Ensuring health-workers are trained and hospitals are able to provide EECC to all patients, would benefit obstetric care, and strengthen emergency obstetric services.

Pediatrics and Emergency Triage, Assessment, and Treatment

Five million children die each year from conditions, such as respiratory infections, diarrhea, malaria, and neonatal conditions.[54] Emergency triage, assessment and treatment (ETAT) is a WHO initiative to identify and treat sick children in low-resource health facilities.[55] Implementing low-cost ETAT is feasible and can halve inpatient mortality among sick children.[56] ETAT recommendations are intended as guidance to frontline workers to ensure that a basic quality of emergency care is maintained. These recommendations involve the same components of care contained in EECC, with the addition of diagnostics and definitive treatments. EECC and ETAT are complementary, and as for obstetric care, a health facility with a workforce and universal systems for the provision of EECC to all patients will be well equipped to provide ETAT, even when health workers rotate between specialties.

Early Warning Systems and Rapid Response Teams

Rapid response teams (RRT) are in-hospital systems for the identification and care of at-risk and deteriorating patients. Such teams use early warning systems (EWS) based on patients' vital signs to identify patients developing critical illness and guide early and effective care.[57] Many of the components of EECC are integral to RRTs to ensure that the basics of identification and care of the critically ill are not missed.[58] EWS uses compound scoring tools to allocate points to each deteriorating vital sign for risk stratification and, above a certain threshold, an RRT may be activated, or another action instituted–the same principle as in the identification domain in EECC. RRTs and EWS must be tailored to the resources available, and challenges in low-resource settings include the incorrect addition of compound scores and insufficient human resources for an effective RRT.[6,59] Through the stabilization of critically ill patients, RRT and EWS in low-resource settings would include the EECC identification and treatment components and, through the stabilizing of critically ill patients, may reduce the number of patients requiring more advanced critical care and improve outcomes.

Infectious Diseases and Sepsis

Infectious diseases leading to sepsis are a common cause of critical illness and death,[60] with an estimated 11 million deaths annually from sepsis.[61] The basis of care for sepsis is supportive, life-saving treatment of vital organ dysfunctions—the same care as in EECC—with the addition of definitive antimicrobials and infectious source-control. The implementation of early identification and resuscitative interventions and other care elements contained in EECC are encouraged in sepsis guidelines and have been seen to improve patient outcomes.[62–64] Although international sepsis guidelines are widely accepted, they cannot be fully implemented in many settings around the world due to resource constraints.[16] Fortunately, EECC provides a feasible approach for the first-tier care of critical illness to all patients with sepsis and other infections complications.

Noncommunicable Diseases

An increasing proportion of the global burden of disease is caused by noncommunicable diseases (NCDs).[65] Hospitalized patients with an NCD, like other patients, may be misdiagnosed, cared for by the wrong specialty (medicine/surgery), suffer from multiple conditions/comorbidities or develop a new condition in hospital (eg, pulmonary embolism or pneumonia). Delivering diagnosis-specific NCD care to all patients is a challenge for any health system around the world, especially in resource-constrained settings. However, patients with NCDs can become critically ill and require urgent lifesaving care. Implementing low-cost EECC across hospitals would add a safety net for patients with NCD who become critically ill, saving lives and gaining time for the definitive care of their underlying condition.

Pandemics and Other Public-Health Emergencies

Pandemics and public-health emergencies lead to surges of patients with critical illnesses. Hospitals and health systems need to be prepared to handle these surges, and the care of critical illnesses has had a pivotal role in outbreaks, such as COVID-19 and Ebola.[66–68] Often, high-resource care for critical illness in ICUs is not sufficiently available and cannot be scaled-up fast enough, as has been seen in the COVID-19 pandemic.[69,70] Provision of essential care is required, and hospitals with implemented EECC systems before a pandemic are likely to be more prepared to scale up services and manage pandemic waves.[71] Providing EECC involves elements central to pandemic preparedness and response, such as a triage system to categorize patients by illness severity, the identification of patients requiring certain therapies, and the prioritization of essential care when demand outstrips supply.

IMPLEMENTING ESSENTIAL EMERGENCY AND CRITICAL CARE
Challenges

It is striking that the simple care contained in EECC, for which there is general agreement, is often not implemented. The primary reasons in this regard are to be understood and overcome if basic life-saving care is to be provided to all patients who need it. The reasons may include a lack of public awareness about critical illness and the potential impact of EECC, a lack of prioritization of acute hospital care within global and public health, and a lack of awareness among policymakers about the unmet need of EECC. Such issues, including a combination of professional and economic interests, draw attention away from the basic, but vitally important, components of essential care and toward research and (attempted) implementation of new, advanced technologies.

Increasing Awareness

There is a strong rationale for prioritizing the essential care that comprises EECC above care with less potential impact. As awareness of the unmet need of EECC and the potential for increasing coverage remains low, increasing awareness may spur implementation efforts. Advocates for improving care for critically ill patients and for EECC must engage with key policymakers at local, national, and global levels, such as governments, the WHO, the World Bank, and development partners. Professional societies should be made aware of EECC and how it aligns with their goals and practices. Interprofessional/multidisciplinary collaborations, such as the growing global EECC Network (www.eeccnetwork.org), can support the dissemination of knowledge with stakeholders at all levels.

Raising public awareness is equally important. Involving patient advocacy organizations, survivors of critical illnesses, and other parts of civil society is needed. The introduction of systems that hold caregivers accountable for the provision of EECC could be a strong incentive for rapid change and promote a positive spiral of media attention, public demand, and EECC implementation.

Implementation

While EECC can be framed as a patient right and thus is universal for all humans and not intended for local adaptation, the *implementation* of EECC is likely to be most effective and successful if adapted to the local context. The coverage of EECC varies largely between settings, and a strategy to implement full EECC coverage will interplay with other local practices. Although implementation in a complex system is difficult and necessitates multifaceted approaches and collaboration across sectors and disciplines, there are a number of elements that may be required or beneficial for success.

Training in EECC at scale will be needed. Both preservice training and in-service refreshers could be mandated to ensure quality and staff confidence. Training would ideally include simulation-based training that is relevant for the local facility,[72] along with mentoring and coaching and a focus on nontechnical skills, such as leadership, teamwork and communication.

The use of guidelines in clinical practice should focus on practice with the highest potential impact. As an overabundance of disease-specific clinical guidelines can result in fatigue among health workers, priorities should be set among guidelines to ensure the most important care is delivered.[73,74] Equity should be a guiding principle, and when there is conflict, the provision of essential care for all, such as EECC, should be prioritized above advanced care for a few. In addition, it should be ensured that essential care is provided at all times—including at night and at weekends. Prioritizing essential care requires that other services might be reduced, demanding strong and brave leadership. The introduction of patient safety and quality assurance units could assist with hospital-wide oversight, monitoring, and quality improvement of essential care.

While implementation of EECC could be attempted within a single department, it should ideally be introduced hospital-wide. Aligning departments and ensuring all health workers are competent in the provision of EECC would increase resilience and raise the chances that the system could cope even when there are surges of patient flow or when staff rotates between departments.

EECC is designed for task sharing. To improve the use of human resources, all health workers should be skilled in EECC. Innovative strategies for this could include the introduction of vital signs assistants—staff or volunteers trained in simple vital sign measurements and initial interpretation. Tools and initiatives, such as triage, EWS, RRT, and vital signs directed therapy (VSDT)[75] could be included in context-appropriate EECC packages. In higher resourced settings, the use of low-cost electronic aids could assist with implementation.

Research and Continuous Learning

To maintain and improve the quality of EECC provision, tools for assessment, implementation, monitoring, and evaluation are required. Robust research into the impact, cost, and potential system-wide side effects of introducing EECC in different settings would assist effective implementation. Implementation success will depend on adaption to the local context, requiring a thorough knowledge of the local processes of change. This could include quantitative bottleneck analyses and an in-depth understanding of the determinants of bottlenecks to guide potential strategies. Moreover, the potential impact of EECC could be better assessed by increased knowledge about the burden of critical illness globally.[76] Changing the processes of care in health facilities and in the health system is complicated, and single approaches to implementation (such as training or guidelines) are unlikely to succeed. Evaluations of successes and learning what works, in which contexts and why, are crucial to the goal of ensuring that all critically ill patients receive the life-saving, EECC that they require.

SUMMARY

EECC is a low-cost solution to a neglected problem with large impact potential. Implementing EECC globally and integrating it with other initiatives and approaches could lead to a substantial reduction in critical illness mortality.

The EECC Network Group

Anuja Abayadeera, Ibrahim Salim Abdullahi, Neill K.J. Adhikari, Asya Agulnik, Theodoros Aslanidis, Lovenish Bains, V. Theodore Barnett, Petronella Bjurling-Sjoberg, Furaha Nzanzu Blaise Pascal, Richard Branson, Dan Brun Petersen, Markus Castegren, Natalie Cobb, Ana Maria Crawford, Patricia Duque, Lorna Guinness, Hampus Ekström, Ahmed Rhassane EL ADIB, Mike English, Rodrigo Genaro Arduini, Martin Gerdin Wärnberg, Dhruva Ghosh, Raúl González-Rodríguez, Rodwell Gundo, Juan Gutierrez-Mejia, Claudia Hanson, Anna Hvarfner, Nemes Iriya, Maria Jirwe, Mtisunge Kachingwe, Shidah S. Kanyika, Raphael Kazidule Kayambankadzanja, Karima Khalid, Haika Kimambo, Teresa B. Kortz, Bharath Kumar, Lisa Kurland, Usha Lalla, Hans-Joerg Lang, Josephine Langton, James S. Lee, Miklos Lipcsey, Lia Ilona Losonczy, Edwin Lugazia, John J. Maiba, Halinder S. Mangat, Janet Martin, Ignacio Martin-Loeches, Janeth Masuma, Juniah Mazeze, Jacob McKnight, Dickson Mkoka, Donald Mlombwa, Amour Mohamed, Elizabeth M. Molyneux, Jolene Moore, Ernesto Moreno, Ben Morton, David Muir, Francis Mupeta, Isihaka Mwandalima, Prashant Nasa, Harrieth Ndumwa, Nathan D. Nielsen, Emmanuel Nsutebu, Jacquie N. Oliwa, Eamon Raith, Halima Salisu-Kabara, Mattias Schedwin, Rebecca Silvers, Juan Silesky- Jiménez, Kapil Dev Soni, Emnet Tesfaye Shimber, Stefan Swartling Peterson, Duyen Thi Hanh Bui, Mpoki Ulisubisya, Wim Van Damme, Ingrid T von der Osten, Richard Peter von Rahden, Thomas Weiser, Tamara Mulenga Willows, Bargo Mahamat Yousif, and Goran Zangana.

CLINICS CARE POINTS

A bulleted list of evidence-based pearls and pitfalls relevant to the point of care. These are more specific statements which are meant to guide the clinician at the point of care, unlike Key Points which are broad statements that summarize the main points of the article.

- All critically ill patients in all wards and units in all hospitals in the world should at least receive the "first tier" of care for their critical illness, defined as Essential Emergency and Critical Care (EECC)
- EECC contains 40 processes including triage, identification of critical illness at arrival to hospital and regularly during care using vital signs, oxygen therapy, intravenous fluids, and patient positioning
- Implementation of EECC is context-dependent, requiring multifaceted approaches and integration with other initiatives including hospital-wide training, guidelines, task-sharing, research and continuous learning.
- EECC is a low-cost solution for a neglected problem and could lead to a substantial reduction of critical illness mortality throughout the world.

DISCLOSURE

C. Owoo declares consultancy fees from the WHO, United States Agency for International Development (USAID), Sanofi, and conference support from Frusenius Kabi, Sanofi and Pfizer, all outside the submitted work. T. Baker declares personal fees from the United Nations Children's Fund, the World Bank, USAID, and the Wellcome Trust, all outside the submitted work. All authors are members of the EECC Network Group. The authors declare no other commercial or financial conflicts of interest.

REFERENCES

1. Adhikari NKJ, Fowler R, Bhagwanjee S, et al. Critical care and the global burden of critical illness in adults. Lancet 2010;376. https://doi.org/10.1016/s0140-6736(10)60446-1.
2. Kayambankadzanja RK, Schell CO, Gerdin Warnberg M, et al. Towards definitions of critical illness and critical care using concept analysis. BMJ open. 2022. Accepted 18th July 2022. https://doi.org/10.1101/2022.01.09.22268917.
3. Kayambankadzanja RK, Schell CO, Namboya F, et al. The prevalence and outcomes of sepsis in adult patients in two hospitals in Malawi. Am J Trop Med Hyg 2020;102(4):896–901.
4. Kayambankadzanja RK, Schell CO, Mbingwani I, et al. Unmet need of essential treatments for critical illness in Malawi. PLoS One 2021;16(9):e0256361.
5. Engdahl Mtango S, Lugazia E, Baker U, et al. Referral and admission to intensive care: a qualitative study of doctors' practices in a Tanzanian university hospital. PLoS One 2019;14(10):e0224355.
6. Friman O, Bell M, Djarv T, et al. National early warning score vs rapid response team criteria-Prevalence, misclassification, and outcome. Acta Anaesthesiol Scand 2019;63(2):215–21.
7. Seymour CW, Liu VX, Iwashyna TJ, et al. Assessment of clinical criteria for sepsis. JAMA 2016;315:762.
8. Sonenthal PD, Nyirenda M, Kasomekera N, et al. The Malawi emergency and critical care survey: a cross-sectional national facility assessment. EClinicalMedicine 2022;44. https://doi.org/10.1016/j.eclinm.2021.101245.
9. Baker T, Lugazia E, Eriksen J, et al. Emergency and critical care services in Tanzania: a survey of ten hospitals. BMC Health Serv Res 2013;13:140. https://doi.org/10.1186/1472-6963-13-140.
10. Coyle RM, Harrison HL. Emergency care capacity in Freetown, Sierra Leone: a service evaluation. BMC Emerg Med 2015;15(1). https://doi.org/10.1186/s12873-015-0027-4.
11. Losonczy LI, Papali A, Kivlehan S, et al. White paper on early critical care services in low resource settings. Ann Glob Health 2021;87(1):1–19.
12. Evans HT, Mahmood N, Fullerton DG, et al. Oxygen saturations of medical inpatients in a Malawian hospital: cross-sectional study of oxygen supply and demand. Pneumonia (Nathan) 2012;1:3–6.
13. King C, Banda M, Bar-Zeev N, et al. Care-seeking patterns amongst suspected paediatric pneumonia deaths in rural Malawi [version 2; peer review: 2 approved]. Gates Open Res 2021;4(178). https://doi.org/10.12688/gatesopenres.13208.2.
14. Hogan H, Healey F, Neale G, et al. Preventable deaths due to problems in care in English acute hospitals: a retrospective case record review study. BMJ Qual Saf 2012;21(9):737–45. https://doi.org/10.1136/bmjqs-2011-001159.
15. McQuillan P, Pilkington S, Allan A, et al. Confidential inquiry into quality of care before admission to intensive care. BMJ 1998;316(7148):1853–8.

16. Baelani I, Jochberger S, Laimer T, et al. Availability of critical care resources to treat patients with severe sepsis or septic shock in Africa: a self-reported, continent-wide survey of anaesthesia providers. Crit Care 2011;15(1):R10.

17. Muttalib F, González-Dambrauskas S, Lee JH, et al. Pediatric emergency and critical care resources and infrastructure in resource-limited settings: a multi-country survey. Crit Care Med 2021;49(4):671–81.

18. Agulnik A, Cárdenas A, Carrillo AK, et al. Clinical and organizational risk factors for mortality during deterioration events among pediatric oncology patients in Latin America: a multicenter prospective cohort. Cancer 2021;127(10):1668–78.

19. Okafor Uv. Challenges in critical care services in Sub-Saharan Africa: perspectives from Nigeria. Indian J Crit Care Med 2009;13(1):25–7.

20. Vincent JL. Critical care–where have we been and where are we going? Crit Care 2013;17(Suppl 1):S2.

21. Bruyneel A, Gallani MC, Tack J, et al. Impact of COVID-19 on nursing time in intensive care units in Belgium. Intensive Crit Care Nurs 2021;62:102967.

22. Graham HR, Bagayana SM, Bakare AA, et al. Improving hospital oxygen systems for COVID-19 in low-resource settings: lessons from the field. Glob Health Sci Pract 2020. https://doi.org/10.9745/GHSP-D-20-00224.

23. Ranney ML, Griffeth V, Jha AK. Critical supply shortages - the need for ventilators and personal protective equipment during the Covid-19 pandemic. N Engl J Med 2020;382(18):e41.

24. Mantena S, Rogo K, Burke TF. Re-Examining the race to send ventilators to low-resource settings. Respir Care 2020;65(9):1378–81.

25. Baker T, Schell CO, Petersen DB, et al. Essential care of critical illness must not be forgotten in the COVID-19 pandemic. Lancet 2020;395(10232):1253–4.

26. Manda-Taylor L, Mndolo S, Baker T. Critical care in Malawi: the ethics of beneficence and justice. Malawi Med J 2017;29(3):268–71.

27. Schell CO, Gerdin Wärnberg M, Hvarfner A, et al. The global need for essential emergency and critical care. Crit Care 2018;22(1):1–5.

28. Schell CO, Khalid K, Wharton-Smith A, et al. Essential emergency and critical care: a consensus among global clinical experts. BMJ Glob Health 2021;6(9):1–12.

29. Duke T, Wandi F, Jonathan M, et al. Improved oxygen systems for childhood pneumonia: a multihospital effectiveness study in Papua New Guinea. Lancet 2008;372(9646):1328–33.

30. Haynes AB, Weiser TG, Berry WR, et al. A surgical safety checklist to reduce morbidity and mortality in a global population. New Engl J Med 2009;360(5):491–9.

31. Salama C, Han J, Yau L, et al. Basic emergency care WHO. NIH 2020;21(1):20–30.

32. Reynolds T, Sawe HR, Rubiano A, et al. Strengthening health systems to provide emergency care: DCP3 disease control priorities. Washington, USA: World Bank.; 2018.

33. Hirshon JM, Risko N, Calvello EJ, et al. Health systems and services: the role of acute care. Bull World Health Organ 2013;91(5):386–8.

34. Kobusingye OC, Hyder AA, Bishai D, et al. Emergency medical systems in low- and middle-income countries: recommendations for action. Bull World Health Organ 2005;83(8):626–31.

35. Marshall JC, Bosco L, Adhikari NK, et al. What is an intensive care unit? A report of the task force of the World Federation of Societies of Intensive and Critical Care Medicine. Journal of critical care 2016;37:270–6.

36. Seidel J, Whiting PC, Edbrooke DL. The costs of intensive care. Continuing Educ Anaesth Crit Care Pain 2006;6(4):160–3.
37. Moerer O, Plock E, Mgbor U, et al. A German national prevalence study on the cost of intensive care: an evaluation from 51 intensive care units. Crit Care 2007;11(3):1–10.
38. WHO. Primary health care. 2022. Available at: https://www.who.int/news-room/fact-sheets/detail/primary-health-care. Accessed March 2, 2022.
39. English M, Lanata C, Ngugi I, et al. The district hospital: DCP3 disease control priorities. Washington, USA: World Bank.; 2018.
40. OMS. The global burden of disease 2004. Geneva, Switzerland: World Health Organization; 2004. p. 146.
41. Krug EG, Sharma GK, Lozano R. The global burden of injuries. Am J Public Health 2000;90(4):523.
42. Jayaraman S, Sethi D, Chinnock P, et al. Advanced trauma life support training for hospital staff. Cochrane Database Syst Rev 2014;2014(8). https://doi.org/10.1002/14651858.CD004173.pub4.
43. Roy N, Kizhakke Veetil D, Khajanchi MU, et al. Learning from 2523 trauma deaths in India- opportunities to prevent in-hospital deaths. BMC Health Serv Res 2017;17(1):1–8.
44. Price R, Makasa E, Hollands M. World Health Assembly Resolution WHA68.15: "Strengthening Emergency and Essential Surgical Care and Anesthesia as a Component of Universal Health Coverage"—Addressing the Public Health Gaps Arising from Lack of Safe, Affordable and Accessible Surgical and Anesthetic Services. World J Surg 2015;39(9):2115–25.
45. Meara JG, Leather AJM, Hagander L, et al. Global Surgery 2030: evidence and solutions for achieving health, welfare, and economic development. The Lancet 2015;386(9993):569–624.
46. McCord C, Kruk ME, Mock CN, et al. Organization of Essential Services and the Role of First-Level Hospitals. In: Debas HT, Donkor P, Gawande A, et al, editors. Essential Surgery: Disease Control Priorities, Third Edition (Volume 1). Washington (DC): The International Bank for Reconstruction and Development / The World Bank; 2015 Apr 2. Chapter 12. Available from: https://www.ncbi.nlm.nih.gov/books/NBK333499/. https://doi.org/10.1596/978-1-4648-0346-8_ch12.
47. Biccard BM, Madiba TE, Kluyts HL, et al. Perioperative patient outcomes in the African Surgical Outcomes Study: a 7-day prospective observational cohort study. Lancet 2018. https://doi.org/10.1016/S0140-6736(18)30001-1.
48. Bainbridge D, Martin J, Arango M, et al. Perioperative and anaesthetic-related mortality in developed and developing countries: a systematic review and meta-analysis. Lancet 2012;380(9847):1075–81.
49. Truché P, Shoman H, Reddy CL, et al. Globalization of national surgical, obstetric and anesthesia plans: the critical link between health policy and action in global surgery. Glob Health 2020;16(1):1.
50. Neligan PJ, Laffey JG. Clinical review: special populations–critical illness and pregnancy. Crit Care 2011;15(4):227.
51. Dasgupta S, Jha T, Bagchi P, et al. Critically ill obstetric patients in a general critical care unit: a 5 years' retrospective study in a public teaching hospital of eastern India. Indian J Crit Care Med 2017;21(5):294–302.
52. O WH. Monitoring emergency obstetric care: a Handbook. WHO; 2009.
53. Pattinson RC, Makin JD, Pillay Y, et al. Basic and comprehensive emergency obstetric and neonatal care in 12 South African health districts. S Afr Med J 2015;105(4):256–60.

54. Global, regional, and national progress towards Sustainable Development Goal 3.2 for neonatal and child health: all-cause and cause-specific mortality findings from the Global Burden of Disease Study 2019. Lancet 2021;398(10303): 870–905. https://doi.org/10.1016/s0140-6736(21)01207-1.

55. World Health Organization.. Emergency triage assessment and treatment (ETAT): manual for participants. Geneva, Switzerland: WHO Press; 2005. p. 78.

56. Molyneux E, Ahmad S, Robertson A. Improved triage and emergency care for children reduces inpatient mortality in a resource-constrained setting. Bull World Health Organ 2006;84(4):314–9.

57. Maharaj R, Raffaele I, Wendon J. Rapid response systems: a systematic review and meta-analysis. Crit Care 2015;19(1):1–15.

58. Na SJ, Ko RE, Ko MG, et al. Automated alert and activation of medical emergency team using early warning score. J Intensive Care 2021;9(1):1–9.

59. Brown SR, Martinez Garcia D, Agulnik A. Scoping review of pediatric early warning systems (PEWS) in resource-limited and humanitarian settings. Front Pediatr 2018;6:410.

60. Vincent JL, Marshall JC, Ñamendys-Silva SA, et al. Assessment of the worldwide burden of critical illness: the intensive care over nations (ICON) audit. Lancet Respir Med 2014;2(5):380–6.

61. Rudd KE, Johnson SC, Agesa KM, et al. Global, regional, and national sepsis incidence and mortality, 1990–2017: analysis for the Global Burden of Disease Study. The Lancet 2020;395(10219):200–11.

62. Evans L, Rhodes A, Alhazzani W, et al. Surviving sepsis campaign: international guidelines for management of sepsis and septic shock 2021. Crit Care Med 2021;49(11):e1063–143.

63. Varon J, Baron RM. A current appraisal of evidence for the approach to sepsis and septic shock. Ther Adv Infect Dis 2019;6. https://doi.org/10.1177/2049936119856517.

64. Jacob ST, Banura P, Baeten JM, et al. The impact of early monitored management on survival in hospitalized adult Ugandan patients with severe sepsis: a prospective intervention study. Crit Care Med 2012;40(7):2050–8.

65. NCD Countdown 2030: worldwide trends in non-communicable disease mortality and progress towards Sustainable Development Goal target 3.4. Lancet 2018; 392(10152):1072–88.

66. Wu Z, McGoogan JM. Characteristics of and important lessons from the coronavirus disease 2019 (COVID-19) outbreak in China: summary of a report of 72314 cases from the Chinese center for disease control and prevention. JAMA 2020. https://doi.org/10.1001/jama.2020.2648.

67. Fowler RA, Fletcher T, Fischer WA, et al. Caring for critically ill patients with ebola virus disease perspectives from west africa. Am J Respir Crit Care Med 2014; 190(7):733–7.

68. Brown C, Kreuels B, Baker P, et al. Ebola and provision of critical care. Lancet 2015;385(9976):1392.

69. Biccard BM, Gopalan PD, Miller M, et al. Patient care and clinical outcomes for patients with COVID-19 infection admitted to African high-care or intensive care units (ACCCOS): a multicentre, prospective, observational cohort study. The Lancet 2021;397(10288):1885–94.

70. Morton B, Banda NP, Nsomba E, et al. Establishment of a high-dependency unit in Malawi. BMJ Glob Health 2020;5(11):e004041.

71. Lamontagne F, Fowler RA, Adhikari NK, et al. Evidence-based guidelines for supportive care of patients with Ebola virus disease. The Lancet 2018;391(10121): 700–8. https://doi.org/10.1016/S0140-6736(17)31795-6.

72. Sørensen JL, Østergaard D, LeBlanc V, et al. Design of simulation-based medical education and advantages and disadvantages of in situ simulation versus off-site simulation. BMC Med Educ 2017;17(1):20.

73. Maaløe N, Ørtved AMR, Sørensen JB, et al. The injustice of unfit clinical practice guidelines in low-resource realities. Lancet Glob Health. doi:10.1016/S2214-109X(21)00059-0

74. Allen D, Harkins KJ. Too much guidance? The Lancet 2005;365(9473):1768.

75. Baker T, Schell CO, Lugazia E, et al. Vital signs directed therapy: improving care in an intensive care unit in a low-income country. PLoS One 2015;10(12): e0144801.

76. Abbas Q, Holloway A, Caporal P, et al. Global PARITY: study design for a multi-centered, international point prevalence study to estimate the burden of pediatric acute critical illness in resource-limited settings. Front Pediatr 2021;9:793326.

Current State of Critical Care Nursing Worldwide

Current Training, Roles, Barriers, and Facilitators

Eunice Ndirangu-Mugo, PhD, MScANP, BScN[a],*,
Lia M. Barros, DNP, AGACNP- BC[b], Benard D. Mutwiri, BSc[a],
Constance S. Shumba, PhD, Msc, BSc[a], Beth Waweru, BScN, MscN[a],
Wangari Waweru Siika, MBChB, MMed, FRCA[c]

KEYWORDS

- Critical care • Intensive care • Nurses • Roles • Responsibilities • Training
- Facilitators • Barriers

KEY POINTS

- Strengthening of professional nurses' competencies targeted at their defined role is important for global critical care capacity. In high-resource settings, critical care nursing is a defined clinical specialty reflecting specific knowledge and clinical competencies. The roles of critical care nurses are clearly understood and generally care is provided in intensive care units. However, in low-resourced settings (low- to middle-income countries) roles and responsibilities of critical care nurses are not well defined.
- Although in high-income countries critical care nurses frequently receive a formal orientation, including critical care consortium with intensive 1 to 3 months of lectures, didactic learning, and one-on-one preceptorship by a more experienced critical care nurse, ongoing professional development in low-resource settings are even fewer.
- Absence of clear national guidelines on critical care nursing practice and a critical care nursing body that sets standards and core competencies to ensure proficiency-based licensure contributes to the limited in-service training and uncertainty about roles and responsibilities.
- Lack of critical care guidelines, insufficient training, high workload, poor training, lack of knowledge, poor technology, limited resources, insufficient exposure to the critical care environment, and ongoing education are the largest barriers to proficient critical care, especially in low-resource settings.

Continued

[a] School of Nursing and Midwifery, Aga Khan University, P O Box 39340-00623, Nairobi, Kenya;
[b] Division of Pulmonary, Critical Care, and Sleep Medicine, University of Washington Medical Center, Campus Box 356522, Seattle 98195-6522, Washington; [c] Department of Anaesthesia, Aga Khan University Hospital, P.O Box 39340-00623, Nairobi, Kenya
* Corresponding author. School of Nursing and Midwifery, Aga Khan University-Kenya, PO Box 39340-00623, Nairobi, Kenya.
E-mail address: eunice.ndirangu@aku.edu
Twitter: @DrENdirangu (E.N.-M.)

Crit Care Clin 38 (2022) 657–693
https://doi.org/10.1016/j.ccc.2022.06.014
0749-0704/22/© 2022 Elsevier Inc. All rights reserved.
criticalcare.theclinics.com

Continued

- Although in-service training, emotional regulations, effective communication, and international partnerships emerge as some of the facilitators of critical care nursing practice, there is a need for a holistic strategy to overcome the existing barriers and improve nursing care of the critically ill in low-resource settings.

BACKGROUND

Over the last several decades our understanding of critical care has evolved. Unlike other specialties of medicine defined by organ system or procedure, new definitions of critical care have tried to broaden the focus to include patients' complexity of illness, the severity of organ dysfunction, and risk of imminent death, irrespective of physical location. Population-based studies suggest that the burden of critical illness is therefore difficult to quantify and likely higher than generally appreciated. This burden is disproportionately affecting low- to middle-income countries (LMICs) and will only continue as populations age,[1] especially with the steady increase in noncommunicable disease incidence in recent years.[2] Understanding this has fed a growing recognition that investing in high-quality critical care is needed. Globally, nurses represent the largest group of health professionals providing critical care and thus are fundamental to achieving this aim. More specifically, recent studies have further suggested that critical care nurses, rationally deployed based on patient load and acuity, improve the quality and efficiency of critical care provision in hospital settings and reduce morbidity and mortality, especially in low resourced settings where inputs are most in short supply.[3,4]

With the expansive provision of critical care services across the globe and the value of critical care nurses in the reduction of patient mortality, it is important to have a shared understanding of the critical care nurse's role, responsibilities, on-the-job training, and key challenges and facilitators.[5] It is thought that although many of these aspects are universal, there are marked differences based on available resourced settings, as well as other key challenges. The purpose of this paper is to identify a shared definition of the critical care nurse's role, their current standard for on-the-job training, the key barriers, and facilitators they face to providing critical care and ultimately to identify any potential solutions to these challenges.

METHODS

The purpose of this review was to provide a holistic understanding of the current state of professional responsibilities, on-the-job training, barriers, and facilitators of critical care nurses across the globe. Thus, although the review was rapid in nature, the study team adopted the Preferred Reporting Items for Systematic Reviews and Meta-Analyses (PRISMA) guidelines[6] to inform the search criteria, articles screening, inclusion and exclusion criteria, data extraction, and the narrative synthesis.

Eligibility Criteria

The population of interest for this review was the nurses working in critical and intensive care units in the hospital and other health care settings. Therefore, among the inclusion criteria, the review team defined critical care setting as any designated health care setting providing pediatric, neonatal, or adult critical care. Moreover, only the studies exploring the preparation, training, roles, and responsibilities of the critical care nurses, as well as the barriers and facilitators of critical care nursing were considered eligible for this review. Although the review did not exclude any study designs, the research team agreed to include only studies published in the English language between 2017 and 2022. The restriction in terms of the publication date was to enhance the review of the most current materials, whereas the English language constraint was to ensure timely synthesis due to the rapid nature of the review.

Search Strategy and Search Terms

The following databases were searched to identify studies reporting the preparation training, roles and responsibilities, barriers, and facilitators of critical care nursing among nurses working in intensive/critical care units: PubMed, CINAHL, Scopus, PsychINFO, Global Index Medicus, and EBSCOhost Academic Search Complete. Relevant unpublished research on the topic was also searched from the OpenGrey database and from institutional electronic resources, mainly from Web sites of the WHO, UNICEF, Centers for Diseases Control and Prevention, and the International Center for Research on Women. The gray literature search was conducted purposively based on the relevance of the Web site and organizations database to provide some relevant review materials. However, although the review team structured specific electronic database search terms and combinations for each database, the search was confined to articles published in English language over the last 5 years.

The search strategy relating to this rapid review comprised of a combination of free terms or key words using controlled descriptors (such as MeSH terms and Boolean operators). The search strategy was guided by the PICO framework. A comprehensive search strategy was developed in PubMed and was adjusted to suit the other databases. The Boolean operators "OR" and "AND" were used to combine the various search terms. The key search terms for this review were as depicted in the following search string: "Intensive Care Nursing" OR "critical care nursing" AND roles OR Duties OR responsibilities OR Barriers OR Facilitators OR education OR "on-the-job training" OR Preparation OR Training ("Intensive Care Nursing" OR "critical care nursing") AND (roles OR Duties OR responsibilities OR Barriers OR Facilitators OR education OR "on-the-job training" OR Preparation OR Training). **Table 1** shows details of the comprehensive search strategy for various databases and the hits.

Selection of the Eligible Studies

Two reviewers (EN, BM) independently conducted the searches on the proposed databases and the gray information sources. Once the database search was completed, the citations titles and abstracts were exported into the Endnote reference management software, which was used to store, organize, cite, and manage the articles during the screening process. After initially identifying and excluding all duplicate articles, 3 members from the research team (LB, BM, WS) reviewed and screened the studies for eligibility. The potentially eligible articles were identified by assessing the titles, abstracts as well as using the search keywords. Full-text copies of all selected studies were obtained to find more details by the 3 reviewers who reviewed the full text of articles and resolve the discrepancies by consensus. Where necessary, the fourth reviewer (EN) helped in the final decision. All the reasons for any exclusion of specific studies at the full-text level were documented. The study inclusion process is presented using a PRISMA flow chart (**Fig. 1**).

Data Extraction and Management

Data extraction was done independently by the 3 members (EN, LB, BM) of the review team. The members comparatively extracted data to attain consensus on the

Table 1
Databases search results

Date	Database	Search String	Applied Filters	Hits/Results
13th Feb, 2022	PubMed	(((("Intensive Care Nursing") OR ("critical care nursing")) AND ((((education) OR ("on-the-job training")) OR (Preparation)) OR (Training)) AND ((y_5[Filter]) AND (english[Filter]))) OR (((("Intensive Care Nursing") OR ("critical care nursing")) AND (((roles) OR (Duties)) OR (responsibilities)) AND ((y_5[Filter]) AND (english[Filter]))) OR ((("Intensive Care Nursing") OR ("critical care nursing")) AND ((Barriers) OR (Facilitators)) AND (y_5[Filter])))	• English • 5 y	1180
14th Feb, 2022	CINAHL	"Intensive Care Nursing" OR "critical care nursing" AND roles OR Duties OR responsibilities OR Barriers OR Facilitators OR education OR "on-the-job training" OR Preparation OR Training AB ("Intensive Care Nursing" OR "critical care nursing") AND AB (roles OR Duties OR responsibilities OR Barriers OR Facilitators OR education OR "on-the-job training" OR Preparation OR Training)	• English • 5 y	115
14th Feb, 2022	Global Index Medicus	"Intensive Care Nursing" OR "critical care nursing" AND roles OR Duties OR responsibilities OR Barriers OR Facilitators OR education OR "on-the-job training" OR Preparation OR Training	• English • 5 y	41
15th Feb, 2022	Scopus	"Intensive Care Nursing" OR "critical care nursing" AND roles OR Duties OR responsibilities OR Barriers OR Facilitators OR education OR "on-the-job training" OR Preparation OR Training	• English • 5 y	779
15th Feb, 2022	EBSCOhost Academic Search Complete	"Critical Care Nursing" OR "Intensive Care Nursing" AND "Facilitators OR Barriers OR Roles OR Responsibilities OR "on-the-Job training" OR Training OR Education"	• English • Academic Journals • 5 y	559
15th Feb, 2022	PyschInfo	"Critical Care Nursing" OR "Intensive Care Nursing" AND "Facilitators OR Barriers OR Roles OR Responsibilities OR "on-the-Job training" OR Training OR Education"	• English • Scholar Journals • 5 y	338
15th Feb, 2022	Other Searches	"Critical Care Nursing" OR "Intensive Care Nursing" AND Facilitators OR Barriers OR Roles OR Responsibilities OR "on-the-Job training"	• English • 5 y	29
Total				3041

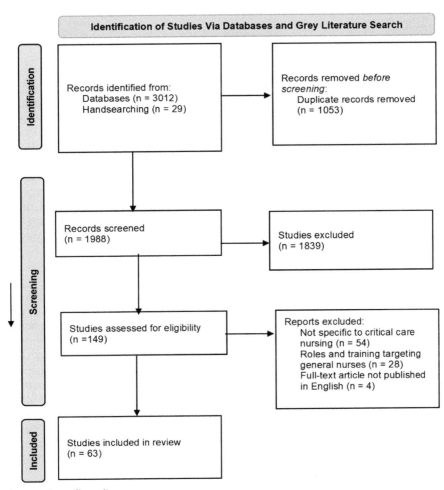

Fig. 1. Prisma flow diagram

results and, where needed, involved the fourth reviewer (BW) to help in the final decision. Specifically, an extraction form (in an Excel spreadsheet) was used for data extraction. The specific data extracted included (1) author and year of publication; (2) country where the study was conducted; (3) study design and methodology; (4) study participants or population characteristics (eg, sample size); (5) study objective; and (6) intensive care unit nurses' preparation, training, roles and responsibilities, barriers, and facilitators in critical care nursing. To avoid double counting or duplicate extraction, the results of studies presented in multiple papers for the same population were included only once.

Data Synthesis

Data from the review were synthesized narratively to address the review question. The review findings were descriptively presented and discussed while elaborating the roles and responsibilities, training and preparation, as well as barriers and facilitators of critical care nursing among the nurses working in intensive care units (ICU)/critical care units. The studies' data findings were presented in tabular form for comparison highlighting country, year of study, study objectives, and the specifics of the review interest.

RESULTS
Study Selection

The complete electronic databases search yielded 3041 articles. After deduplication, 1988 article were subjected to title and abstracts screening. Based on the inclusion and exclusion criteria only 149 studies were found eligible, thus subjected to full-text review. Three reviewers (EN, LB, BM) assessed the remaining articles based on the inclusion criteria while consulting with the fourth reviewer where consensus was not reached. The final synthesis included 63 articles that met the inclusion and exclusion criteria (see **Fig. 1**). The rationale for the exclusion of the 86 articles were incorrect topic area, incorrect setting, inappropriate population, ineligible document type, document is a duplicate, and no primary data on ICU/ critical care unit nurses' preparation, training, roles and responsibilities, barriers, and facilitators in ICU/ critical care unit nurses.

Characteristics of the Included Studies

Table 2 results provide a summary of the characteristics of the 65 studies on role and responsibilities, on-the-job training, as well as, barriers, and facilitators faced by critical care nurses included in this review. Seemingly, most of the studies were conducted in high-income countries (HICs), such as United states (n = 15), Canada (n = 4), Spain (n = 3), Romania, Sweden (n = 4), Poland (n = 2), Turkey (n = 3), Southern California, Jordan (n = 2), Iran (n = 3), Korea, Scotland, Nepal, Japan, Singapore, Denmark, Norway, China, Austria, London, New Zealand, Sydney, NSW Australia, Sydney, Italy, and Pakistan. Only 4 studies were conducted in sub-Saharan Africa, that is, Ethiopia, Rwanda, and Zambia (n = 2). In addition, most of the studies were conducted in hospital settings with majority using qualitative research design (n = 29), cross-sectional design (n = 8), descriptive survey design (n = 12), literature (n = 4), systematic and integrative reviews (n = 6), quasi-experimental study, and pre-interventional and postinterventional design.

Table 2 results highlight various aspects relative to roles, responsibilities, barriers, and facilitators of critical care nursing across the globe. Interestingly, the findings indicate a significant gap in literature on critical care nursing between the high-income and LMICs, especially on the role definition, on-the-job training, as well as the barriers, and facilitators of the critical care delivery.

Roles and Responsibilities of Critical Care Nurses

We identified only 6 studies discussing the roles and responsibilities of critical care nurses,[7–12] and only one was conducted in an LMIC.[12] In high-income settings, the critical care nursing roles were deemed to provide the 4 C's role, that is, convening, checking, caring, and continuing.[7] Besides, in addition to providing care for acutely ill patients with high potential life-threatening problems, the critical care nurses are expected to provide expert and specialist care, work as a part of multidisciplinary team, monitor and initiate timely treatment, and also provide psychosocial support and advanced system treatment.[9] In addition, critical care nurses are involved in facilitation and preparation of family conference for terminally ill patients,[10] provision of complex medical procedures, such as ventilation, and consistent nursing assessments to ensure survival.[11] On the other hand, a scoping review conducted to assess the execution of critical care nursing in LMIC revealed that, although various skills and

Table 2
Characteristics of the included studies

Author (Year) [Citation]	Country	Objective	Study Design & Sample Size	Key Findings (Roles, Training, Barriers, and Facilitators)
Roles and Responsibilities of Critical Care Nurses				
Anderson & Turner,[7] 2020	USA	To provide a comprehensive description of the central role of nurses in providing primary palliative care	Webinar series	The 4 Cs • Convening, checking, caring, and continuing
Bloomer et al,[8] 2019	Global Review	To provide international recommendations to inform and assist critical care nursing associations, health services, governments, and other interested stakeholders in the development and provision of an appropriate critical care nursing workforce	Literature review	• A critical care unit nurse leader should have a recognized postregistration critical care qualification with significant clinical and leadership experience • Units' leaders need critical care training and should be senior and experienced registered nurses (RNs) with appropriate expertise to lead the clinical team • RNs are expected to work toward a postregistration qualification or certification in critical care.

(continued on next page)

Table 2
(continued)

Author (Year) [Citation]	Country	Objective	Study Design & Sample Size	Key Findings (Roles, Training, Barriers, and Facilitators)
Credland et al,[9] 2021	USA	Introduce the role of critical care nursing and what it involves, as well as looking at how critical care nurses can support the whole patient.	Review	• Provide expert and specialist care to the most severely ill or injured patient (technical skill and knowledge) • Highly trained and skilled safety working as part of a multidisciplinary team. • Undertake postgraduate study and ongoing training • Identify, monitor, and initiate timely treatment to prevent clinical deterioration and support ward nurses • Advance system assessment • Rescue patients BEFORE irretrievable and/or cardiac arrest takes place • Gather accurate data on physiologic parameters to provide real-time feedback to help evaluate critical care interventions and detect any deterioration promptly • Provide psychosocial care, family care

Kawashima et al,[10] 2020	Japan	To clarify nurse' contribution to family conferences for terminally ill patients in critical care and their families and examine the priority of each used	Modified Delphi method	• Nurses are involved in preparation, facilitation, and follow-up after a family conference
Kurth et al,[11] 2021	USA	To discuss the crucial role and dearth of critical care nurses in the United States highlighted during the COVID-19 pandemic.	Review	• Critical care RNs are educated and trained to care for "acutely/critically ill patients who are at high risk for actual or potential life-threatening health problems, regardless of the setting for their nursing care • Requires vigilance, critical thinking, and rapid responsiveness in high-intensity and clinically complex situations. These patients typically require a variety of complex medications and procedures as well as frequent and thorough nursing assessments to ensure survival.

(continued on next page)

Table 2
(continued)

Author (Year) [Citation]	Country	Objective	Study Design & Sample Size	Key Findings (Roles, Training, Barriers, and Facilitators)
Macey et al,[12] 2022	LMIC	A scoping review of how critical care nursing is performed in low-income countries and lower middle-income countries	Scoping review guided by the JBI Manual for Evidence Synthesis	Roles • Care of the ventilated patient, medication management, and clinical education • Post basic critical care trained nurses have responsibilities to provide care to deteriorating patients in the wider hospital • Care of mechanically ventilated patients, health care assistants, ancillary staff Training • Nurses have a range of formal and informal training • In Kenya 50% of nurses working in ICUs were reported as holding post basic qualification • India recommends that all nurses working in critical care areas hold formal post basic qualifications

Training for Critical Care Nurses

Author	Country	Study type	Purpose	Findings
Carter et al,[13] 2020	Zambia	Literature review	To review the literature relating to critical care nursing in sub-Saharan Africa to support a review and validation of the current critical care nursing course and to prepare a framework for a Bachelor of Science (BSc) in critical care nursing program in Zambia.	Barriers • Staff shortages a barrier • Inadequate resourcing • No standard; a variety of nursing practices and nonclinical responsibilities • Paucity of research on critical care education • Critical care course, certificate program
Cunnington,[14] 2018	USA	Literature review	To establish aspects of transition programs that best support new graduate nurses improve competence and confidence to transition into critical care nursing specialties.	• Transition programs exist to support transition of nurses into practice • Differ in effectiveness (duration, structure, components, rotations, financial support, and content)
McBride,[15] 2017	USA	Expert opinion	Brief essays that summarize major elements of the Education and Training Plenary for critical care nurses	• Rigorous orientation and meaningful continuing education may augment that

(continued on next page)

Table 2
(continued)

Author (Year) [Citation]	Country	Objective	Study Design & Sample Size	Key Findings (Roles, Training, Barriers, and Facilitators)
Monesi,[16] 2021	Italy	This short communication describes our experience of an "in-situ" simulation training course in an Italian tertiary level hospital.	Descriptive study	• Short lectures on fundamental principles of intensive care nursing and brief hands-on sessions, and a set of simulated scenarios, based on the most common situations to be faced in the ICU
Padhya,[17] 2021	USA	To determine the feasibility and effectiveness of remote training of international critical care providers that included physicians and nurses.	Ancillary analysis of prospective observational study	• Remote simulation training of international partners • Resulted in improvement in compliance for measures determined as best practice guidelines in simulation rounding and overall improvement in critical tasks for simulated admission cases after remote training.
Short,[18] 2019	USA	Evaluate a critical care skills program for newly hired nurses	Program evaluation with qualitative and quantitative analysis	• Shows CNS may increase nursing competencies and mentorship

Author	Country	Purpose	Study Type	Findings
Stephens,[19] 2017	Sri Lanka	To deliver and evaluate a short critical care nurse training course while simultaneously building local training capacity	Program evaluation	• Short-period training may increase critical care capacity • International partners for capacity building creates train the trainer models
Barriers				
Beckstrand et al,[20] 2021	America	To gather first-hand data from CCNs regarding obstacles related to EOL care	Qualitative Study (n = 104 CCN)	• Poor communication among physicians • Insufficient nurse staffing • Inadequate EOL care education for nurses
Bahramnezhad & Dolatabadi,[21] 2019	Iran	Identify role of ICU in disaster preparedness.	Letter to the editor	ICU nurses found they lack: • Inappropriate equipment management • No skilled personnel • Inappropriate management and leadership • Lack of awareness about triage of patients • No adequate financial support • Lack of fire management • High number of requests to provide equipment from these units • Unsafety of the units • Devices and equipment falling down • No power and water

(continued on next page)

Table 2
(continued)

Author (Year) [Citation]	Country	Objective	Study Design & Sample Size	Key Findings (Roles, Training, Barriers, and Facilitators)
				• Excessive presence of personnel in the unit and lack of its appropriate management • Lack of possibility to replace skilled personnel when needed • Lack of attention to the comfort of personnel regarding safety of their family members • The lack of training courses for families about providing care at home during emergencies and disasters.
Begerow et al,[22] 2020		To understand how intensive care nurses perceive their working conditions and the consequences for patient care	Qualitative survey (n = 397 nurses)	• Limited knowledge, professional demand, and family pressure
Castellà-Creus et al,[23] 2019	Barcelona (Catalonia)	To identify and classify the barriers and facilitators of the individualization process of the standardized care plan in hospitalization wards	Qualitative study (n = 39 nurses)	• Lack of interest and knowledge • Traditional narrative records • Wards routines requirements

Çelik et al,[24] 2017	Turkey	To determine the level of fatigue among nurses working in ICUs and the related factors	Descriptive study (n = 102 nurses)	• Fatigue and anxiety
Coleman & Angosta,[25] 2017	Western USA	To explore the lived experiences of acute-care bedside nurses caring for patients and their families with limited English proficiency	Phenomenology research (n = 40 nurses)	• Caring for patients with limited English proficiency is a challenge
Cotrău et al,[26] 2019	Romania	To determine the occupational stress levels, burnout syndrome, and work satisfaction among ICU nurses	Survey design (n = 29)	• Workload stress • Conflict with other health professionals
DeGrande et al,[27] 2018	Texas	To explore the experiences of nurses who were hired into adult intensive care as a new graduate and survived their transition from novice to competent, starting the third year of practice	Hermeneutic phenomenology research approach (n = 11)	• Stress & difficulties
Falk et al,[28] 2019	Sweden	To identify barriers to patient participation in the critical care unit, as identified by critical care nurses	Qualitative study (n = 17)	• Nurses' attitude toward caring • Patient's health condition • Organization of the critical care unit
Fernández-Castillo et al,[29] 2021	Spain	To explore and describe the experiences and perceptions of nurses working in an ICU during the COVID-19 global pandemic	A qualitative study (n = 17)	• Fear and isolation

(continued on next page)

Table 2
(continued)

Author (Year) [Citation]	Country	Objective	Study Design & Sample Size	Key Findings (Roles, Training, Barriers, and Facilitators)
Ghazanchaie et al,[30] 2020	Isfahan (Iran)	To explain the nurses' experiences of barriers to palliative care in NICUs	A qualitative study (n = 12)	• Unfavorable conditions, such as "unsuitable physical environment" and "shortage of nurses" • Nurse's mental problems, doctors, and parental presence challenges
Ghezeljeh et al,[31] 2021	Iran	To explore factors affecting error communication in ICUs	Qualitative study (n = 17)	• Fear over being stigmatized as incompetent • Fear over punishment and fear over negative judgments about nursing
González-Gil et al,[32] 2021	Spain	To identify needs related to safety, organization, decision-making, communication, and psycho-socio-emotional needs perceived by critical care and emergency nurses in the region of Madrid, Spain, during the acute phase of the epidemic crisis	Cross-sectional study (n = 557)	• Poor communication with middle management • Inability to provide psychosocial care to patients • Emotional exhaustion
Gordon et al,[33] 2021	United States	To examine their experiences caring for patients with COVID-19	Qualitative study (n = 11)	• Intense psychological and physical effects as a result of caring for patients diagnosed with COVID-19 (anxiety/stress, helplessness, worry, fear)

Author/Year	Country	Purpose	Study design	Findings
Habiballah,[34] 2017	Jordan	To investigate barriers toward pressure ulcer prevention as perceived by Jordanian nurses who work in critical care units	Cross-sectional study (n = 103)	• Lack of staff • Insufficient time • Uncooperative or severely ill patient
Jackson et al,[35] 2018	Canada	To investigate burnout and resilience in critical care nurses	Qualitative grounded theory (n = 11)	• Burnout
Jakimowicz et al,[36] 2017	NA	To systematically review the literature describing factors perceived by nurses as affecting the provision of patient-centered nursing in the ICU	Integrative review (n = 23)	• Emotional and physical demands of critical care
Kim et al,[37] 2019	Korea	To identify barriers perceived by critical care nurses, corresponding educational needs, and provide useful information for program implementation in Korea	Cross-sectional study (n = 151)	• High workload • Patients' inability to exercise • Inadequate time • Insufficient nurse/patient ratio • Lack of relevant education
Kiwanuka et al,[38] 2019	NA	To assess the barriers to patient-and family centered care among health care providers, patients, and family members in adult ICUs	Systematic review	• Lack of knowledge on the requirements for patient- and family centered care • Individual and family barriers • Organizational constraints

(continued on next page)

Table 2
(continued)

Author (Year) [Citation]	Country	Objective	Study Design & Sample Size	Key Findings (Roles, Training, Barriers, and Facilitators)
Kydonaki et al,[39] 2019	Scotland	To understand the challenges to optimizing sedation in the Scottish ICU settings before the trial	A qualitative exploratory design	• Uncertainty in decision-making • System-level factors including the ICU environment • Organizational aspects and educational gaps
Limbu et al,[40] 2019	Nepal	Describe the lived experiences of intensive care nurses in caring for critically ill patients in ICUs	A hermeneutic phenomenological study (n = 13)	• Low technology of care and insufficient resources • Physical and psychological distress
Liyew et al,[41] 2021	Northwest Ethiopia	To assess the nurses' practice and barriers to physical assessment among critically ill patients	Multicenter cross-sectional study (n = 299)	• Reliance on others and technology toward physical assessment practice • Culture and specialty issues
Meilando et al,[42] 2022		To identify barriers and challenges of end-of-life care implementation in the ICU	Literature review (n = 11)	• Lack of knowledge and communication during end-of-life care
Nankundwa & Brysiewicz,[43] 2017	Rwanda	To explore the lived experiences of nurses caring for a patient with a DNR order in an ICU (ICU) in Kigali, Rwanda	Phenomenological approach (n = 6)	• Feeling emotional distress

Ong et al,[44] 2018	Singapore	To understand the perceptions of critical care nurses toward providing end-of-life care	A qualitative descriptive study (n = 10)	• Nurses tension in care
Pastores et al,[45] 2019	NA	To assess—by literature review and expert consensus—workforce, workload, and burnout considerations among intensivists and advanced practice providers	Literature review	• Workforce, workload, and burnout
Petersen et al,[46] 2017	Denmark	To determine barriers and facilitating factors related to 3 aspects of the EWS protocol	Qualitative study (n = 18)	• High workload • Limited collaboration and communication between doctors and nurses
Rababa et al,[47] 2021	NA	To examine nurses' perceived barriers to and facilitators of pain assessment and management in adult critical care patients	Systematic review (n = 20)	• Nurses' lack of knowledge regarding the use of pain assessment tools • Patients' inability to communicate • Absence of standardized guidelines and protocols for pain evaluation and control
Robstad et al,[48] 2018	Norway	To obtain a deeper understanding of qualified intensive care nurses' experiences of caring for obese patients in intensive care	A qualitative hermeneutic approach (n = 13)	• Physically demanding care situations • Unwillingness to care

(continued on next page)

Table 2
(*continued*)

Author (Year) [Citation]	Country	Objective	Study Design & Sample Size	Key Findings (Roles, Training, Barriers, and Facilitators)
Tume et al,[49] 2020	57 countries (Europe, North America, Latin America, Asia, Oceania, & Africa)	To explore the perceived barriers by pediatric intensive care health care professionals (nurses, dieticians, and physicians) in delivering enteral nutrition to critically ill children across the world	Cross-sectional survey (n = 920)	• Withholding of the enteral feeds in advance of procedures • Inadequate or lack of dietitian coverage on weekends and evenings • Lack of knowledge, training, time, and education on optimal feeding of the patients
Velarde-García et al,[50] 2017		To describe the difficulties perceived by nursing staff in the delivery of end-of-life care to critically ill patients within ICUs	Descriptive phenomenological qualitative study (n = 22)	• Lack of training in end-of-life care • Inadequate space and privacy for the patient and family • Psychoemotional barriers
Wang et al,[51] 2020	China	To investigate the knowledge, attitudes, and perceived barriers of ICU nurses regarding the early mobilization of ICU patients	Cross-sectional design (n = 227)	• Heavy workload • Insufficient resources • Lack of written guidelines • Insufficient training • Limited staffing and potential work risks
Weare et al,[52] 2019	Austria	To examine the knowledge, skills, and attitudes of a cohort of Australian nurses toward caring for patients with mental illness in the ICU	Survey design (n = 112)	• Training and education to care for patients with mental illness • Negative stereotypes and stigma • Pressure of the environment

Weisgerber,[53] 2018	United States, Canada	To explore what critical care nurses perceive as facilitators of and barriers to providing quality palliative care in critical care	Qualitative descriptive study (n = 12 critical care nurses)	Barriers • Ineffective communication • Challenges with end-of-life decision-making • Lack of palliative care education • Barriers related to the critical care environment Facilitators • Advanced care planning • Effective communication • Palliative care education • Contribution of the interdisciplinary team • Palliative order sets • Provision of a conducive environment
Yaman et al,[54] 2017	Turkey and Poland	To determine the problems related to nurse-patient communication in the ICU	Descriptive survey (n = 102 critical care nurses)	• Communication problems • Patient-to-nurse ratio in ICUs
Facilitators				
Alkhawaldeh et al,[55] 2020	NA	To summarize and appraise the methodological quality of primary studies on interventions for the management of occupational stress among intensive and critical care nurses	Systematic reviews 12 eligible studies	• Cognitive-behavioral skills training • Mindfulness-based intervention

(continued on next page)

Table 2
(*continued*)

Author (Year) [Citation]	Country	Objective	Study Design & Sample Size	Key Findings (Roles, Training, Barriers, and Facilitators)
Anderson,[56] 2021	Central London NHS Trust	To explore the effects of a mindfulness-based stress reduction intervention on a cohort of critical care nurses in terms of quality of life, perceived stress, mindfulness awareness, and sickness and absence rates	Pre-/postinterventional design n = 25 nurses working within a critical care unit	• Mindfulness-based stress reduction intervention
Babanataj et al,[57] 2019	Sari City, Iran	To determine the effect of training for resilience on the ICU nurses' occupational stress and resilience level	Quasi-experimental intervention n = 30 nurses selected from critical care units	• Resilience training
Bourgault et al,[58] 2022	America	To explore sources of evidence sought by critical care nurses during a pandemic and to explore nurses' perceptions of EBP	A qualitative exploratory study	• Formal and informal sources supporting evolving clinical practices, for example, social media
Bourgault et al,[59] 2018	Central Florida	To explore the use of Gemba boards and Gemba huddles to facilitate practice change	Qualitative, descriptive study (n = 22 critical care nurses)	• Utilization of Gemba boards
Breen,[60] 2019	Canada	To examine the impact of education on palliative and end-of-life (EOL) care in normalizing and mitigating nursing grief and promoting resilience	Quasi-experimental study	• Palliative and end-of-life education to ease the grief experiences

Carter et al,[61] 2021	Zambia	To develop and evaluate a Zambian context-specific mentorship model that supports registered nurses completing emergency, trauma, and critical care programs in Zambia	Qualitative study	• Mentorship program of critical care nurses
Crowe,[62] 2017	NA	To examine recent relevant literature for the purpose of developing and creating support for ICU nursing practice for the withdrawal of life-sustaining therapies and end-of-life care	Literature review (n = 119 articles)	• Open communication • Family centered care model & engagement in decision-making • Guidelines for the withdrawal of life care and withdrawal of life-sustaining therapies
Forsberg & Engström,[63] 2018	Northern Sweden	To describe the experiences of critical care nurses (CCNs) when performing successful peripheral intravenous catheterization (PIVC) on adult inpatients in difficult situations	Qualitative approach (n = 22)	• Releasing time and creating peace • Feeling self-confidence in the role of expert nurse • Technical interventions
Jakimowicz et al,[36] 2017	NA	To systematically review the literature describing factors perceived by nurses as affecting the provision of patient-centered nursing in the ICU	An integrative literature review (n = 23)	• Positive values • Colleagues and significant others • Family • Technology

(continued on next page)

Table 2
(continued)

Author (Year) [Citation]	Country	Objective	Study Design & Sample Size	Key Findings (Roles, Training, Barriers, and Facilitators)
Jarden et al,[64] 2019	New Zealand	Identify intensive care nurses' perspectives of strategies that strengthen their workplace well-being	An inductive descriptive qualitative (n = 65)	• Personal resources, such as mindfulness and yoga • Peer supervision • Formal debriefing • Nurses working as a team to support each other
Johansson et al,[65] 2019	Sweden	To explore how nursing staff experienced the use of ICU patient diaries	A qualitative study (n = 27)	• Use of ICU diaries
Kharatzadeh et al,[66] 2020	Sweden	To evaluate the effectiveness of emotional regulation training on depression, anxiety and stress, and professional quality of life for intensive and critical care nurses	Experimental comparison trial (n = 60) Treatment group (n = 30) or a wait-list control group (n = 30)	• Emotional regulation training programs
Lord et al,[67] 2021	Sydney, NSW Australia	To explore ICU nurses' willingness to care during the COVID-19 pandemic	A prospective cross-sectional study (n = 83)	• Timely/effective communication
Wei et al,[68] 2020	United States	To determine perceptions of self-care strategies to combat professional burnout among nurses and physicians in pediatric critical care settings	Qualitative descriptive study (n = 20)	Self-care strategies: • Finding meaning in work • Connecting with an energy source • Nurturing interpersonal connections

			• Developing an attitude of positivity • Performing emotional hygiene • Recognizing one's uniqueness and contributions at work
Zulfiqar & Rafiq,[69] 2020	Pakistan	To explore the experiences and coping strategies of nurses working in pediatric ICUs in a public sector hospital of Lahore, Pakistan	A qualitative study (n = 5)	Coping strategies: • Diet charts • Sharing with colleagues • Religious coping

resources were lacking, ICU nurses doubled as health care assistants and technical or ancillary staff, managed medications, cared for mechanically ventilated patients, provided care to deteriorating patients, and also conducted clinical education.[12] Indeed, although the critical care nursing roles are universal, the outbreak of coronavirus disease 2019 (COVID-19) exposed the lack of preparedness and poor resources to support critical care nurses, especially in low-resource settings.

Training and Orientation

Although professional nursing roles capacity strength relies on initial training, refreshers, workshops, and the institutional on-the-job training frameworks, the review findings indicated undefined standardization of the critical care nursing training and orientation in both HICs and low-resource settings. In HICs, the results indicated that critical care nurses require to have postregistration critical care qualification or critical care training.[8] They also have transition training programs for critical care nurses, continued education, short-period training sessions, short lecture simulations for hands-on skills, and orientation sessions to support critical care nurses.[14,15,17–19] However, although the 2 studies executed in LMIC alluded to similar capacity enhancement trainings for critical care nurses, such as postbasic formal qualifications and informal training,[12] a review conducted in Zambia to validate a critical care nursing course and develop a framework for a Bachelor of Science (BSc) in critical care nursing program revealed a dearth of research on critical care education and lack of standard guidelines to inform critical care nursing.[12,13]

Barriers to Critical Care Nursing Practice

The most abundant literature describing the state of critical care nursing has focused on the existing barriers and facilitators to practice (see **Table 2**). These barriers are inherently different based on resource availabilities. In HICs, some of the most cited barriers to critical care nursing were system level factors, such as ICU environment, poor collaboration between doctors and nurses, emotional distress, posttraumatic stress, anxiety, emotional exhaustion, fear of isolation during COVID-19, and workload stress among the psychosocial challenges experienced by critical care nurses.[23,24,29,33,35,70,71]

Because of heterogeneous nature of the environment in which critical care is provided in both HICs and LMICs, there was an evident variation in reported barriers to critical care nursing. The most dominant barriers in LMIC were lack of critical care guidelines, poor training, lack of knowledge, poor technology, limited resources, and insufficient exposure to the critical care environment[38,39,42,47,52] (see **Table 2**). Equally reported barriers were poor communication in critical care delivery process evident among nurses, doctors, and patients who are challenged by language and also between the management and nurses regarding critical care and work design issues.[53,54] Several studies also identified insufficient staff and high workload for nurses, which caused physical and emotional distress among patients. Fatigue, exhaustion, and burnout resulting from lower nurse patient ratio as well as poor organizational design of the ICU environment were also adduced as barriers to critical care.[51] Other challenges include organizational constraints, such as absence of standards and lack of resources, family challenges, cultural issues, negative stereotypes of the nursing role, and unsuitable or uncomfortable physical environment.

Facilitators for Critical Care Nursing

Regarding supporting framework for critical care nurses, the review had several studies discussing different facilitators for critical care nursing: effective communication,[53,57,62,67] family or colleague support,[36,62,64,69] and cognitive behavioral skills training on mindfulness-based intervention for stress reduction,[55–57] as carried out by institutions such as Britain's National Health Service (NHS).[56] Nurses have also undergone emotional resilience training in places such as Iran.[57] Indeed, mindfulness-based intervention, resilience training, and emotional regulation training programs have capacity to effectively address psychosocial challenges that nurses experience and enhance their emotional capability to cope with stress and other challenges. The critical care environment exposes nurses to posttraumatic stress challenges, and the long working hours could lead to exhaustion and burnout. Effective stress management and coping interventions are necessary to improve the health and well-being of nurses and the quality of outcomes. Other significant facilitators for critical care nurses evidenced in this review were utilization of Gemba Boards, simulation training, use of diet charts, and ICU diaries by nurses to track the critical care service delivery processes.[59,65,69]

Enhancing hands-on skills is critical in strengthening critical care nurses' skills. The review findings found that in both HIC and LMIC simulation training for ICU nurses, utilization of formal and informal sources to support clinical practice, such as social media and technical interventions, is an essential facilitator for critical care.[63,72] Mentorship programs and positive values were reported as some of the mechanisms that nurses have adopted to enhance safety and quality. Other facilitators include self-confidence, interprofessional communication and engagement, teamwork, and self-care strategies. For instance, Wei and colleagues[68,73] identified self-care practices such as finding meaning and purpose in work, nurturing interpersonal connections, and recognizing one's uniqueness and contributions to the workplace. Equally essential in enhancement of success in critical care nursing was the palliative education, advance care planning, and the creation of a conducive environment.[53,74]

DISCUSSION

To the best of our knowledge, this is the first global review providing insights on the current state of roles and responsibilities, on-the-job training, barriers, and facilitators of critical care nurses. Subject to the review's objectives, the findings expounded the defining roles of critical care nurses and the on-the-job training as well as the barriers and facilitators of critical care nursing. Some of the key roles and trainings of critical care nurses identified were providing care for acutely ill patients, delivering expert and specialist care, working as a part of a multidisciplinary team, monitoring and initiate timely treatment, and also providing psychosocial support and advanced system treatment especially in HIC. In LMIC, critical care nurses worked as health care assistants, technical or ancillary staff, and clinical educators, managed medications, cared for mechanically ventilated patients, and provided care to deteriorating patients. Postregistration critical care qualification or critical care training, transition training programs for critical care nurses, continued education, short period refresher and simulation lecture, and orientation sessions were the evident competencies' enhancement initiative for critical care nurses. With regard to barriers and facilitators of critical care nursing in both HIC and LMIC, the study found that system level factors, such as ICU environment, poor collaboration between doctors and nurses, emotional distress, posttraumatic stress, anxiety, emotional exhaustion, fear of isolation during COVID-19, and workload stress were most common barriers in HIC. On the other hand, LMIC-based studies identified lack of critical care guidelines, poor training, lack of knowledge, poor technology, limited resources, and insufficient exposure to the critical care environment. Further, the key facilitators for critical care nursing process among most of the nurses were identified as the provision of necessary resources, defined roles and responsibilities guidelines, technological support, on-the-job trainings and educational skills, cognitive behavioral skills training on mindfulness-based intervention for stress reduction and burnout, timely and effective communication, family or colleague support, emotional resilience training, and utilization of simulation training as well as advanced care plans.

Roles and Responsibilities of Critical Care Nurses

In high-resource settings, critical care nursing is a defined clinical specialty reflecting specific knowledge and clinical competencies. The roles of critical care nurses are clearly understood and generally care is provided in ICUs.[1] Literature describes the role as experts who require vigilance, critical thinking, and rapid responsiveness in high intensity and clinically complex situations. They identify, monitor, and initiate timely treatment to prevent clinical deterioration.[11] They accomplish this through performing regular advanced system assessments, delivering complex medications and procedures.[11] Several publications have described critical care nurses taking on additional roles such as delivering hemodialysis, observing continuous hemodynamic monitoring, and performing mechanical ventilation support. Lastly, it is clear that within high-resource settings, they work within multidisciplinary teams and play a significant role in family and patient communication. They are involved in preparation, facilitation, and follow-up after family care conferences.[10,56] In addition to their responsibilities within the ICU setting, in high-resource countries critical care nurses often lead many outreach teams that identify, monitor, and initiate timely treatment to prevent clinical deterioration and support of non-ICU staff.[75]

In contrast, in low-resource settings roles and responsibilities of critical care nurses are not well defined.[12] Despite being poorly understood, it can be assumed their roles and responsibilities in managing critical illness are inherently different compared with that of their colleagues in high-resource settings. Sparce literature on critical care nursing in LMIC settings highlights several key differences that help shape the nurse's roll. First, critical care is provided across heterogeneous contexts. ICUs are sparse, and many critically ill patients are cared for outside ICUs by nurses with no formal training in critical care.[1,21] The nurses who do work in the few existing ICUs in LMIC settings generally have not received specialized training and often rotate regularly between the ICU and general wards, making it challenging to hone necessary ICU skills[12]; this may cultivate into roles of critical care nurses within a health care institution not being explicitly defined. Often responsibilities of critical care nurses within LMICs not only differ across various ICUs but also tend to include functions and duties devolved from physicians.[12] Lastly, unlike their colleagues in high-resource settings, critical care nurses often lack the technology for continuous monitoring, as technology equipment is either not available or donations of equipment accepted by hospitals without accompanying capacity building leads to limitations in the utility of these well-intentioned gifts, amplified by lack of financial resources for recurrent costs and maintenance. All these challenges confront low-resourced health care systems and make on-the-job training difficult to target critical care nurses, thus hindering the critical care delivery.

Strengthening of Critical Care Capacity

The strengthening of professional nurses' competencies targeted at their defined role is important for global critical care capacity. Unfortunately, even less is understood about the standardization of critical care orientation and continued education. In high-resource countries, it seems critical care nurses frequently receive a formal orientation that may include a critical care consortium with intensive 1 to 3 months of lectures, didactic learning, and one-on-one preceptorship by a more experienced critical care nurse.[14,15] These programs are often facilitated by specialized trained Clinical Nurse Specialists who increase mentorship and staff competencies.[18] And yet, even in environments with clearly defined critical care nursing roles, financial capacity, and staff availability, the orientation programs have been found to differ in duration, structure, components, content, and financial support.[13,15] Continued education (CE) also varies. Although high-income settings often have national nursing body that sets standards and core competencies to ensure proficiency-based licensure, CE is not consistent nationally. Some investigators have tried to describe the efficacy of such programs and found that short lectures on fundamental principles or intensive care nursing, brief hands-on sessions, and simulation training may be an effective CE.[15,16]

Ongoing professional development in low-resource settings are even fewer. Unlike high-resource settings, many LMICs lack a national nursing body that sets standards and core competencies ensuring proficiency-based licensure. Poorly defined roles, lack of financial support for educational time, and a dearth of specialized nurse educators, all contribute to the lack of formal orientation and ongoing education. Orientation is either nonformal or does not exist, and ongoing education is often heavily dependent on partnerships with high-resource international collaborations. The unique responsibilities and knowledge of critical care nursing are instead a nonformal process where knowledge and skill are transferred from more experienced nurses to novice nurses through experiential learning and a patchwork of often north-south training strategies.[13,19]

Our review also identified insufficient knowledge among the barriers for critical care nurses; this results from poor education, lack of training programs, unpreparedness for the critical care environment, poor regulation of critical care nurses competencies, and limited resource.[24,35,38,39,49,52–54,76,77] Poor training contributes to lack of confidence and the negative attitude to nursing and critical care, thus hindering quality and safe care to critically ill patients. The nurse mentorship program in Zambia[13] can be effective in addressing the barriers resulting from lack of education and proper training. The mentorship program focuses on emergency, trauma, and critical care programs, which is aimed at enhancing nurse competency and improving confidence in their abilities to offer safe and quality care. Health institutions need to invest in continuous training and development of their staff to enhance their competence and professional readiness for critical care tasks.[78] Continuous professional development is also necessary to improve nurse confidence motivation and attitude toward critical care practice. The simulation training discussed by Bond and Hallmark[79] can be effective in enhancing nurse competence, and health care institutions also need to use technological interventions that would improve health outcomes. However, these interventions are expensive and their access in LMICs would be limited in view of the existing resource constraints. Nonetheless, investments in simulation and technological interventions have the potential to expand competencies and expertise sharing between and across geographies; hence, while leveraging on advancement in HICs, organizations need to adopt technical interventions to improve nurse competence and clinical practice.

Psychosocial Well-Being of Critical Care Nurses

Further, our review adduced mental health issues resulting from anxiety and burnout as one of the major indicators of the success or failure of critical care nurses. Health care workers are exposed to emotional and psychosocial health challenges arising from the workplace environment and need effective psychological preparedness to cope. Researchers such as DeGrand and colleagues[27,71] identified workplace stress in places such as Texas to be among the key challenges to critical care nursing. Fernandez and colleagues[29] identified fear and isolation in Spain, with nurses fearing punishment, negative judgment, and being stigmatized as incompetent.[31] The researchers also identified psychosocial factors such as worry, anxiety, and stress resulting from caring for patients diagnosed with COVID-19.[33] The evidence shows that critical care nurses are prone to mental health challenges, and health care institutions need proper interventions to stem such challenges. Kharatzadeh and colleagues[66] identified emotional regulation training programs in Sweden as among the facilitators of critical care nurses. Such programs, together with the mindfulness-based stress reduction program offered by the NHS and resilience training offered to Iranian critical care nurses, could be effective in enhancing emotional resilience among nurses.[56,57] In addition, there is need for critical care nurses to adopt coping and self-care strategies, such as finding meaning and purpose in work, nurturing interpersonal connections, and recognizing one's uniqueness and contributions to the workplace.[68] In certain cultures, such as Pakistan, religion can provide an effective coping strategy for critical care nurses.[69] Breen and colleagues[60] also identified palliative and end-of-life education to ease grief experiences among critical care nurses. Jarden and colleagues[64] identified teamwork, formal debriefing peer supervision, and mindfulness and yoga as among the strategies to strengthen the well-being of critical care nurses.

Inadequate Staffing in Critical Care Environments

Related to the psychosocial well-being of critical care nurses, workload, burnout, and emotional fatigue result from insufficient staffing, especially in low-resource settings. Critical care environments require highly trained and experienced nurses to maintain quality and safety standards required to realize favorable outcomes. Limited staffing creates workload challenges, resulting in long working hours, the absence of work-life balance for nurses, and emotional and physical exhaustion of nurses. Organizations need effective mapping of their human resource gap and the development and implementation of the strategies required to address the human resource needs of the organization. Continuous recruitment and selection, performance improvement and management, and nurse retention strategies are critical in stemming staff shortage, which affects the quality and safety of patient care.[80–82] Sufficient staffing will solve the physical challenges experienced by nurses, such as fatigue and exhaustion, as well as the psychological challenges, such as anxiety, fear, and worry.

Organizational Design Challenges

Organizational design challenges such as poor communication and uncomfortable working environments hinder effective delivery of critical care nursing. The review synthesis indicated that nurses reported various communication challenges when handling patients who are not versed with English and those who could not communicate at all. Furthermore, poor communication with colleagues and unstructured communication flow from management was a key issue in critical care settings. Poor design of the ICU environment and other organizational challenges such as the absence of modern facilities for safe and quality care were also identified. Effective and open communication enhances critical care nursing services.[53,62,67] Nurses work in wide environments requiring collaboration and coordination; hence, health care institutions need to establish proper communication frameworks among nurses. Effective interprofessional communication and engagement has been identified as among the most effective strategies for enhancing safety and improving quality within the critical care environment. Weisgerber[53] also identified conducive work environment as an important facilitator of safety and quality in critical care nursing. Health care institutions should use effective work-life balance strategies and improve organizational aspects such as leadership, peer supervision, teamwork, and employee engagement to make the workplace environment more conducive for critical care nurses.

Implications of the Findings

Overall, although this review informs on the existing health care gaps in critical care nursing across the globe, it is evident that the LMIC nurses face a myriad of challenges. In our understanding, in low-resource settings, critical care is provided across heterogeneous contexts. ICUs are sparse, and many critically ill patients are cared for outside ICUs by nurses with no formal training in critical care. Nurses who work in the few existing ICUs in LMIC settings generally have not received specialized training and often rotate regularly between the ICU and general wards, making it challenging to hone necessary ICU skills. Furthermore, the roles of critical care nurses within a health care institution may not be explicitly defined, and responsibilities of critical care nurses may not only be different across various ICUs but often include functions and duties devolved from physicians. Besides, ongoing professional development in low-resource settings are few due to lack of a national nursing body that sets standards and core competencies ensuring proficiency-based licensure that contributes to the limited in-service training and uncertainty about roles and responsibilities. Lack of human resources results in inappropriate task shifting and significantly higher patient:nurse ratios than in HIC where there are laws that limit these ratios. Indeed, lack of defined roles, responsibilities, and the on-the-job training calls for development of clear guides to inform care practices among low-resource setting ICU nurses. There is a significant need to address the technological knowhow, resources issues, educational training, better-staffing, basic monitoring, and ventilation management skills, as well as standardization of the onboarding process for critical care nurses in LMIC. The fundamental voicing of the ICU nurses by enhancing their competencies is significant in advancing the care practice and improving the quality of life among the critically ill patients.

A holistic strategy is required to overcome these existing barriers and improve nursing care of the critically ill in low-resource settings. For example, it is important to recognize where critically ill patients are managed and by whom in the health care structure. This facilitates the definition of nursing roles and delineation of responsibilities within the system. Perhaps the most central element, however, is to enhance nurse training. This is an important and cost-effective strategy to meet the health care needs of a population.

One model frequently used in LMIC settings is in-service training provided by groups from high-resource settings, usually teams from nonprofit organizations or schools of nursing in wealthy countries. Successful implementation of these collaborative initiatives requires a comprehensive understanding of the nurse's role and previous training. Visiting teams must recognize their limitations when different languages are used, and they need to be familiar with local contexts and have studied the cultural norms and customs in order to effectively engage key stakeholders in the health care and government sectors. Adequate financial support is necessary for the development, implementation, and sustainment of educational collaborations. Funding models should leverage existing resources while minimizing the financial burden on LMICs, making sure to be adding to the dearth of resources and not taking. Many current strategies depend on nurses from HIC to pay significant funds and volunteer their time. One unique approach to improve financial sustainability is twinning mixed resourced hospitals where employers support their nurses to work with their LMIC partners as part of their professional practice. Training formats should also recognize and accommodate LMIC provider challenges including the time and cost burden (such as, transportation, time away from the bedside), which can make nurse participation difficult. To date, north-south training strategies have been ineffective because they are based in didactic classroom settings, rather than in the clinical setting, making it difficult for nurses to translate their learning into practice. Applied training creates long-term system improvements and ensures content meets the needs of local nursing practice. Foreign educators who are not immersed in a culture and do not base their training on detailed needs assessments often find it difficult to address the challenges and meet the training needs of their students.

The well-being of ICU nurses is crucial in health care delivery. Therefore, it is essential for health care to address the organizational challenges that affect quality and health outcomes. Health care institutions should also identify the professional challenges that nurses face and implement strategies to improve the health and well-being of their nurses. Cognitive behavior training on mindfulness and resilience for stress reduction are critical in addressing the psychological challenges that critical care nurses experience, such as stress, anxiety, worry, and fear. In addition, institutions require nurse mentorship programs aimed at boosting confidence and enhancing critical care outcomes. Organizations also require effective interprofessional communication and engagement among nurses to encourage teamwork and peer support among critical care nurses. Health care institutions will also need effective organizational design and development to provide the right human and material resources required to enhance quality, safety, and critical care outcomes. At individual level, critical care nurses should improve their skills and competence, adopt appropriate coping strategies, engage colleagues, and establish conducive environments for critical care practice. However, the major driver is to steer development of policy and regulatory framework for enhancing and standardizing competencies and role clarity for ICU nurses in LMICs through guidelines on scopes of practice for critical care nurses and harmonizing education and training.

CLINICS CARE POINTS

- Although critical care nursing is an essential service in the health care system, the absence of a cross-cutting definition and clear national guidelines on critical care nursing practice and a critical care nursing body that sets standards and core competencies to ensure proficiency-based licensure contributes to the limited in-service training and uncertainty about roles and responsibilities.

- While in-service training, emotional regulations, effective communication, and international partnerships emerge as some of the facilitators of critical care nursing practice, there is a need for a holistic strategy to overcome the existing barriers and improve nursing care of the critically ill in low-resource settings.

DISCLOSURE

The authors have nothing to disclose.

REFERENCES

1. Aitken LM, Chaboyer W, Schuetz M, et al. Health status of critically ill trauma patients. J Clin Nurs 2014;23(5–6):704–15.

2. Gyasi RM, Phillips DR. Aging and the rising burden of noncommunicable diseases in sub-Saharan Africa and other low-and middle-income countries: a call for holistic action. Gerontologist 2020;60(5):806–11.

3. Aiken LH, Sloane DM, Bruyneel L, et al. Nurse staffing and education and hospital mortality in nine European countries: a retrospective observational study. Lancet 2014;383(9931):1824–30.

4. Chamberlain D, Pollock W, Fulbrook P. ACCCN Workforce standards for intensive care nursing: systematic and evidence review, development, and appraisal. Aust Crit Care 2018;31(5):292–302.

5. Murthy S, Wunsch H. Clinical review: international comparisons in critical care - lessons learned. Crit Care 2012;16(2):218.

6. Page MJ, McKenzie JE, Bossuyt PM, et al. The PRISMA 2020 statement: an updated guideline for reporting systematic reviews. Bmj 2021;372.

7. Anderson W, Turner K. Palliative care in the ICU: a 360° view of the nurse's role. Crit Care Nurse 2020;40(5):84.

8. Bloomer MJ, Fulbrook P, Goldsworthy S, et al. World Federation of critical care nurses 2019 position statement: provision of a critical care nursing Workforce. Connect 2019;13(1):3–7.

9. Credland N, Stayt L, Plowright C, et al. Essential critical care skills 1: what is critical care nursing? Nurs Times 2021;117(11):18–21.

10. Kawashima T, Tanaka M, Kawakami A, et al. Nurses' contribution to end-of-life family conferences in critical care: a Delphi study. Nurs Crit Care 2020;25(5): 305–12.

11. Kurth A, Pinker E, Martinello RA, et al. Critical care nursing: a key constraint to COVID-19 Response and healthcare Now and in the Future. J Nurs Adm 2021; 51(3):E6–12.

12. Macey A, O'Reilly G, Williams G, et al. Critical care nursing role in low and lower middle-income settings: a scoping review. BMJ Open 2022;12(1):e055585.

13. Carter C, Mukonka PJ, Sitwala LJ, et al. The development of critical care nursing education in Zambia. Br J Nurs 2020;29(9):499–505.

14. Cunnington T, Calleja P. Transition support for new graduate and novice nurses in critical care settings: an integrative review of the literature. Nurse Education Pract 2018;30:62–72.

15. McBride ME, Beke DM, Fortenberry JD, et al. Education and training in pediatric Cardiac critical care. World J Pediatr Congenit Heart Surg 2017;8(6):707–14.

16. Monesi A, Imbriaco G, Mazzoli CA, et al. In-situ simulation for intensive care nurses during the COVID-19 pandemic in Italy: Advantages and challenges. Clin Simul Nurs 2022;62:52–6.

17. Padhya D, Tripathi S, Kashyap R, et al. Training of pediatric critical care providers in developing countries in evidence based medicine utilizing Remote simulation sessions. Glob Pediatr Health 2021;8. 2333794X211007473.

18. Short K, Freedman K, Matays J, et al. Making the transition: a critical care skills program to support newly hired nurses. Clin Nurse Spec 2019;33(3):123–7.

19. Stephens T, De Silva AP, Beane A, et al. Capacity building for critical care training delivery: development and evaluation of the Network for Improving Critical care Skills Training (NICST) programme in Sri Lanka. Intensive Crit Care Nurs 2017; 39:28–36.

20. Beckstrand RL, Willmore EE, Macintosh JL, et al. Critical care nurses' qualitative Reports of experiences with physician behaviors, nursing issues, and other Obstacles in end-of-life care. Dimensions Crit Care Nurs 2021;40(4):237–47.

21. Bahramnezhad F, Dolatabadi ZA. Letter to editor: a report on the first meeting on the role of the nurses working in the intensive care units in emergencies and disasters in Iran. Health Emergencies Disasters Q 2019;5(1):1–3.

22. Begerow A, Michaelis U, Gaidys U. Wahrnehmungen von Pflegenden im Bereich der Intensivpflege während der COVID-19-Pandemie. Pflege 2020;33(4):229–36.

23. Castellà-Creus M, Delgado-Hito P, Casanovas-Cuellar C, et al. Barriers and facilitators involved in standardised care plan individualisation process in acute hospitalisation wards: a grounded theory approach. J Clin Nurs 2019;28(23–24):4606–20.

24. Çelik S, Taşdemir N, Kurt A, et al. Fatigue in intensive care nurses and related factors. Int J Occup Environ Med 2017;8(4):199–206.

25. Coleman JS, Angosta AD. The lived experiences of acute-care bedside registered nurses caring for patients and their families with limited English proficiency: a silent shift. J Clin Nurs 2017;26(5–6):678–89.

26. CotrĂU P, Hodosan V, Vladu A, et al. Burnout, perceived stress and work satisfaction of intensive care unit nurses. Appl Med Inform 2019;41:38.

27. DeGrande H, Liu F, Greene P, et al. Developing professional competence among critical care nurses: an integrative review of literature. Intensive Crit Care Nurs 2018;49:65–71.

28. Falk AC, Schandl A, Frank C. Barriers in achieving patient participation in the critical care unit. Intensive Crit Care Nurs 2019;51:15–9.

29. Fernández-Castillo RJ, González-Caro MD, Fernández-García E, et al. Intensive care nurses' experiences during the COVID-19 pandemic: a qualitative study. Nurs Crit Care 2021;26(5):397–406.

30. Ghazanchaie Z, Nourian M, Khanali MAjan L, et al. Nurses' toward palliative care and its barriers in neonatal intensive care Units. J Crit Care Nurs 2020;13(3):20–30.

31. Ghezeljeh TN, Farahani MA, Ladani FK. Factors affecting nursing error communication in intensive care units: a qualitative study. Nurs Ethics 2021;28(1):131–44.

32. González-Gil MT, González-Blázquez C, Parro-Moreno AI, et al. Nurses' perceptions and demands regarding COVID-19 care delivery in critical care units and hospital emergency services. Intensive Crit Care Nurs 2021;62:102966.

33. Gordon JM, Magbee T, Yoder LH. The experiences of critical care nurses caring for patients with COVID-19 during the 2020 pandemic: a qualitative study. Appl Nurs Res 2021;59:151418.

34. Habiballah L. Nurses perceived barriers toward pressure ulcer prevention in critical care units in Jordan. Pakistan J Med Health Sci 2017;11(4):1623–8.

35. Jackson J, Vandall-Walker V, Vanderspank-Wright B, et al. Burnout and resilience in critical care nurses: a grounded theory of Managing Exposure. Intensive Crit Care Nurs 2018;48:28–35.

36. Jakimowicz S, Perry L, Lewis J. An integrative review of supports, facilitators and barriers to patient-centred nursing in the intensive care unit. J Clin Nurs 2017;26(23–24):4153–71.

37. Kim H, Chang SJ. Implementing an educational program to improve critical care nurses' enteral nutritional support. Aust Crit Care 2019;32(3):218–22.

38. Kiwanuka F, Shayan SJ, Tolulope AA. Barriers to patient and family-centred care in adult intensive care units: a systematic review. Nurs Open 2019;6(3):676–84.

39. Kydonaki K, Hanley J, Huby G, et al. Challenges and barriers to optimising sedation in intensive care: a qualitative study in eight Scottish intensive care units. BMJ Open 2019;9(5):e024549.

40. Limbu S, Kongsuwan W, Yodchai K. Lived experiences of intensive care nurses in caring for critically ill patients. Nurs Crit Care 2019;24(1):9–14.

41. Liyew B, Tilahun AD, Kassew T. Practices and barriers towards physical assessment among nurses working in intensive care Units: Multicenter cross-sectional study. Biomed Res Int 2021;2021:5524676.

42. Meilando R, Kosasih CE, Emaliyawati E. Barriers and challenges of end-of-life care implementation in the intensive care Unit: literature review. Jurnal Keperawatan Komprehensif (Comprehensive Nurs Journal) 2022;8(1):1–125.

43. Nankundwa E, Brysiewicz P. Lived experiences of Rwandan ICU nurses caring for patients with a do-not-resuscitate order. South Afr J Crit Care 2017;33(1): 19–22.

44. Ong KK, Ting KC, Chow YL. The trajectory of experience of critical care nurses in providing end-of-life care: a qualitative descriptive study. J Clin Nurs 2018; 27(1–2):257–68.

45. Pastores SM, Kvetan V, Coopersmith CM, et al. Workforce, workload, and burnout among intensivists and advanced practice providers: a narrative review. Crit Care Med 2019;47(4):550–7.

46. Petersen JA, Rasmussen LS, Rydahl-Hansen S. Barriers and facilitating factors related to use of early warning score among acute care nurses: a qualitative study. BMC Emerg Med 2017;17(1):36.

47. Rababa M, Al-Sabbah S, Hayajneh AA. Nurses' perceived barriers to and facilitators of pain assessment and management in critical care patients: a systematic review. J Pain Res 2021;14:3475–91.

48. Robstad N, Söderhamn U, Fegran L. Intensive care nurses' experiences of caring for obese intensive care patients: a hermeneutic study. J Clin Nurs 2018;27(1–2): 386–95.

49. Tume LN, Eveleens RD, Verbruggen S, et al. Barriers to delivery of enteral Nutrition in pediatric intensive care: a World survey. Pediatr Crit Care Med 2020;21(9): e661–71.

50. Velarde-García JF, Espejo MM, González-Hervías R, et al. [End of life care difficulties in intensive care units. The nurses' perspective]. Gac Sanit 2017;31(4): 299–304.

51. Wang J, Xiao Q, Zhang C, et al. Intensive care unit nurses' knowledge, attitudes, and perceived barriers regarding early mobilization of patients. Nurs Crit Care 2020;25(6):339–45.

52. Weare R, Green C, Olasoji R, et al. ICU nurses feel unprepared to care for patients with mental illness: a survey of nurses' attitudes, knowledge, and skills. Intensive Crit Care Nurs 2019;53:37–42.

53. Weisgerber, L., Barriers and Facilitators in the Provision of Quality Palliative Critical Care: Critical Care Nurse's Perspectives. 2018.

54. Yaman Aktas Y, Nagórska M, Karabulut N. Problems in critical care nurse-patient communication: examples of Poland and Turkey. Acta Clin Croat 2017;56(3): 437–45.

55. Alkhawaldeh JMA, Soh KL, Mukhtar FBM, et al. Stress management interventions for intensive and critical care nurses: a systematic review. Nurs Crit Care 2020; 25(2):84–92.

56. Anderson N. An evaluation of a mindfulness-based stress reduction intervention for critical care nursing staff: a quality improvement project. Nurs Crit Care 2021; 26(6):441–8.

57. Babanataj R, Mazdarani S, Hesamzadeh A, et al. Resilience training: Effects on occupational stress and resilience of critical care nurses. Int J Nurs Pract 2019;25(1):e12697.
58. Bourgault AM, Davis JW, Peach BC, et al. Use of social media to exchange critical care practice evidence during the pandemic. Dimensions Crit Care Nurs 2022;41(1):36–45.
59. Bourgault AM, Upvall MJ, Graham A. Using Gemba Boards to facilitate evidence-based practice in critical care. Crit Care Nurse 2018;38(3):e1–7.
60. Breen C. Easing the grief of pediatric critical care nurses through education on palliative and end-of-life (EOL) care...Canadian Association of critical care nurses' Dynamics of critical care conference 2019, September 16-18, 2019, Halifax, Nova Scotia. Can J Crit Care Nurs 2019;30(2):25.
61. Carter C, Mukonka PS, Sitwala LJ, et al. The 'sleeping elephant': the role of mentorship of critical care nurses in Zambia. Int Nurs Rev 2021;68(4):543–50.
62. Crowe S. End-of-life care in the ICU: supporting nurses to provide high-quality care. Can J Crit Care Nurs 2017;28(1):30–3.
63. Forsberg A, Engström Å. Critical care nurses' experiences of performing successful peripheral intravenous catheterization in difficult situations. J Vasc Nurs 2018;36(2):64–70.
64. Jarden RJ, Sandham M, Siegert RJ, et al. Strengthening workplace well-being: perceptions of intensive care nurses. Nurs Crit Care 2019;24(1):15–23.
65. Johansson M, Wåhlin I, Magnusson L, et al. Nursing staff's experiences of intensive care unit diaries: a qualitative study. Nurs Crit Care 2019;24(6):407–13.
66. Kharatzadeh H, Alavi M, Mohammadi A, et al. Emotional regulation training for intensive and critical care nurses. Nurs Health Sci 2020;22(2):445–53.
67. Lord H, Loveday C, Moxham L, et al. Effective communication is key to intensive care nurses' willingness to provide nursing care amidst the COVID-19 pandemic. Intensive Crit Care Nurs 2021;62:102946.
68. Wei H, Kifner H, Dawes E, et al. Self-care strategies to Combat burnout among pediatric critical care nurses and physicians. Crit Care Nurse 2020;40(2):44–53.
69. Zulfiqar L, Rafiq M. Exploring experiences and coping strategies of nurses working in intensive care unit: a qualitative study. Anaesth Pain Intensive Care 2020;24(1):42–9.
70. Al-Majid S, Carlson N, Kiyohara M, et al. Assessing the Degree of Compassion satisfaction and Compassion fatigue among critical care, Oncology, and Charge nurses. J Nurs Adm 2018;48(6):310–5.
71. DeGrande H, Liu F, Greene P, et al. The experiences of new graduate nurses hired and retained in adult intensive care units. Intensive Crit Care Nurs 2018;49:72–8.
72. Bourgault AM. Critical care nurse and the Editors who shaped the Journal's history. Crit Care Nurse 2021;41(4):12–4.
73. Wei W, Niu Y, Ge X. Core competencies for nurses in Chinese intensive care units: a cross-sectional study. Nurs Crit Care 2019;24(5):276–82.
74. Breen SJ, Rees S. Barriers to implementing the Sepsis Six guidelines in an acute hospital setting. Br J Nurs 2018;27(9):473–8.
75. Credland N, Gerber K. The BACCN and COVID: what have we learned? Nurs Crit Care 2020;25(4):201–2.
76. Alberto L, Pawlowicz RG, Barrionuevo E, et al. Critical care in critical times of COVID-19 in Argentina: a Viewpoint. Connect 2020;14(3):147–53.
77. Kim C, Kim S, Yang J, et al. Nurses' perceived barriers and educational needs for early mobilisation of critical ill patients. Aust Crit Care 2019;32(6):451–7.

78. Viljoen M, Coetzee I, Heyns T. Critical care nurses' reasons for poor attendance at a continuous professional development program. Am J Crit Care 2017; 26(1):70–6.
79. Bond L, Hallmark B. Educating nurses in the intensive care Unit about Gastrointestinal Complications: using an Algorithm Embedded into simulation. Crit Care Nurs Clin North Am 2018;30(1):75–85.
80. Martin J, Kumar K. Education needs of Australian Flight nurses: a qualitative study. Air Med J 2020;39(3):178–82.
81. Martin JB, Badeaux JE. Beyond the intensive care Unit: Posttraumatic stress Disorder in critically ill patients. Crit Care Nurs Clin North Am 2018;30(3):333–42.
82. Martinez R, Rogado MIC, Serondo DJF, et al. Critical care nursing in the Philippines: Historical Past, current practices, and Future Directions. Crit Care Nurs Clin North Am 2021;33(1):75–87.

The State of Global Trauma and Acute Care Surgery/ Surgical Critical Care

Kapil Dev Soni, MD[a], Varun Bansal, MBBS[b],
Harshit Arora, MBBS (Dayanand Medical College & Hospital)[c],
Sukriti Verma, MBBS (Himalayan Institute of Medical Sciences)[d,e],
Martin Gerdin Wärnberg, MD, PhD[f,g,1],
Nobhojit Roy, MD, MPH, PhD[e,h,*]

KEYWORDS

- Global trauma • Acute care surgery • Surgical critical care
- Trauma economic burden • Trauma systems • Global trauma solutions
- Trauma registries

KEY POINTS

- Trauma is a leading cause of morbidity and mortality globally, with a significant burden attributable to the low- and middle-income countries.
- Road injuries are the major contributors to trauma-related economic burden, with the United States, China, and India being the highest impacted countries.
- Many injured patients are treated in critical care units, and timely intervention may improve the overall prognosis.
- Strengthening existing care mechanisms can help develop efficient and cost-effective trauma systems.

[a] Critical & Intensive Care, Jai Prakash Narayan Apex Trauma Center, All India Institute of Medical Sciences, Ring Road, Raj Nagar, Safdarjung Enclave, New Delhi, Delhi 110029, India; [b] Department of General Surgery, 2nd Floor Registration Building, Seth G.S.M.C. and K.E.M. Hospital, Parel, Mumbai 400012, India; [c] Department of Surgery, Punjab Institute of Medical Sciences, Gadha Road, Jalandhar, Punjab 144006, India; [d] Department of Blood Bank, Guru Teg Bahadur Hospital, Tahirpur Rd, GTB Enclave, Dilshad Garden, New Delhi, Delhi 110095, India; [e] WHO Collaborating Center for Research on Surgical Care Delivery in LMICs, Department of Surgery, BARC Hospital, Anushaktinagar, Mumbai 400094, India; [f] Department of Global Public Health, Karolinska Institutet, Tomtebodavägen 18, 171 65 Solna, Stockholm 171 65, Sweden; [g] Function Perioperative Medicine and Intensive Care, Karolinska University Hospital Solna, SE - 171 76, Stockholm, Sweden; [h] The George Institute of Global Health India, F-BLOCK, 311-312, Third Floor, Jasola Vihar, New Delhi, Delhi 110025, India
[1] Shared senior co-author with Roy.
* Corresponding author. The George Insitute of Global Health, New Delhi, India.
E-mail address: nobsroy@gmail.com

Crit Care Clin 38 (2022) 695–706
https://doi.org/10.1016/j.ccc.2022.06.011
0749-0704/22/© 2022 Elsevier Inc. All rights reserved.

INTRODUCTION

Trauma is a global health problem with an unevenly distributed impact, the major brunt borne by low- and middle-income countries (LMICs), where more than 90% of worldwide trauma-related deaths occur[1] (**Fig. 1**). Furthermore, countries belonging to lower socioeconomic strata have proportionally greater age-standardized injury-related death rates (**Fig. 2**). Within these regions, people from poor backgrounds are more vulnerable, making poverty a risk factor for trauma-related morbidity and mortality. In this review, we describe the worldwide distribution of trauma and critical care facilities and discuss solutions for mitigating the burden in LMICs.

TRAUMA AND GLOBAL BURDEN OF DISEASE

In 2019, 714 million people suffered, and 4.3 million died from injuries, accounting for 7.6% of the worldwide mortality.[2] Over the last 30 years, trauma has been consistently ranked as the leading cause of death in the 10–49-year age group and overall, the third most common cause of global deaths and disability-adjusted life years (DALYs). Although the incidence of trauma has increased by 12.5% between the years 2010 and 2019, the age-standardized death rates (see **Fig. 2**) and DALY rates (**Fig. 3**) have decreased by 19.4% and 18.6%, respectively. Since 1990, there has been a marked shift toward a greater proportion of the burden of DALYs due to years lost due to disability (YLDs) from noncommunicable diseases and injuries, compared with communicable, maternal, neonatal, and nutritional diseases, the epidemiological transition being most noticeable in high-income countries (HICs).

Unintentional injuries are a major contributor to the 4.3 million annual trauma-related deaths, with road traffic injuries (RTIs) being prevalent among adolescents and young adults and falls in the elderly. Geographic variations in fatal trauma mechanisms result from a higher proportion of penetrating injuries in HICs, which contribute significantly to the burden of self-harm and interpersonal violence.[2] Apart from leading to deaths, nonfatal trauma is associated with increased acute care hospital visits and disabilities requiring long-term rehabilitation. Hence, preventing injuries has been included in Sustainable Development Goal targets, focusing on unintentional injuries.[3]

It is difficult to characterize the burden of severe trauma in LMICs owing to a paucity of resources for quantifying outcome measures and the limited availability of critical care facilities,[4] because of which first-hand intensive care unit (ICU)-based data are likely to underestimate the true magnitude of the population at risk. However, mortality from critical illnesses in LMICs is reported to be higher than that in HICs and has been shown to affect younger age groups.[5,6]

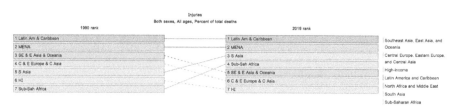

Fig. 1. Ranking based on percentage of total injury-related deaths with respect to Global Burden of Disease region in 1990 and 2019, showing that the least proportion of deaths occurred in HICs (5.48%) in 2019. (Institute for Health Metrics Evaluation. Used with permission. All rights reserved.)

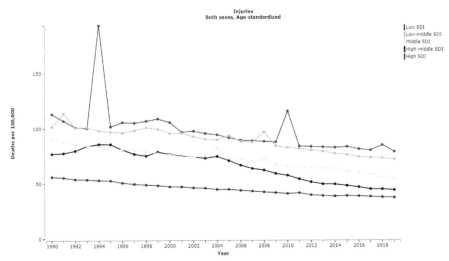

Fig. 2. Declining trend of age-standardized death rates from 1990 to 2019 categorized by Sociodemographic Index (SDI), a composite indicator of income per capita, years of schooling, and fertility rate in females under 25 years of age. (Institute for Health Metrics Evaluation. Used with permission. All rights reserved.)

ECONOMIC COSTS TO NATIONS

In addition to their direct medical consequences, trauma and critical illnesses have major economic implications. In a simulation study, Chen and colleagues[7] estimated that road injuries will cost the world economy about US$1.8 trillion (measured in constant prices as of 2010) in 2015–2030. The United States, China, and India will be the highest

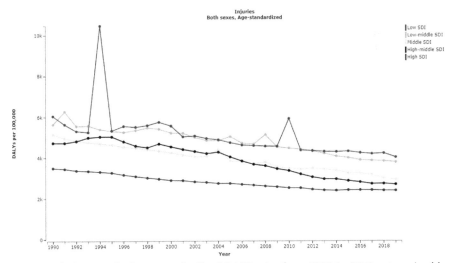

Fig. 3. Declining trend of age-standardized DALY rates from 1990 to 2019 categorized by Sociodemographic Index (SDI). (Institute for Health Metrics Evaluation. Used with permission. All rights reserved.)

impacted countries. Despite the large share of road injury-related DALYs contributed by LMICs, their share of the economic burden is only 46.4% of the global loss. This study suggested that though LMICs have the highest trauma burden, HICs share the largest economic fallout of road injuries. The macroeconomic burden among LMICs is expected to rise owing to increased motorization and infrastructure development.[8]

Trauma Systems Worldwide

A trauma system is a comprehensive and coordinated injury response network equipped with the facilities to care for an injured patient.[9] It includes emergency medical services (EMS) dispatch and pre-arrival instructions, EMS field triage and transport, trauma system hospital, inter-facility transfer, trauma team activation, operating room and interventional radiology, ICU, and general unit care, early rehabilitation, and injury prevention.[10] The World Health Organization (WHO) proposed a Trauma System Maturity Index which classified trauma centers from Level I to Level IV with the former being the least mature or unorganized and the latter being the most mature and well equipped.[11] This is contrary to the classification proposed by the American College of Surgeons/Committee on Trauma (ACS/COT), which classified centers from Level I to Level III.[11,12] The higher number of Level I and II trauma centers in LMICs as compared with Level III and IV systems in HICs is explained by the greater availability of trained personnel, ambulances, and better adherence to trauma management protocols supported by advanced facilities in HICs.[11]

The lacunae in trauma care at various stages likely account for the higher injury-related mortality in LMICs, which is approximately twice that in HICs.[13] To begin with, most LMICs lack organized prehospital care and triage, without systematic communication between the EMS team and hospital personnel before the transfer, leading to unpreparedness for critically injured patients.[14,15] Most emergency personnel in LMICs lack training in Basic Life Support (BLS) and Advanced Trauma Life Support (ATLS), as a consequence of which patients do not receive prehospital life-saving treatment.[14,16] Delays in seeking definitive care are prevalent among patients injured in smaller cities; many of whom clock unnecessary distances and receive nontherapeutic interventions at inadequately equipped basic and intermediate level health centers before arriving at tertiary care centers. The time from injury to receiving care varies widely within these countries, ranging from approximately 9–10 h in poorly resourced regions[17,18] to less than an hour in metropolitan cities.[19] Lack of training, equipment and drugs, and hospital policy-related issues contribute to the failure of provision of essential functions such as cervical spine and limb fracture immobilization, pelvic fixation, and immediate dressing of burns at peripheral and some district-level health centers.[20,21] District and central tertiary care centers experience a significant shortage of staff and resources needed round the clock for patient care, including laboratory and imaging investigations, and personal protection.[22,23] Lastly, long-term patient care services are not addressed adequately, with referral and transportation delays resulting in deficient patient rehabilitation via occupation and physical therapy.[24]

Acute Care Surgery

Acute care surgery applies similar principles of trauma care – team approach, processes, and quality improvement – to other time-sensitive non-trauma surgical conditions. It encompasses the management of critically ill patients developing shock, organ failure, sepsis, and requiring advanced organ support following acute non-trauma surgical conditions. This broadened scope of surgical care has led to the development of this specific field in surgical care. Initially in most places model started as on call surgeon for all emergency surgeries. This often-caused overburdening of the emergency surgical sphere and restriction or cancellation of elective surgeries. To optimize the resources and efficient organized systems of surgical care delivery, the models of Acute Care Surgeries were developed and implemented across the healthcare system in North America. The model ensemble dedicated surgical teams – surgeons, residents, and nursing staff with expertise in surgical critical care as well. The essential structural components of ACS models are- ED, Trauma, and Critical Care coverage. The surgeons with such training are accountable for the Acute care chain, beginning from the emergency department, Operating room, and critical care of patients. This development of Acute care surgery and critical care enabled the rekindling of acute care surgery compared to other elective surgical branches. The adoption of acute care surgical models within the healthcare systems has been shown to improve patient outcomes and cost-effectiveness within the North American healthcare system[25]. However, there is considerable variation in the development and adoption of these ACS models worldwide due to nonuniform resources and priorities. In the recent systematic review, the authors investigated the essential components of the ACS model and their adoption worldwide.[26] They found that most developed ACS models were chiefly in North America and to some extent in Australia. While within Europe and in a few countries in Asia the studies reported either partial adoption of the model or the initial phases of adoption. The heterogeneous adoption of ACS models reflects larger variation in the healthcare environment, resources, needs, and competing priorities or it may be reflective of the time lag of the development of healthcare systems overall. In LMIC the focus is on overall access to emergency healthcare rather than acute care surgery, thus restricting the development.Of all the three components – ED, Acute Surgery, and Critical Care – the adherence to availability of dedicated surgical care for all non-trauma emergency surgery was highest in hospitals that adopted the ACS models, though the round–clock site attending coverage was found only in centers from US and Taiwan. Critical care services, which are integral to ACS models, have been largely confined to US models and have not been reported from other parts of the world. Though ACS models have shown improvement in the care of non-trauma acute care surgical practices, the widespread adoption in different health care environments remains little. Whether the adoption of ACS models in different health care settings would have a similar effect as in North American settings, is yet to be evaluated. Though the potential benefit can not be excluded, the ineffectiveness with wastage of resources, overburdening of healthcare system is also a possibility, given the mismatch between demand and availability of resources. The adoption of ACS models worldwide would require flexibility in approach and would need need to be context specific integrating the essential components of ACS with available resources.

THE INTERPLAY BETWEEN TRAUMA AND CRITICAL CARE

Critical care emphasizes life-saving and supportive therapies that maintain vital organ functions rather than the definitive treatment, which is the focus of other medical specialties. The core interventions for trauma management, similar to critical care, encompass physiologic monitoring and stabilization to allow specific therapies to improve the underlying condition causing acute deterioration. Most measures in acute trauma management rely upon timely interventions, beginning with securing the airway, breathing, and circulation, which if delayed or performed unsatisfactorily reduce the efficacy of the intervention. Khajanchi and colleagues[27] reported that only 15% of patients with severe isolated traumatic brain injury (Glasgow Coma Scale score < 9) received a definite airway before arriving at tertiary care centers in an Indian trauma registry, in contrast with Level 1 recommendations for intubation by various trauma guidelines.[28,29] Deficiencies in fluids, vasopressors, and inotropes for maintaining circulation are common, exacerbated by a failure to display cardiopulmonary resuscitation (CPR) algorithms in resuscitation trolleys, even in tertiary care hospitals in LMICs.[30,31] Many trauma-related deaths occur in the first week, after 24 h in the ICU.[32] The delayed deaths are often attributed to post-injury complications such as acute respiratory distress syndrome, pneumonia, coagulopathy, and acute kidney injury.[33] The impact of post-injury intensive care complications is unknown owing to deficient data in LMIC settings.

Considering the urgent needs of critically injured patients, it is hypothesized that treating them in dedicated trauma units may improve outcomes compared with general care in emergency departments and ICUs catering to trauma and non-trauma patients simultaneously.[34,35] However, the availability of the former is variable, albeit negligible worldwide, especially in LMICs. Furthermore, a survey of trauma centers in the United States revealed distinct variability in managing patients in trauma ICUs, with many beds being occupied by non-trauma surgical patients.[36]

Global Trauma Management in Intensive Care Units

The availability of ICUs varies globally, irrespective of disease epidemiology. Although approximately 5–30 ICU beds are available per 100,000 people in HICs, only 0.1–2.5 ICU beds are available per 100,000 people in LMICs.[37] Fundamentally, the provision of critical care should be standardized as many trauma-related deaths are preventable. However, disparities exist and are multifactorial.

First, ICUs are resource-intensive, and despite using substantial resources, outcomes may be unfavorable. Compared with critical illnesses, fewer resources are needed for treating non-acute illnesses, which also provide favorable outcomes. Thus, it may not be cost-effective to set up ICUs. Costing studies from HICs report average daily costs of ICU care between US\$230 and 4915 (as per costs in 2020).[38] Though the average cost reported in an LMIC-based study was US\$109, it is not covered by insurance in many LMICs.[39–41] The severity of illness, mechanical ventilation, hemodialysis, and longer length of stay are associated with escalation of charges.[38,42,43] Although the growth of private-care hospitals in LMICs may partially offset the demand for critical care services, the quality of care is variable, and only a small subset of the population can afford the associated expenses.[8] This deficit is further compounded by reductions in international health care aids as countries transition from lower-income to lower-middle-income status.[44] Thus, there is an unmet need for an affordable critical care model and restructuring organization.

Second, most ICU interventions are technologically demanding, which hampers uniform availability and adoption, thus leading to a large variation in the quality of ICUs.[37] Although overall ICU-running costs are lower in LMICs, equipment costs can be significantly higher because of importation taxes and noncompetitive pricing structures resulting from a dearth of local manufacturers and indigenous products.[37,45]

Third, in low-resource settings, hospitals are often burdened with an influx of critically ill patients beyond their ICU capacity. This limited availability of ICU beds leads to spill over of acutely ill patients in the wards and other settings, compromising their care. Improvement in organizational structure, hospital-wide triage models, training and empowerment of nurses, and generation of local guidelines may help in providing critical care outside of ICU and improved triaging of patients requiring ICU care.

Lastly, the lack of reliable estimates of critical illnesses in resource-limited settings complicates the extrapolation of clinical management guidelines originating from HICs.[46] However, because of the absence of reliable data, the guidelines are adapted with local modifications to incorporate variations in disease frequencies and available resources. It would be prudent to formulate critical care guidelines based on reliable estimates from local studies that will provide more effective solutions.

Trauma and Acute Care Surgery Solutions

Implementing well-structured protocols from prehospital settings to a designated care facility, culminating in meticulous rehabilitation for chronic sequelae, is necessary to reduce the global burden from injuries and critical illnesses.

A delay in seeking care for the trauma victim (first delay), untimely transportation of the victim to the nearest trauma center (second delay), and longer time taken for medical interventions (third delay) are some deficiencies that need to be highlighted in the LMIC setting. Factors such as illiteracy of the public, insufficient ambulances and health care personnel, and a scarcity of nearby trauma centers contribute to these delays.[47] Although HICs have road and air emergency transport systems, most patients in LMICs rely on private or commercial vehicles for transportation to the nearest trauma center.[48] Establishing prehospital care systems and formally training first responders through the assessment of knowledge and provision of basic equipment may help halve injury-related mortality in LMICs.[49,50]

Training health care workers, especially resident/postgraduate doctors involved in delivering trauma and critical care services, is of paramount importance as they form the pillars of care delivery in teaching hospitals. Although 51 of 79 LMICs offer surgical postgraduate medical education, only 34 of these include traumatology in their curriculum.[51] Masters and fellowship in trauma programs designed to facilitate acute care surgery systems in LMICs can help sensitize young trainees to limitations in resource-restricted settings and maximize and generate future leaders in the field.[52] Trauma life support training courses have been shown to improve the overall skill of health care workers.[49] Although ATLS training is variable among resident doctors in LMICs, owing potentially to its cost, alternate options such as the primary trauma care (PTC) course and its modules are available for free and have significant potential for implementation in LMIC settings.[53,54] Trauma team training is a novel approach that may reduce the time taken to administer critical interventions by directing training toward a group rather than an individual solely.[55] It must, however, be emphasized that training programs alone may not directly improve outcomes for injury victims, reiterating the importance of a multifaceted approach to strengthen trauma systems.[56]

Although there are various deficiencies in trauma and critical care delivery in LMICs, it must be acknowledged that several well-functioning informal mechanisms already exist and could serve as the foundation for a more robust system.[15,57] Gwaram and colleagues[58] elucidated numerous benefits of establishing a trauma center in a tertiary hospital in Nigeria. Equipped with dedicated trauma teams and resources over the clock, the center could address complex multisystem injuries and was pivotal in managing mass casualty situations from RTIs, fires, civil unrest, and bomb explosions. Requiring police officers to inform the hospital about crash victims beforehand promoted trauma team preparedness. The center also provided the infrastructure for developing fellowships in trauma and critical care and ATLS training and enabled fellows to engage in research activities. Modifying trauma systems in line with local needs helps individualize care delivery while adhering to basic protocols. The Hamad Trauma Center in Qatar besides maintaining trauma care units also offers clinical psychological services, efficient rehabilitation programs, and an Injury Prevention Program aimed at increasing awareness about trauma prevention among civilians.[59] Integrating major trauma centers with peripheral hospitals by strengthening referral systems improves the efficiency and cost-effectiveness of patient transfer.[60] Mobile phone and WhatsApp-based groups are still being used widely in LMICs to coordinate the transfer of COVID-positive patients during the pandemic by communicating the patient status and the availability of beds and ventilators.[61] Multiple stakeholders are updated about the problems faced to plan for the subsequent work period via online video-based meeting platforms such as Zoom, serving as surrogates for quality control and assurance, which are necessary to build sustainable care capacity. Such features can be emulated into trauma systems at a smaller scale.[62,63] In 2019, the WHO launched "The WHO Global and Trauma Care Initiative" (GETI), aiming to increase capacities for quality emergency and trauma care worldwide and foster awareness about life-saving measures.[63]

Trauma rehabilitation plays an important role in improving functional outcomes. Although rehabilitation is usually offered in a hospital environment under medical regulation, the same is not easily accessible to most patients in LMICs.[64] Trauma patients can gain significant support in their journey toward attaining physical and psychological health by involving their community.[65,66] Carefully considering the health priorities of victims and fostering community engagement improves acceptability of interventions, aiding not only in the recovery of function but also prevention of injuries such as falls in the elderly.[67]

Role of Trauma Registries

Trauma registries enable service evaluation, surveillance, research, and quality improvement activities. Most critical care registries encompass a broad group of patients, producing a heterogeneous case-mix that increases the complexities in evaluating a particular cohort of disease, more so for trauma patients arriving in the ICU. Therefore, disease-specific registries may provide better quality information. However, there are certain limitations, such as variability of data elements, absence of data regarding ICU admission and complications, and long-term functional outcomes.[68] Given the above deficiencies, developing a Trauma Critical Care Registry can help bridge the knowledge gap.[69]

SUMMARY

Trauma and critical illnesses lead to significant mortality and impairment of functional and psychological outcomes among survivors, with consequential economic strain exerted on patients and hospital services, more so in LMICs. Development and implementation of management protocols in line with existing systems at the prehospital, in-hospital, and post-injury rehabilitation levels can help address local needs resulting from heterogeneity in disease burden and resources.

CLINICS CARE POINTS

- Most trauma-related deaths occur in low- and middle-income countries (LMICs), and poor patients living in rural areas in these regions are more severely affected than those in metropolitan cities

- Delays at various levels in seeking, reaching, and receiving life-saving treatment lead to higher injury and critical illness-related mortality in LMICs than high-income countries (HICs)

- Measures taken to address these delays may decrease mortality and improve functional outcomes

- Developing trauma and critical care registries in LMICs can help formulate guidelines and protocols in line with local needs by providing crucial data

DISCLOSURE

The article is original, has not been published before, and is not being considered for publication anywhere else. All authors have sufficiently contributed for the article. There is no conflict of interests and financial support involved. The article has been read and approved for submission by all authors.

REFERENCES

1. Alonge O, Agrawal P, Talab A, et al. Fatal and non-fatal injury outcomes: results from a purposively sampled census of seven rural sub districts in Bangladesh. Lancet Glob Health 2017;5(8):818–27.
2. GBD 2019 Diseases and Injuries Collaborators. Global burden of 369 diseases and injuries in 204 countries and territories, 1990-2019: a systematic analysis for the Global Burden of Disease Study 2019. Lancet 2020;396(10258): 1204–22. Erratum in: Lancet. 2020 Nov 14;396(10262):1562.
3. Ma T, Peden AE, Peden M, et al. Out of the silos: embedding injury prevention into the Sustainable Development. Goals Inj Prev 2021;27(2):166–71.
4. Vukoja M, Riviello ED, Schultz MJ. Critical care outcomes in resource-limited settings. Curr Opin Crit Care 2018;24(5):421–7.
5. Baker T, Khalid K, Acicbe O, et al. Council of the world federation of societies of intensive &; critical care medicine. Critical care of tropical disease in low income countries: report from the task force on tropical diseases by the world federation of societies of intensive and critical care medicine. J Crit Care 2017;42:351–4.
6. Murthy S, Adhikari NK. Global health care of the critically ill in low-resource settings. Ann Am Thorac Soc 2013;10(5):509–13.
7. Chen S, Kuhn M, Prettner K, et al. The global macroeconomic burden of road injuries: estimates and projections for 166 countries. Lancet Planet Health 2019; 3(9):e390–8.
8. Yadav J, Menon G, Agarwal A, et al. Burden of injuries and its associated hospitalization expenditure in India. Int J Inj Contr Saf Promot 2021;28(2):153–61.
9. Anagnostou E, Larentzakis A, Vassiliu P. Trauma system in Greece: quo vadis? Injury 2018;49(7):1243–50.
10. American College of Surgeons. Available at: https://www.facs.org/Quality-Programs/Trauma/TQP/systems-programs/TSCP/components. Accessed February 22, 2022.
11. Dijkink S, Nederpelt CJ, Krijnen P, et al. Trauma systems around the world: a systematic overview. J Trauma Acute Care Surg 2017;83(5):917–25.
12. Latifi R, Ziemba M, Leppäniemi A, et al. Trauma system evaluation in developing countries: applicability of American College of Surgeons/Committee on Trauma (ACS/COT) basic criteria. World J Surg 2014;38(8):1898–904.
13. Roy N, Gerdin M, Ghosh S, et al. 30-Day in-hospital trauma mortality in four urban university hospitals using an Indian trauma registry. World J Surg 2016;40(6): 1299–307.
14. Uthkarsh PS, Gururaj G, Reddy SS, et al. Assessment and availability of trauma care services in a district hospital of south India; a field observational study. Bull Emerg Trauma 2016;4(2):93–100.
15. Kim J, Barreix M, Babcock C, et al. Acute care referral systems in Liberia: transfer and referral capabilities in a low-income country. Prehosp Disaster Med 2017; 32(6):642–50.

16. Moore L, Champion H, Tardif PA, et al. International injury care improvement initiative. impact of trauma system structure on injury outcomes: a systematic review and meta-analysis. World J Surg 2018;42(5):1327–39.

17. Lin N, Nwanna-Nzewunwa O, Carvalho M, et al. Geospatial analysis of trauma burden and surgical care capacity in teso sub-region of eastern Uganda. World J Surg 2019;43(11):2666–73.

18. Radjou AN, Mahajan P, Baliga DK. Where do I go? A trauma victim's plea in an informal trauma system. J Emerg Trauma Shock 2013;6(3):164–70.

19. Ahuja R, Tiwari G, Bhalla K. Going to the nearest hospital vs. designated trauma centre for road traffic crashes: estimating the time difference in Delhi, India. Int J Inj Contr Saf Promot 2019;26(3):271–82.

20. Lucumay NJ, Sawe HR, Mohamed A, et al. Pre-referral stabilization and compliance with WHO guidelines for trauma care among adult patients referred to an urban emergency department of a tertiary referral hospital in Tanzania. BMC Emerg Med 2019;19(1):22.

21. Seo DH, Kim H, Kim KH, et al. Status of emergency signal functions in Myanmar hospitals: a cross-sectional survey. West J Emerg Med 2019;20(6):903–9.

22. Agarwal-Harding KJ, Chokotho L, Young S, et al. Assessing the capacity of Malawi's district and central hospitals to manage traumatic diaphyseal femoral fractures in adults. PLoS One 2019;14(11):e0225254.

23. Chokotho L, Mulwafu W, Singini I, et al. Improving hospital-based trauma care for road traffic injuries in Malawi. World J Emerg Med 2017;8(2):85–90.

24. Fuhs AK, LaGrone LN, Moscoso Porras MG, et al. Assessment of rehabilitation infrastructure in Peru. Arch Phys Med Rehabil 2018;99(6):1116–23. https://doi.org/10.1016/j.apmr.2017.10.020.

25. Chana P, Burns EM, Arora S, Darzi AW, Faiz OD. A systematic review of the impact of dedicated emergency surgical services on patient outcomes. Annals of Surgery 2016;263(1):20–7.

26. van der Wee MJL, van der Wilden G, Hoencamp R. Acute care surgery models worldwide: A systematic review. World Journal of Surgery 2020;44(8):2622–37.

27. Khajanchi MU, Kumar V, Wärnberg Gerdin L, et al. Prevalence of a definitive airway in patients with severe traumatic brain injury received at four urban public university hospitals in India: a cohort study. Inj Prev 2019;25(5):428–32.

28. Committee on Trauma, American College of Surgeons. Advanced trauma life support student course manual. Chicago (IL): American College of Surgeons; 2018.

29. Mayglothling J, Duane TM, Gibbs M, et al. Emergency tracheal intubation immediately following traumatic injury: an Eastern Association for the Surgery of Trauma practice management guideline. J Trauma Acute Care Surg 2012;73(5 Suppl 4):S333–40.

30. Tsima BM, Rajeswaran L, Cox M. Assessment of cardiopulmonary resuscitation equipment in resuscitation trolleys in district hospitals in Botswana: a cross-sectional study. Afr J Prim Health Care Fam Med 2019;11(1):e1–7.

31. Latifi R, Gunn JK, Stroster JA, et al. The readiness of emergency and trauma care in low- and middle-income countries: a cross-sectional descriptive study of 42 public hospitals in Albania. Int J Emerg Med 2016;9(1):26.

32. Bhandarkar P, Patil P, Soni KD, et al. An analysis of 30-day in-hospital trauma mortality in four urban university hospitals using the Australia india trauma registry. World J Surg 2021;45:380–9. https://doi.org/10.1007/s00268-020-05805-7.

33. Prin M, Li G. Complications and in-hospital mortality in trauma patients treated in intensive care units in the United States, 2013. Inj Epidemiol 2016;3(1):18.

34. Lombardo S, Scalea T, Sperry J, et al. Neuro, trauma, or med/surg intensive care unit: does it matter where multiple injuries patients with traumatic brain injury are admitted? Secondary analysis of the American Association for the Surgery of Trauma Multi-Institutional Trials Committee decompressive craniectomy study. J Trauma Acute Care Surg 2017;82(3):489–96.

35. Duane TM, Rao IR, Aboutanos MB, et al. Are trauma patients better off in a trauma ICU? J Emerg Trauma Shock 2008;1(2):74–7.

36. Michetti CP, Fakhry SM, Brasel K, et al. TRIPP study group. Trauma ICU Prevalence Project: the diversity of surgical critical care. Trauma Surg Acute Care Open 2019;4(1):e000288.

37. Turner HC, Hao NV, Yacoub S, et al. Achieving affordable critical care in low-income and middle-income countries. BMJ Glob Health 2019;4:e001675.

38. Mastrogianni M, Galanis P, Kaitelidou D, et al. Factors affecting adult intensive care units costs by using the bottom-up and top-down costing methodology in OECD countries: a systematic review. Intensive Crit Care Nurs 2021;66:103080.

39. Agrawal A, Gandhe MB, Gandhe S, et al. Study of length of stay and average cost of treatment in Medicine Intensive Care Unit at tertiary care center. J Health Res Rev 2017;4:24–9.

40. Riviello ED, Letchford S, Achieng L, et al. Critical care in resource-poor settings: lessons learned and future directions. Crit Care Med 2011;39(4):860–7.

41. Tan SS, Bakker J, Hoogendoorn ME, et al. Direct cost analysis of intensive care unit stay in four European countries: applying a standardized costing methodology. Value Health 2012;15(1):81–6.

42. Mahomed S, Mahomed OH. Cost of intensive care services at a central hospital in South Africa. S Afr Med J 2018;109(1):35–9.

43. Karabatsou D, Tsironi M, Tsigou E, et al. Variable cost of ICU care, a microcosting analysis. Intensive Crit Care Nurs 2016;35:66–73.

44. Mekontso Dessap A. Frugal innovation for critical care. Intensive Care Med 2019; 45:252–4. https://doi.org/10.1007/s00134-018-5391-6.

45. Kundury KK, Mamatha HK, Rao D. Comparative assessment of patient care expenses among intensive care units of a tertiary care teaching hospital using cost block method. Indian J Crit Care Med 2017;21(2):85–8.

46. Diaz JV, Riviello ED, Papali A, et al. Global critical care: moving forward in resource-limited settings. Ann Glob Health 2019;85(1):3.

47. Patel A, Vissoci JRN, Hocker M, et al. Qualitative evaluation of trauma delays in road traffic injury patients in Maringá, Brazil. BMC Health Serv Res 2017; 17(1):804.

48. Moore L, Champion H, Tardif PA, et al. Impact of trauma system structure on injury outcomes: a systematic review and meta-analysis. World J Surg 2018;42: 1327–39. https://doi.org/10.1007/s00268-017-4292-0.

49. Jin J, Akau'ola S, Yip CH, et al. International society of surgery (ISS) and the G4 alliance international standards and guidelines for quality safe surgery and anesthesia (ISG-QSSA) group. Effectiveness of quality improvement processes, interventions, and structure in trauma systems in low- and middle-income countries: a systematic review and meta-analysis. World J Surg 2021;45(7):1982–98.

50. Callese TE, Richards CT, Shaw P, et al. Layperson trauma training in low- and middle-income countries: a review. J Surg Res 2014;190(1):104–10.

51. Livergant RJ, Demetrick S, Cravetchi X, et al. Trauma training courses and programs in low- and lower middle-income countries: a scoping review. World J Surg 2021;45(12):3543–57.

52. Merchant AI, Walters CB, Valenzuela J, et al. Creating a global acute care surgery fellowship to meet international need. J Surg Educ 2017;74(5):780–6.

53. Kadhum M, Sinclair P, Lavy C. Are Primary Trauma Care (PTC) courses beneficial in low- and middle-income countries - a systematic review. Injury 2020;51(2):136–41.

54. Muzzammil M, Minhas MS, Ramzan Ali SAA, et al. Primary trauma care course: alternative basic trauma course in developing countries. "The Need of the Hour". Int J Clin Pract 2021;75(8):e14327.

55. Noonan M, Olaussen A, Mathew J, et al. What is the clinical evidence supporting trauma team training (TTT): a systematic review and meta-analysis. Medicina (Kaunas) 2019;55(9):551.

56. Jayaraman S, Sethi D, Chinnock P, et al. Advanced trauma life support training for hospital staff. Cochrane Database Syst Rev 2014;(8):CD004173. https://doi.org/10.1002/14651858.CD004173.pub4.

57. Mwandri MB, Hardcastle TC. Evaluation of resources necessary for provision of trauma care in Botswana: an initiative for a local system. World J Surg 2018;42(6):1629–38.

58. Gwaram UA, Okoye OG, Olaomi OO. Observed benefits of a major trauma centre in a tertiary hospital in Nigeria. Afr J Emerg Med 2021;11(2):311–4.

59. Al-Thani H, El-Menyar A, Asim M, et al. Evolution of the Qatar trauma system: the journey from inception to verification. J Emerg Trauma Shock 2019;12(3):209–17.

60. Okereke IC, Zahoor U, Ramadan O. Trauma care in Nigeria: time for an integrated trauma system. Cureus 2022;14(1):e20880.

61. Salman S, Saleem SG, Shaikh Q, et al. Epidemiology and outcomes of trauma patients at the indus hospital, karachi, Pakistan, 2017 - 2018. Pakistan J Med Sci 2020;36(1):S9–13.

62. Blair KJ, Paladino L, Shaw PL, et al. Surgical and trauma care in low- and middle-income countries: a review of capacity assessments. J Surg Res 2017;210:139–51.

63. World Health Organization. (n.d. Global emergency and trauma care initiative. World Health Organization. Avaiable at: https://www.who.int/initiatives/global-emergency-and-trauma-care-initiative#:~:text=The%20WHO%20Global%20Emergency%20and,its%20potential%20to%20save%20lives.   Accessed February 18, 2022.

64. Schrieff-Elson LE, Steenkamp N, Hendricks MI, et al. Local and global challenges in pediatric traumatic brain injury outcome and rehabilitation assessment. Childs Nerv Syst 2017;33(10):1775–84.

65. Glancy D, Reilly L, Cobbe C, et al. Lockdown in a specialised rehabilitation unit: the best of times. Ir J Psychol Med 2020;37(3):169–71.

66. Kamenov K, Mills JA, Chatterji S, et al. Needs and unmet needs for rehabilitation services: a scoping review. Disabil Rehabil 2019;41(10):1227–37.

67. Jagnoor J, Keay L, Jaswal N, et al. A qualitative study on the perceptions of preventing falls as a health priority among older people in Northern India. Inj Prev 2014;20(1):29–34.

68. Shivasabesan G, O'Reilly GM, Mathew J, et al. Australia-India Trauma Systems Collaboration (AITSC). Establishing a multicentre trauma registry in India: an evaluation of data completeness. World J Surg 2019;43(10):2426–37.

69. Bommakanti K, Feldhaus I, Motwani G, et al. Trauma registry implementation in low- and middle-income countries: challenges and opportunities. J Surg Res 2018;223:72–86.

Factors to be Considered in Advancing Pediatric Critical Care Across the World

Andrew C. Argent, MB, BCh, MMed(Paeds), MD(Paeds), DCH(SA), FCPaeds(SA), FRCPCH(UK), Cert Crit Care (Paeds) (SA)[a],*, Suchitra Ranjit, MD, FCCM[b], Mark J. Peters, MBChB, MRCP, FRCPCH, FFICM, PhD[c,d], Amelie von Saint Andre-von Arnim, MD[e,f], Md Jobayer Chisti, MD, PhD[g], Roberto Jabornisky, MD[h], Ndidiamaka L. Musa, MD[i], Niranjan Kissoon, MB, BS, FRCP(C), FAAP, MCCM, FACPE[j]

KEYWORDS

- Pediatric critical care • Global health • Development

KEY POINTS

- Pediatric critical care encompasses the care of critically ill or injured children, or those recovering from major surgery, from first point of care with health services to full rehabilitation at home.
- Pediatric critical care involves multiple disciplines and segments of society and should be fully integrated within overall healthcare services.
- The management of post-intensive care symptoms is developing, and with it comes a refocus on how to assess outcomes of critical illness episodes.

Continued

[a] Department of Paediatrics and Child Health, University of Cape Town, Red Cross War Memorial Children's Hospital, Klipfontein Road, Rondebosch, Cape Town, 7700, South Africa; [b] Pediatric ICU, Apollo Children's Hospital, 15, Shafee Mhd Road, Chennai 600006, India; [c] University College London Great Ormond Street Institute of Child Health, London, WC1N 3JH, UK; [d] Paediatric Intensive Care Unit, Great Ormond Street Hospital NHS Foundation Trust, London, WC1N 1EH, UK; [e] Department of Pediatrics, Division of Pediatric Critical Care, University of Washington, Seattle Children's, 4800 Sand Point Way NorthEast, Seattle, WA 98105, USA; [f] Department of Global Health, University of Washington, Seattle Children's, 4800 Sand Point Way NorthEast, Seattle, WA 98105, USA; [g] ARI Ward, Dhaka Hospital, Nutrition and Clinical Services Division, icddr,b, Dhaka 1212, Bangladesh; [h] Universidad Nacional Del Nordeste, Argentina. Pediatric Intensive Care Unit (Hospital Juan Pablo II and Hospital Olga Stuky) Argentina, Sociedad Latinoamericana de Cuidados Intensivos Pediátricos, LARed Network, Universidad Nacional Del Nordeste, 1420 Mariano Moreno, Corrientes 3400, Argentina; [i] Paediatric Critical Care, University of Washington, 4800 Sand Point Way NorthEast, Seattle, WA 98105, USA; [j] British Columbia Children's Hospital and The University of British Columbia, Vancouver, 4480 Oak Street, Vancouver, BC V6H 3V4, Canada
* Corresponding author.
E-mail address: Andrew.Argent@uct.ac.za

Crit Care Clin 38 (2022) 707–720
https://doi.org/10.1016/j.ccc.2022.07.001
0749-0704/22/© 2022 Elsevier Inc. All rights reserved.

criticalcare.theclinics.com

Continued

- As we start to understand the risks and benefits of even basic interventions, there is a growing body of research focussed on the need to tritrate all therapies to the needs of specific patients.
- There is a tension between providing optimal care to all individuals in high income areas and providing as much care as possible to as many children as possible in lower income areas.

INTRODUCTION

Pediatric intensive care is a relatively new discipline, as outlined in several publications.[1–3] With the development of pediatric intensive care has come the conceptualization of pediatric critical care (PCC). One perspective is that PCC encompasses the care of children with a life-threatening illness or injury, or who require major elective surgery; this care includes everything from the first point of contact with health care services through to full rehabilitation at home.[4] The Pediatric Acute Lung Injury and Sepsis Initiative (PALISI) group have recently been addressing this issue via a systematic review and a Delphi study, whereas the World Health Organization (WHO) has been focusing on what constitutes essential emergency and critical care medicine.[5] These initiatives underline the need for a lexicon of terms relating to the management of critically ill or injured children and an understanding of the interventions and standards of care that can and should be expected at each level of a health care system.

Across the world, there is a constant tension between the realities and aspirations of critical care in high-income countries (HIC), versus those in the low- and middle-income countries (LMICs). To add to the complexity, there are communities in HIC that have very limited access to PCC and communities in low-income countries (LICs) that have access to highly-resourced advanced care. Regardless of resource limitations, ensuring that resources are used to achieve the most good is important. However, an overarching principle should be that critical care involves many other disciplines and segments of society and should not be practiced in isolation but in the context of overall care in society (**Fig. 1**).

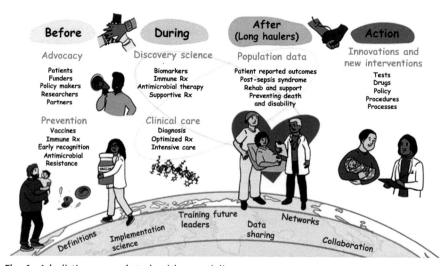

Fig. 1. A holistic approach to health care delivery.

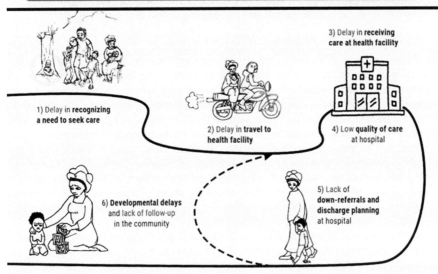

Fig. 2. Journey of a mother and sick child: areas in need of intervention to improve pediatric critical care.

WHERE DOES PEDIATRIC CRITICAL CARE BEGIN AND END?

There is increasing recognition that critical care should not be limited within the walls of an institution but should include care delivered in the community, the pre-intensive care setting, as well as the care of children following discharge from pediatric intensive care units. There has thus been a proliferation of triage tools (for use in emergency departments or in mass casualty events[6]), early warning systems (to identify sick children in wards and health care systems[7]), and criticality indices[8] (to identify critically ill children within health care systems). Not all systems have been successfully implemented, and substantial change may be required within systems to ensure that critically ill children are identified and treated expeditiously **(Fig. 2)**.

There is a growing realization that patients (and families) who survive intensive care (and PCC) admission and treatment may develop long-term challenges related specifically to that experience. This realization is leading to increased research into the post-PCC discharge outcomes and quality of life; this has included a refocus of outcomes assessment (from pediatric intensive care unit [PICU] survival to hospital survival and on toward outcomes years later), from survival through to quality-of-life outcomes,[9] and impact of pediatric critical illness on the family[10,11] (and possibly the extended community). Adult and pediatric intensive care services are increasingly recognizing the post-intensive care syndrome[12] and are developing long-term follow-up clinics to provide support and specialist care to "graduates" of those services.

There is recognition of the postdischarge mortality of critically ill children, particularly in LMICs.[13–15] The causes of the mortality may relate to what has happened within the hospital and the PICU, but may also relate to multiple factors that increase the risk of severe illness including the child,[16,17] the home environment, social structures, and the interactions of all these. There is increasing interest, but limited data, on the contribution of the "child context" to ongoing morbidity and mortality. Indeed, in some settings, PICU has also played the role of the "canary in the coalmine" in alerting health care systems about problems that are developing within communities.[18,19]

Who is Cared for in the Pediatric Critical Care Environment?

In the early years of PCC, there was a heavy preponderance of patients with acute infections and trauma. Across the world, the incidence of infections in previously well children has decreased dramatically as a result of improved living conditions, and immunization against many common childhood illnesses.[20] In poorer countries, the impact of these measures has been substantial, but there are still areas of the world where previously well children suffer critical illness as a result of infections such as pneumonia, malaria, dengue, tuberculosis, and diseases due to zoonotic pathogens (including cysticercosis and a range of bacterial pathogens). Although the use of antibody preparations has reduced the impact of infections such as respiratory syncytial virus (RSV) in preterm infants in richer countries, the global burden of RSV remains substantial (particularly in LMICs) and the development of effective maternal and/or pediatric vaccines would have significant impact.[21]

The development of disciplines such as pediatric oncology and transplant services has led to increasing numbers of children who develop complications related to their underlying disease processes and management, and are admitted to PICU with complex medical conditions and associated infections. In addition, disciplines such as pediatric cardiac surgery are undertaking ever more complex procedures (often in neonates or very young infants) resulting in patient populations in which appropriate therapy can only be provided by teams with detailed knowledge of those conditions and the associated physiology, and with access to sophisticated imaging and monitoring technologies. This situation is in contrast to poorer countries in which most of the PICU admissions are related to either infection or trauma in previously well children (despite the increasingly recognized burden of pediatric congenital heart disease in these regions[22]).

Medical advances in the recognition of "rare diseases"[23] especially in richer parts of the world have led to an increasing proportion of patients admitted to the PICU—often for long stays—suffering from these conditions. These conditions pose substantial challenges to the PCC team because of the limited experience of treating patients with those conditions. Inevitably adequate clinical management relies on the development and experience of multidisciplinary teams[24] working in innovative ways. Related to the diagnosis and management of rare diseases is the increasing utilization of genomic studies to provide potential diagnoses in these children[25–27] (particularly in critically ill infants). The use of these technologies raises new ethical dilemmas[28] regarding issues such as consent for these studies, dealing with unexpected results, and dealing with results in which the significance of the abnormalities detected is not known or understood. At present, access to and utilization of many of these tests are limited to HICs.

An ongoing challenge in the PCC environment relates to the availability or nonavailability of PCC bed spaces, particularly in LMICs. Processes to prioritize admission to the limited beds available are an ongoing consideration.[29,30] Long-stay patients raise challenging issues in the PCC. Although some of the long-stay patients may have good long-term outcomes, in general, they have worse outcomes than those admitted for short periods.[31–34] The underlying reality is that access to PCC beds requires the allocation of substantial resources.

The coronavirus disease 2019 pandemic has overwhelmed adult critical care re-sources leading to PCC communities caring for adolescents and young adults. At the other end of the age spectrum, neonatal care has frequently overlapped with PCC, particularly in the management of infants requiring surgical intervention (for many years most neonatal cardiac intensive care has taken place under the ambit of pediatric intensivists). There is a growing need to provide advanced neonatal ser-vices including respiratory support,[35] and particularly to provide neonatal surgical and anesthetic support in LIMCs.[36] This need creates an opportunity to integrate the neonatal and pediatric perisurgical services and PCC.

Generally, adolescents in LMICs are cared for in adult intensive care units; this is problematic because their specific needs are not being met. A particular concern is that the adult units may not be attuned to the physiology of congenital heart disease. This concern becomes increasingly relevant as the global population of "grown-up pa-tients with congenital heart disease" now exceeds the population of children with congenital heart disease.

The Treatment and Technology Advances in Pediatric Critical Care

Over time, the technology available for diagnostic and therapeutic purposes in the PICU has become increasingly sophisticated; this provides wonderful opportunities to optimize therapy, and also carries inevitable associated costs to provide mainte-nance, supply ongoing consumables (usually disposable and not for repeat use), and train all the PICU staff to the appropriate levels of competence and expertise with that equipment.

There is growing realization that interventions to support organ systems can cause injury to patients. This injury might be a direct one, for example, from excessive airway pressures or tidal volume,[37] or an indirect one from medication (sedative drugs)[38] and procedures (vascular access)[39] that facilitate these therapies.

We are starting to understand the complexity of the risks and benefits of even basic interventions for critical illness. Formal, larger-scale clinical trials in acutely unwell chil-dren are refining our practice. It is now understood that less aggressive blood trans-fusion[40] or glycemic control[41] and conservative use of parenteral nutrition[42] are not associated with worse outcomes. More conservative use of oxygen therapy,[43–48] fluid administration,[49–53] vascular access, and antibiotic therapies[54] all have evidence to support them. There is growing awareness to titrate all these therapies to the needs of specific patients, to specific and appropriate end points and goals, and with aware-ness of the associated adverse effects of all these interventions.

Across the board there has been a move toward the "minimum safe intervention" with the wider use of less-invasive therapies, particularly respiratory support, in which technologies such as high-flow humidified nasal oxygen, nasal continuous positive air-ways pressure (nCPAP), and noninvasive ventilation strategies with physician-supervised monitoring[55–58] seem to have been effective in some groups of patients (eg, bronchiolitis, WHO-defined severe pneumonia with hypoxemia, undifferentiated respiratory distress) and associated with reduced complications. Several major collaborative research networks are investigating options for less-aggressive thera-pies in formal trials.[58] However, there is substantial work required to determine how these therapies should be implemented.

The development of collaborative research networks (eg, the PALISI) across the world has increased research output significantly with developing focus on random-ized controlled trials. A recurrent theme in multiple structured literature reviews on a wide range of topics has been the lack of robust evidence on which to base treatment recommendations for PCC. Unfortunately there remain concerns about the relationship between regions of high PCC mortality and those of high research interest and output. There are concerns about the very high rate of negative results from costly randomized controlled studies,[59] and there are ongoing concerns about the processes and priorities in research in LMICs.[60]

Over the last decades, there has been a huge focus on the development of definitions and guidelines for conditions such as sepsis[61,62] and pediatric acute respiratory distress syndome (ARDS).[63] This approach has been associated with substantial improvements in outcomes for patients with these clinical syndromes in some parts of the world. However, there is increasing realization that these syndromes may have considerable heterogeneity, and may include several different phenotypes[64,65] each of which requires different treatment, and may have different outcomes. We may need to consider moving away from the large categories of conditions to focus on the characteristics and needs of individual patients,[66] or at least smaller groups of patients. With the development of new genomic, metabolomic, and proteomic technologies for the diagnosis of specific conditions and the identification of patients with particular responses (to the illness but also to the therapy), there is growing hope that we might be able to individualize care and deliver personalized medicine.

In many ways, this issue highlights the different challenges across the world. In many parts of the world, the focus (justifiably) has to be on getting things right most of the time for most of the patients (the 80:20 rule; **Table 1**). In the absence of multiple highly trained professionals with sophisticated diagnostic and therapeutic resources, we have to find protocols and processes that can be implemented effectively by teams with less training and resources; this will have the most positive impact on most patients (but inevitably compromise the care of some individuals). By contrast in HICs, the resources and skills are available to recognize relatively subtle differences between groups, to apply a wide range of contrasting therapies. PCC will serve fewer patients and save fewer lives in that setting but will do a better job for individuals.

What Supporting Structures and Systems Are Required?

PCC cannot function in isolation. In many parts of the world infrastructure such as transport systems, stable power supplies, consistent clean water supplies, appropriate waste disposal systems, and communication systems are taken for granted. Unfortunately, in many (if not most) LMICs many of these structures are not reliably in place, and that places great stress on the team to provide bridges to overcome these difficulties.

From a medical equipment perspective, reliable implementation of high-technology services relies on well-established and functional supply chains (for both capital equipment and consumables),[67] support and maintenance infrastructure (particularly the presence of trained technologists), financial structures, and controls. It is surprisingly difficult to introduce innovations in equipment and processes in an environment in which there is little established infrastructure to validate and license the use of new equipment and systems.

From the medical consumable perspective, access to consumables and pharmaceuticals (such as essential antibiotics[68]) may be extremely limited in LMICs, and, to make financial pressures even worse, many medications are relatively expensive in these countries.

Provision of PCC may be challenging without optimal laboratory and medical imaging services together with blood transfusion services. Unfortunately, many of these services are substantially suboptimal in LMICs.[69] There is considerable opportunity developing in the current era with the development of point-of-care laboratory systems and particularly with the use of ultrasound systems (which have become

Table 1
Examples of the 80/20 rules in prioritizing pediatric critical care delivery

1	*Identify the top conditions that pose acute life threats in that region* For example, in many poorer countries, the commonest diagnosis at PICU admission is previously healthy children with acute life threats that can be treated with relatively low resources: infections, pneumonia, severe acute malnutrition, poisoning, seizures, head trauma	Identify simultaneously the "resource suckers": where 80% of treatment options/health care costs are attributed to and only help 20% of patients?
2	*Enable task sharing between health professionals* to bridge the quality gap in settings with restricted human resources *(essential emergency and critical care (EECC)concept)*	Identify the top 20% of basic life-saving actions that must be performed by 80% of health professions in the facility (irrespective of primary role)
3	*Manage equipment/technology wisely* Higher volume of low tech and lower volumes of high tech may be preferred in LMIC *Factor in service and support availability, consumables*	Identify the 20% of equipment/ technology can aid in the management of 80% of patients admitted to the health facility
4	*Prevention* Depending on the region, create a plan of top 3 *actionables* that can be marketed to educate public to do more and bring more impact (vaccination/ clean water/helmets)	Identify which 20% of public actions can decrease 80% of the region's preventable child illness

portable, relatively robust, and affordable). Unfortunately, there will be pressure on scarce staff to become competent in the utilization of this sort of technology.

One of the consequences of relatively easy access to antibiotics, extremely limited resources for microbiological services, and poor implementation of infection control is the looming menace of antibiotic resistance across the world;[68] this is a real threat to PCC in the future.

The development of electronic health care records (EHCR) for PCC has already had a huge impact in HICs (not always positive). EHCR have the potential to support PCC with data collection and optimization of multiple processes. Unfortunately, implementation has not always been successful, and inevitably requires a substantial infrastructure to support the system. However, innovative use of computer records in areas such as East Africa has shown some remarkable benefits at low cost.[70]

How do We Know that Our Staff Are Competent?

The issue of competence in PICU has become increasingly formalized in richer countries, whereas in poorer countries (and also often in the private sectors of rich countries) the level of surveillance over levels of staff competence is minimal. Defining and maintaining competence is potentially a complex field. There is a need to ensure that new staff working in the PCC environment are given comprehensive training to use the equipment and the procedures that are available to them; this requires theoretic education, practical training and experience, and ongoing evaluation, both at the time of initial training and during ongoing clinical practice. Detailed licensing and credentialing processes have been developed in many areas, for example, point-of-care ultrasonography.[71]

How Are Pediatric Critical Care Services Organized?

PCC services have developed along multiple different pathways. In some centers PCC developed in close association with anesthetic and perioperative services, and in those settings surgical patients (particularly related to disciplines such as neurosurgery and cardiothoracic surgery) have predominated in the patient population while the staff are predominantly from those disciplines. In other settings PCC has developed within the pediatric services, and many of these centers have focused primarily on the care of patients with "medical" conditions, particularly infections. Over time these units have gone through amalgamations and divisions into organ system-specific units.

There is substantial evidence to suggest that children are best cared for within PCC services (vs mixed services with adults),[72] but there is also evidence that optimal patient outcomes may be achieved in specialist units (with the proviso that there is adequate allocation of staffing and resources) when there is adequate patient turnover to ensure appropriate training and experience for all cadres of staff.

One recent development has been the introduction of telemedicine as a tool to bring expertise and services to the children who are cared for in more remote areas of the world.[73]

Who Works in Pediatric Critical Care?

From initial units in HICs that were staffed with small numbers of nurses and doctors (relative to patients) PICUs have developed to include large multidisciplinary teams with high ratios of staff to patients. In the words of an editorial "it takes a well-educated village"[74] to staff and maintain the levels of care required in PCC.

Unfortunately poorer countries have not been able to emulate that growth, and so there is growing interest in the possibilities of incorporating the child caregivers (predominantly mothers) into the monitoring and caring team.[75] This particular process may be facilitated by the use of mobile devices to improve patient monitoring.[76]

There has been substantial evidence over time (and in a variety of settings[77]) to show that the presence of pediatric intensivists in PCC is associated with improved patient outcomes. Some years ago there was evidence that (although training is essential) the presence of inexperienced residents in PCC was associated with worse outcomes.[78] More recently there has been increased emphasis in HICs on 24-hour intensivist presence in the PICU[79] that perhaps offsets this inexperience. On the other hand, in most LMICs, the presence of even a single trained intensivist is a luxury, and it may be impossible to ensure that there is 24-hour in-house subspecialist presence. New developments in telemedicine are opening opportunities to "spread expertise" and make scarce, experienced intensivists virtually available to clinicians in less well staffed areas.[73]

There is also substantial training required for nursing personnel, at all levels including advanced nurse practitioners[80] (who play a substantial role in management of the PCC environment in many HICs).

Apart from rigorous and ongoing training substantial clinical experience[81] makes a significant contribution to clinical care and patient outcomes. In addition there is evidence that limiting the resources available to train PCC nurses may be associated with worse outcomes. The development of training programs for PCC nurses is a challenge in LMICs and one that is potentially a rate-limiting factor for the development of PCC services across the world. To that is added the complication of significant "brain drain" of trained nursing and medical personnel from LMICs to richer countries.

A major concern relates to the sustainability of professional careers in the PCC environment. There are persistent reports of high levels of stress, moral distress,[82] burnout,[83,84] and poor mental health among nurses and doctors working in the PCC environment. Most of this information comes from HICs, but as PCC expands in LMICs (where there are much lower staff numbers) burnout is likely to become a greater problem.

Since its inception PCC has been associated with expectations that health care workers will work long shifts and extended hours on duty. There are cultural shifts in expectations from both health care workers and their families about what hours and conditions of work are acceptable. Inevitably it seems that for many reasons many health care workers will no longer be prepared to work extraordinarily long hours, and this will affect the workforce requirements, as well as the time taken to complete clinical training. Although there is evidence that shorter shifts from nursing staff may be associated with improved patient outcomes, there are parts of the world where changing to shorter shifts is limited by concerns about the safety of staff traveling to and from work at different times of day. Failure to address these matters will inevitably lead to ongoing concerns about PCC development and sustainability.

Is Pediatric Critical Care Sustainable?

The sustainability of PCC in LMICs is a considerable concern. In a financial environment in which national annual per capita expenditure may be less than $30, it is extremely difficult to justify the high daily costs of PCC, particularly if the outcomes are poor. In poorer countries, individuals and their families bear a substantial part of the burden of health care costs, and in countries such as India and neighboring Bangladesh, it is possible to reduce entire families to debt and extreme poverty with the bills related to PCC. Financial systems will need to be put in place to ensure that individuals and their families are protected, while at the same time providing financial resources to support the care of critically ill children.

Even in richer countries there are major concerns regarding the amount of waste that is produced by large intensive care units, with largely disposable consumable equipment (which may amount to a substantial burden of waste per patient per day[85]). In the light of current concerns about climate change and pollution, these issues will have to be addressed.

What Are the Implications of Global Climate Change for Pediatric Critical Care?

Global climate change may adversely affect the resources needed and the delivery of PCC. It is known that global climate change has been associated with increased weather instability with more frequent extreme weather events and disasters across the world,[86] with increasing food insecurity, population displacement, and considerable human costs (lives, morbidity, financial, and social). Children especially in poorer parts of the world are deeply affected by these events, and the need for PCC will follow.[87] Changing weather patterns have also been associated with changes in the geographic distribution of insect-borne diseases such as dengue,[88] malaria, and chikungunya, and this is likely to continue.

SUMMARY

As we look to the future of PCC across the world, we are faced with multiple challenges, some that must be faced by all practitioners in PCC, and others that are widely divergent in different settings. It is hoped that we will be able to learn from each other as a community and address these challenges in ways that benefit children in all settings.

CLINICS CARE POINTS

- Formal, larger-scale clinical trials in acutely unwell children are necessary to refine many aspects of pediatric critical care.
- Training programs are required across the world to equip critical care practitioners with the skills required to care for patients in their settings.
- Telemedicine has the potential to ameliorate some of the shortages of skilled pediatric critical care practitioners, particularly in LMICs.
- A new focus in pediatric critical care is the need for "sustainable" critical care. The sustainability ranges from adequate staffing, through funding to support families of critically ill children, to processes that minimize the generation of waste in critical care.
- Critical care cannot happen in the absence of adequate supporting structures and systems. This includes human resources, imaging and diagnostic services as well as blood product availability.

REFERENCES

1. Slusher TM, Kiragu AW, Day LT, et al. Pediatric Critical Care in Resource-Limited Settings-Overview and Lessons Learned. Front Pediatr 2018;6:49.
2. Levin DL, Downes JJ, Todres ID. History of pediatric critical care medicine. J Pediatr Intensive Care 2013;2:147–67.
3. Epstein D, Brill JE. A history of pediatric critical care medicine. Pediatr Res 2005; 58:987–96.
4. Kissoon N, Argent A, Devictor D, et al. World Federation of Pediatric Intensive and Critical Care Societies-its global agenda. Pediatr Crit Care Med 2009; 10(5):597–600.
5. Schell CO, Khalid K, Wharton-Smith A, et al. Essential Emergency and Critical Care: a consensus among global clinical experts. BMJ Glob Health 2021;6(9).
6. Christian MD, Toltzis P, Kanter RK, et al. Treatment and triage recommendations for pediatric emergency mass critical care. Pediatr Crit Care Med 2011;12(6 Suppl):S109–19.
7. Duncan H, Hutchison J, Parshuram CS. The Pediatric Early Warning System score: a severity of illness score to predict urgent medical need in hospitalized children. J Crit Care 2006;21:271–8.
8. Rivera EAT, Patel AK, Chamberlain JM, et al. Criticality: A New Concept of Severity of Illness for Hospitalized Children. Pediatr Crit Care Med 2021;22(1): e33–43.
9. Carlton EF, Pinto N, Smith M, et al. Overall Health Following Pediatric Critical Illness: A Scoping Review of Instruments and Methodology. Pediatr Crit Care Med 2021;22(12):1061–71.
10. Ducharme-Crevier L, La KA, Francois T, et al. PICU Follow-Up Clinic: Patient and Family Outcomes 2 Months After Discharge. Pediatr Crit Care Med 2021;22(11): 935–43.
11. Chandran A, Sikka K, Thakar A, et al. The impact of pediatric tracheostomy on the quality of life of caregivers. Int J Pediatr Otorhinolaryngol 2021;149:110854.
12. Grieshop S. Post-intensive care syndrome. Am J Crit Care 2022;31:145.
13. English L, Kumbakumba E, Larson CP, et al. Pediatric out-of-hospital deaths following hospital discharge: a mixed-methods study. Afr Health Sci 2016; 16(4):883–91.

14. Wiens MO, Kumbakumba E, Larson CP, et al. Postdischarge mortality in children with acute infectious diseases: derivation of postdischarge mortality prediction models. BMJ Open 2015;5(11):e009449.

15. Chisti MJ, Salam MA, Bardhan PK, et al. Treatment Failure and Mortality amongst Children with Severe Acute Malnutrition Presenting with Cough or Respiratory Difficulty and Radiological Pneumonia. PLoS One 2015;10(10):e0140327.

16. Chisti MJ, Salam MA, Bardhan PK, et al. Treatment Failure and Mortality amongst Children with Severe Acute Malnutrition Presenting with Cough or Respiratory Difficulty and Radiological Pneumonia. PLoS One 2015;10(10):e0140327.

17. Wahl B, O'Brien KL, Greenbaum A, et al. Burden of Streptococcus pneumoniae and Haemophilus influenzae type b disease in children in the era of conjugate vaccines: global, regional, and national estimates for 2000–15. The Lancet Glob Health 2018;6(7):e744–57.

18. Reynolds LG, Klein M. Iron poisoning–a preventable hazard of childhood. South Afr Med Je 1985;67:680–3.

19. Coetzee S, Morrow BM, Argent AC. Measles in a South African paediatric intensive care unit: again. J Paediatr Child Health 2014;50:379–85.

20. Wahl B, et al. Burden of Streptococcus pneumoniae and Haemophilus influenzae type b disease in children in the era of conjugate vaccines: global, regional, and national estimates for 2000–15. Lancet Glob Health 2018;6:e744–57.

21. Shi T, Denouel A, Tietjen AK, et al. Global Disease Burden Estimates of Respiratory Syncytial Virus-Associated Acute Respiratory Infection in Older Adults in 2015: A Systematic Review and Meta-Analysis. J Infect Dis 2020;222(Suppl 7): S577–83.

22. Zimmerman MS, Smith AGC, Sable CA, et al. Global, regional, and national burden of congenital heart disease, 1990–2017: a systematic analysis for the Global Burden of Disease Study 2017. The Lancet Child Adolesc Health 2020; 4(3):185–200.

23. Elliott E, Zurynski Y. Rare diseases are a 'common' problem for clinicians. Aust Fam Physician 2015;44:630–3.

24. Trabacca A, Russo L. Children's rare disease rehabilitation: from multidisciplinarity to the transdisciplinarity approach. Eur J Phys Rehabil Med 2019;55:136–7.

25. Wise AL, Manolio TA, Mensah GA, et al. Genomic medicine for undiagnosed diseases. Lancet 2019;394(10197):533–40.

26. Carey AS, Chung WK. Genomic sequencing for infants and children in intensive care units. Curr Pediatr Rep 2019;7:78–82.

27. Wilkinson DJ, Barnett C, Savulescu J, et al. Genomic intensive care: should we perform genome testing in critically ill newborns? Arch Dis Child Fetal Neonatal Ed 2016;101:F94–8.

28. Sanderson SC, Lewis C, Hill M, et al. Decision-making, attitudes, and understanding among patients and relatives invited to undergo genome sequencing in the 100,000 Genomes Project: A multisite survey study. Genet Med 2022; 24(1):61–74.

29. Argent AC, Ahrens J, Morrow BM, et al. Pediatric intensive care in South Africa: an account of making optimum use of limited resources at the Red Cross War Memorial Children's Hospital. Pediatr Crit Care Med 2014;15(1):7–14.

30. Argent AC. PICU in Mozambique-the real challenge of pediatric intensive care when resources are less than what you might want (or need). Pediatr Crit Care Med 2018;19:1094–5.

31. Geoghegan S, Oulton K, Bull C, et al. The Experience of Long-Stay Parents in the ICU: A Qualitative Study of Parent and Staff Perspectives. Pediatr Crit Care Med 2016;17(11):e496–501.

32. Geoghegan S, Oulton K, Bull C, et al. The Challenges of Caring for Long-Stay Patients in the PICU. Pediatr Crit Care Med 2016;17(6):e266–71.

33. Namachivayam P, Taylor A, Montague T, et al. Long-stay children in intensive care: Long-term functional outcome and quality of life from a 20-yr institutional study. Pediatr Crit Care Med 2012;13(5):520–8.

34. Naghib S, van der Starre C, Gischler SJ, et al. Mortality in very long-stay pediatric intensive care unit patients and incidence of withdrawal of treatment. Intensive Care Med 2010;36(1):131–6.

35. Tooke L, Ehret DEY, Okolo A, et al. Limited resources restrict the provision of adequate neonatal respiratory care in the countries of Africa. Acta Paediatr 2021;111(2):275–83.

36. Cvetkovic M. Challenges in pediatric cardiac anesthesia in developing countries. Front Pediatr 2018;6:254.

37. Koopman AA, de Jager P, Blokpoel RGT, et al. Ventilator-induced lung injury in children: a reality? Ann Transl Med 2019;7(19):506.

38. Vet NJ, Kleiber N, Ista E, et al. Sedation in Critically Ill Children with Respiratory Failure. Front Pediatr 2016;4:89.

39. Patel N, Petersen TL, Simpson PM, et al. Rates of Venous Thromboembolism and Central Line-Associated Bloodstream Infections Among Types of Central Venous Access Devices in Critically Ill Children. Crit Care Med 2020;48(9):1340–8.

40. Lacroix J, Hebert PC, Hutchison JS, et al. Transfusion strategies for patients in pediatric intensive care units. The New Engl J Med 2007;356(16):1609–19.

41. Macrae D, Grieve R, Allen E, et al. A randomized trial of hyperglycemic control in pediatric intensive care. N Engl J Med 2014;370(2):107–18.

42. Fivez T, Kerklaan D, Mesotten D, et al. Early versus Late Parenteral Nutrition in Critically Ill Children. N Engl J Med 2016;374(12):1111–22.

43. Peters MJ, Jones GAL, Wiley D, et al. Conservative versus liberal oxygenation targets in critically ill children: the randomised multiple-centre pilot Oxy-PICU trial. Intensive Care Med 2018;44(8):1240–8.

44. Maitland K, Kiguli S, Olupot-Olupot P, et al. Randomised controlled trial of oxygen therapy and high-flow nasal therapy in African children with pneumonia. Intensive Care Med 2021;47(5):566–76.

45. Singer M, Young PJ, Laffey JG, et al. Dangers of hyperoxia. Crit Care 2021; 25(1):440.

46. Hochberg CH, Semler MW, Brower RG. Oxygen toxicity in critically ill adults. Am J Respir Crit Care Med 2021;204:632–41.

47. Barrot L, Asfar P, Mauny F, et al. Liberal or Conservative Oxygen Therapy for Acute Respiratory Distress Syndrome. N Engl J Med 2020;382(11):999–1008.

48. Angus DC. Oxygen therapy for the critically ill. New Engl J Med 2020;382:1054.

49. Maitland K, Kiguli S, Opoka RO, et al. Mortality after fluid bolus in African children with severe infection. N Engl J Med 2011;364(26):2483–95.

50. Inwald DP, Canter R, Woolfall K, et al. Restricted fluid bolus volume in early septic shock: results of the Fluids in Shock pilot trial. Arch Dis Child 2019;104(5):426–31.

51. Sinott Lopes CL, Eckert GU, da Rocha TS, et al. Early fluid overload was associated with prolonged mechanical ventilation and more aggressive parameters in critically ill paediatric patients. Acta Paediatr 2019.

52. Alobaidi R, Morgan C, Basu RK, et al. Association Between Fluid Balance and Outcomes in Critically Ill Children: A Systematic Review and Meta-analysis. JAMA Pediatr 2018;172(3):257–68.
53. Lopes CLS, Piva JP. Fluid overload in children undergoing mechanical ventilation. Rev Bras Ter Intensiva 2017;29:346–53.
54. Willems J, Hermans E, Schelstraete P, et al. Optimizing the Use of Antibiotic Agents in the Pediatric Intensive Care Unit: A Narrative Review. Paediatr Drugs 2021;23(1):39–53.
55. Sessions KL, Smith AG, Holmberg PJ, et al. Continuous positive airway pressure for children in resource-limited settings, effect on mortality and adverse events: systematic review and meta-analysis. Arch Dis Child 2021.
56. Sessions KL, et al. Bubble CPAP and oxygen for child pneumonia care in Malawi: a CPAP IMPACT time motion study. BMC Health Serv Res 2019;19:533.
57. Perkins GD, Ji C, Connolly BA, et al. Effect of Noninvasive Respiratory Strategies on Intubation or Mortality Among Patients With Acute Hypoxemic Respiratory Failure and COVID-19: The RECOVERY-RS Randomized Clinical Trial. Jama 2022; 327(6):546–58.
58. Richards-Belle A, Davis P, Drikite L, et al. FIRST-line support for assistance in breathing in children (FIRST-ABC): a master protocol of two randomised trials to evaluate the non-inferiority of high-flow nasal cannula (HFNC) versus continuous positive airway pressure (CPAP) for non-invasive respiratory support in paediatric critical care. BMJ Open 2020;10(8):e038002.
59. Laffey JG, Kavanagh BP. Negative trials in critical care: why most research is probably wrong. Lancet Respir Med 2018;6(9):659–60.
60. von Saint Andre-von Arnim AO, et al. Challenges and Priorities for pediatric critical care clinician-researchers in low- and middle-income countries. Front Pediatr 2017;5:277.
61. Weiss SL, Peters MJ, Alhazzani W, et al. Surviving Sepsis Campaign International Guidelines for the Management of Septic Shock and Sepsis-Associated Organ Dysfunction in Children. Pediatr Crit Care Med 2020;21(2):e52–106.
62. Weiss SL, Peters MJ, Agus MSD, et al. Perspective of the Surviving Sepsis Campaign on the Management of Pediatric Sepsis in the Era of Coronavirus Disease 2019. Pediatr Crit Care Med 2020;21(11):e1031–7.
63. Laffey JG, Kavanagh BP. Negative trials in critical care: why most research is probably wrong. Lancet Respir Med 2018;6(9):659–60.
64. Dahmer MK, Yang G, Zhang M, et al. Identification of phenotypes in paediatric patients with acute respiratory distress syndrome: a latent class analysis. The Lancet Respir Med 2022;10(3):289–97.
65. Shankar-Hari M, Santhakumaran S, Prevost AT, et al. Defining phenotypes and treatment effect heterogeneity to inform acute respiratory distress syndrome and sepsis trials: secondary analyses of three RCTs. Efficacy Mech Eval 2021;8.
66. Gattinoni L, Marini JJ. Isn't it time to abandon ARDS? The COVID-19 lesson. Crit Care 2021;25.
67. Yadav. Health P. Product supply chains in developing countries: diagnosis of the root causes of underperformance and an agenda for reform. Health Syst Reform 2015;1:142–54.
68. Shafiq N, Pandey AK, Malhotra S, et al. Shortage of essential antimicrobials: a major challenge to global health security. BMJ Glob Health 2021;6(11).
69. Roberts DJ, Field S, Delaney M, et al. Problems and Approaches for Blood Transfusion in the Developing Countries. Hematol Oncol Clin North Am 2016;30(2): 477–95.

70. English M, Irimu G, Agweyu A, et al. Building Learning Health Systems to Accelerate Research and Improve Outcomes of Clinical Care in Low- and Middle-Income Countries. Plos Med 2016;13(4):e1001991.

71. Wells MG, LN, Beringer C. Emergency Medicine Society of South Africaguidelines for the training and credentialingin emergency point-of-care ultrasound. South Africa Med J 2021;111:491–512.

72. Pearson G, Shann F, Barry P, et al. Should paediatric intensive care be centralised? Trent versus Victoria. Lancet 1997;349(9060):1213–7.

73. Truszkowski MPS, Fain J, Sauer E, et al. Telemedicine in Pediatric Intensive Care Units: Development of a new care modality. Children's Med 2020;XXVII:138–44.

74. Karsies TJ, Brilli RJ. Pediatric intensive care unit care–it takes a well-educated village. Pediatr Crit Care Med 2010;11:303–4.

75. von Saint Andre-von Arnim AO, Kumar RK, Oron AP, et al. Feasibility of Family-Assisted Severity of Illness Monitoring for Hospitalized Children in Low-Income Settings. Pediatr Crit Care Med 2021;22(2):e115–24.

76. Vaughn J, et al. Mobile Health technology for pediatric symptom monitoring: a feasibility Study. Nurs Res 2020;69:142–8.

77. Goh AY, Lum LC, Abdel-Latif ME. Impact of 24 hour critical care physician staffing on case-mix adjusted mortality in paediatric intensive care. Lancet 2001;357:445–6.

78. Pollack MM, Patel KM, Ruttimann E. Pediatric critical care training programs have a positive effect on pediatric intensive care mortality. Crit Care Med 1997;25:1637–42.

79. Nishisaki A, Pines JM, Lin R, et al. The impact of 24-hr, in-hospital pediatric critical care attending physician presence on process of care and patient outcomes. Crit Care Med 2012;40(7):2190–5.

80. Sorce L, Simone S, Madden M. Educational preparation and postgraduate training curriculum for pediatric critical care nurse practitioners. Pediatr Crit Care Med 2010;11:205–12.

81. Hickey PA, Pasquali SK, Gaynor JW, et al. Critical Care Nursing's Impact on Pediatric Patient Outcomes. Ann Thorac Surg 2016;102(4):1375–80.

82. Larson CP, Dryden-Palmer KD, Gibbons C, et al. Moral Distress in PICU and Neonatal ICU Practitioners: A Cross-Sectional Evaluation. Pediatr Crit Care Med 2017;18(8):e318–26.

83. Lin TC, Lin HS, Cheng SF, et al. Work stress, occupational burnout and depression levels: a clinical study of paediatric intensive care unit nurses in Taiwan. J Clin Nurs 2016;25(7–8):1120–30.

84. Rushton CH, Batcheller J, Schroeder K, et al. Burnout and Resilience Among Nurses Practicing in High-Intensity Settings. Am J Crit Care 2015;24(5):412–20.

85. Ghersin ZJ, Flaherty MR, Yager P, et al. Going green: decreasing medical waste in a paediatric intensive care unit in the United States. New Bioeth 2020;26(2):98–110.

86. UN Office for Risk Reduction. Human cost of disasters: and Overview of the last 20 years. 2000-2019; 2020.

87. Helldén D, Andersson C, Nilsson M, et al. Climate change and child health: a scoping review and an expanded conceptual framework. The Lancet Planet Health 2021;5(3):e164–75.

88. Campbell LP, Luther C, Moo-Llanes D, et al. Climate change influences on global distributions of dengue and chikungunya virus vectors. Philos Trans R Soc Lond B Biol Sci 2015;370(1665).

The Next Frontier in Neurocritical Care in Resource-Constrained Settings

Madiha Raees, MD[a],*, Beverly Cheserem, BM[b],
Benjamin Mutiso, MBChB[c], Tsegazeab Laeke, MD[d,e,f],
Brian Jason Brotherton, MD, MS[g,h]

KEYWORDS

- Trauma • Stroke • Infection • Seizures • Asphyxia neonatorum • Critical care
- Global health • Neurocritical care

KEY POINTS

- The burden of neurocritical illness (NCI) in resource-limited settings (RLS) is high and is projected to increase over the coming years.
- Evidence-based management guidelines for the burgeoning field of neurocritical care (NCC) are developed in resource-rich environments (RRS) assuming access to expensive equipment and subspecialty skills.
- Many RLS lack resources to effectively implement these guidelines, including intensive care units (ICUs) with trained physicians, nursing, and rehabilitation staff, equipment, and protocols; thus, the next frontier in NCC in RLS will require investing in the education and recruitment of staff and adaptation of guidelines designed for RRS.

[a] Division of Critical Care Medicine, Department of Anesthesia and Critical Care Medicine, Children's Hospital of Philadelphia, 3401 Civic Center Boulevard, Wood Building 6107, Philadelphia, PA 19104, USA; [b] Department of Neurosurgery, Aga Khan University Hospital, 3rd Parklands Avenue, Limuru Road, P.O. Box 30270 - 00100. Nairobi, Kenya; [c] Department of Neurosurgery, University of Nairobi, Kenyatta National Hospital, Ngong Road, P O BOX 20, Nairobi, Kijabe 00220, Kenya; [d] Division of Neurosurgery, Department of Surgery, College of Health Sciences, Addis Ababa University, 0000 0001 1250 5688, grid.7123.7, P.O. Box 9086, Churchill Avenue, Addis Ababa, Ethiopia; [e] Department of Clinical Medicine, Faculty of Medicine, University of Bergen, Jonas Lies veg 87, N-5021 Bergen, Norway; [f] NIHR Global Health Research Group on Neurotrauma, Division of Neurosurgery, Box 167, Cambridge Biomedical Campus, Addenbrooke's Hospital, University of Cambridge, Cambridge, UK, CB2 0QQ; [g] Department of Critical Care, AIC Kijabe Hospital, PO Box 20, Kijabe 00220, Kenya; [h] Department of Critical Care Medicine, University of Pittsburgh School of Medicine, 3550 Terrace Street, Scaife Hall Suite 600, Pittsburgh, PA 15213, USA
* Corresponding author.
E-mail address: raeesm@chop.edu

Crit Care Clin 38 (2022) 721–745
https://doi.org/10.1016/j.ccc.2022.06.016
0749-0704/22/© 2022 Elsevier Inc. All rights reserved.
criticalcare.theclinics.com

Abbreviations	
NCC	Neurocritical Care
RLS	Resource-Limited Settings
RRS	Resource-Rich Settings
NCI	Neurocritical Illness
LMIC	Low- and Middle-Income Country
HIC	High-Income Country
CNS	Central Nervous System
TBI	Traumatic Brain Injury
SCI	Spinal Cord Injury
CT	Computed Tomography
ICP	Intracranial Pressure
NC	Neurocysticercosis
TM	Tuberculous Meningitis
LP	Lumbar Puncture
CSF	Cerebrospinal Fluid
HIV	Human Immunodeficiency Virus
CM	Human Immunodeficiency Virus
SE	Status Epilepticus
EEG	Electroencephalography
NE	Neonatal Encephalopathy

INTRODUCTION

Neurocritical care (NCC) emerged as a distinct specialty with the advent of advanced neurosurgical techniques, improved understanding of resuscitation, and major technological advances, such as bedside invasive neuromonitoring. Much of the pioneering work was carried out by dedicated neurosurgeons such as Walter Dandy and Donald Munro, who established neurologically focused intensive care units (ICUs) in 1932 and 1936, respectively. Further advancements were made by neurologists such as Fred Plum and Jerome Posner with anesthesiology and neurosurgery support in the 1970 to 80s.[1] Today, NCC is a vibrant, diverse field that includes trauma, infectious diseases, congenital and genetic syndromes, and postsurgical conditions across the entire age continuum focused on the stabilization of primary brain injury and prevention of secondary brain insults.

The establishment of NCC as a unique area of practice was in direct response to the wide prevalence of neurologic injury among critically ill patients. A survey of 2876 ICUs in 1993 reported primary neurocritical illness (NCI) in 5% of ICU admissions.[2] This number continues to rise, exemplified by a reported prevalence of 11.5% in an adult cohort followed from 2009 to 2013 in 160 ICUs[3] and 16.2% in an international pediatric cohort from 107 ICUs established in 2011 to 2012.[4] Reports in the literature suggest even higher proportions of NCI in resource-limited settings (RLS).[5]

Following the development of protocols focused on reducing secondary brain injury, outcomes from NCI have improved in resource-rich settings (RRS). Zimmerman and colleagues reported a significant reduction in hospital mortality in an adult cohort from seizures (72%), stroke (47%), and head trauma (10%) over the course of 30 years in 14 ICUs in the United States.[6] Unfortunately, these trends have not been reproduced in RLS. Practitioners in RLS are faced with a higher burden of communicable diseases that cause NCI, such as malaria, coupled with a global rise in noncommunicable disease.[7] As an example, death from strokes in high-income countries (HICs) has reduced by 16%, while in low- and middle-income countries (LMICs), the incidence has only increased, resulting in even more demands placed on clinicians in RLS who are challenged by limited prehospital care systems, variable access to diagnostics and therapeutics, and a lack of specialty-trained medical staff.[8] The burden of NCI in RLS is only projected to rise in the future,[9] and critical care capacity has not kept up with demand.[10,11]

Evidence generated from RLS is desperately needed to develop management strategies that can be tailored to local resource availability. In this review, we report the epidemiology, management, and outcomes of traumatic central nervous system (CNS) injury, acute stroke, CNS infection, acute seizures and status epilepticus (SE), and birth asphyxia in RLS. These pathologies were chosen as they have been delineated as the most common causes of critical illness of neurologic etiology and remain a significant burden within RLS.[12–14] We reflect on advances made to date in NCC in RLS and propose future directions to strive toward in the next frontier of NCC.

Traumatic Brain and Spinal Cord Injury

Injuries result in more than 4 million deaths per year, with road traffic accidents, falls, and violence as the most common causes worldwide. Ninety percent of these deaths occur in LMICs. Even within HICs, disadvantaged socioeconomic classes bear a higher burden of injury-related death and disability, suggesting the strong impact of resource allocation and other social determinants of health.[15–18] In the realm of NCC, traumatic brain injury (TBI) and spinal cord injury (SCI) remain significant causes of morbidity and mortality. An international study involving 46 different countries demonstrated that the burden of TBI was significantly higher in RLS, and patients with severe TBI in LMICs were twice as likely to die as those in HICs.[19] Similarly, SCI was proportionally higher in RLS with a 5-fold higher mortality rate reported in LMICs.[20]

RRS have established standards of care that have led to significantly improved outcomes from traumatic CNS injury in the preceding decades. This success is contingent on the presence of trauma-focused triage systems, physical rehabilitation, and eventual integration back into society, including specialized and expensive equipment and trauma-trained staff, which represent challenging hurdles for RLS.[21–23] Only about one-quarter of the population in sub-Saharan Africa can access urgent neurosurgical services, largely comprised of populations around urban referral centers.[24] Many centers in RLS lack resources to implement first-tier therapies as outlined by the Brain Trauma Foundation Guidelines for the management of TBI, such as intracranial pressure monitoring systems and hyperosmolar therapies.[25–27] Where equipment and medications are available, progress can be hampered by lack of education and trained staffing.[28] Further, simply attempting to implement what has been successful in RRS without larger change imparts increased stress on already heavily burdened trauma systems without necessarily improving outcomes, demonstrating the critical need for RLS-generated evidence and guidelines.[29,30]

Many clinicians in RLS have come up with original solutions tailored to available resources. For example, models in Iraq, Cambodia, and Ghana have successfully trained lay providers to serve as front line trauma care providers to deliver evidence-based prehospital care at low cost with improvement in outcomes.[31] Clinicians in Latin America have managed patients with severe TBI with serial head computed tomography (CT) and examination findings with similar outcomes in those managed with intracranial pressure monitors, allowing for the publication of consensus-based guidelines tailored to RLS.[32,33] Trauma registries are being created, guidelines are being developed, and epidemiologic studies are being published.[34–36] Low-cost alternatives to advanced imaging such as optic nerve sheath diameter via ultrasound are also being explored.[37] Along with established predictors of mortality such as hypotension and hypoxia, delay in receiving definitive care has been recognized as independently associated with mortality.[38,39] Single centers in RLS have reported successful improvement in outcomes with timely surgical intervention and intensive NCC.[40–42] However, this represents care at higher resourced tertiary centers. Many patients in RLS continue to struggle with access to neurosurgeons[43] and NCC to prevent secondary CNS injury, leading to continued high rates of mortality.[44] Additionally, survivors of severe TBI or SCI in RLS face significant challenges with access to rehabilitation and reintegration into society without support outside of their families.[45]

International neurosurgical and trauma societies have taken note of the trends and have established nongovernmental organizations to address this unmet need. One example is the Foundation for International Education in Neurosurgery. This organization has facilitated the training of neurosurgeons from numerous RLS and has active projects in more than 20 countries.[46] This program is one of several dedicated to expanding trauma and surgical capacity in RLS and represents a global focus on increasing numbers of trained staff with eventual decentralization of resources from city centers.[47] Further, globally minded physicians and researchers have released public policy recommendations, emphasizing the need for governments to invest in the primary prevention of traumatic CNS injury and enhancement of trauma systems throughout the spectrum of care.[48] Until these unmet needs are addressed on a macro level, telemedicine and educational partnerships can be used to bridge the gap in certain areas. For example, telerehabilitation has been explored as a low-cost alternative to traditional intensive outpatient neurorehabilitation for patients with TBI and SCI.[49–51] Successful partnerships with RRS have led to the training of local surgical personnel in completing life-saving emergency procedures such as burr holes, along with the systematic redirection of surplus equipment to particularly austere settings.[52] A combination of systemic change with creative solutions to address gaps in care are key in continuing to improve outcomes for patients with traumatic CNS injury in RLS.

As mentioned, primary management of TBI and SCI focuses on the prevention of secondary injury. There is significant support in the literature for avoiding hypotension, hypoxia, and aberrations in blood carbon dioxide levels.[53] Other aims of preventing secondary brain injury involve preventing elevations in intracranial pressure (ICP). While the placement of externalized ventricular drains (EVDs), intraparenchymal monitors, or microdialysis catheters are outside the capabilities of most RLS, there are other noninvasive modalities of monitoring ICP. Monitoring pupil size and reactiveness (ie, neurologic pupil index (NPI)) with pupillometers rather than conventional inspection with a light, has been shown to reduce errors in evaluation and interoperator dependency. NPI has also been shown to correlate with sustained elevations in ICP.[54] Additionally, the use of bedside ultrasound for transcranial doppler measurement and optic nerve sheath diameter has been shown to be helpful in assessing for increased ICP.[55,56]

Regardless of setting, there are a number of TBI care initiatives that can be performed to improve the outcome for these patients. **Fig. 1** details high yield areas of therapeutic importance and can also provide a means for elevating the local quality of care delivery.

While the prevention of secondary injury SCI is similar to that of TBI, there are several distinct differences to highlight. One is the need for surgical decompression in the setting of cord impingement.[57,58] The second is the implementation of a mean arterial pressure (MAP) floor (ie, aiming to keep MAP above a set number). Hypotension and neurogenic shock are common complications of SCI and require adequate volume resuscitation and intravenous vasopressors.[59,60] Despite the common practice of maintaining a MAP goal, the evidence is not strong and remains Level III.[61] Lastly, the evidence surrounding glucocorticoid use in SCI has been

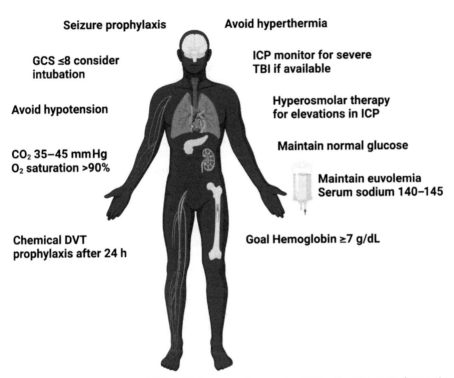

Seizure prophylaxis

Avoid hyperthermia

GCS ≤8 consider intubation

ICP monitor for severe TBI if available

Avoid hypotension

Hyperosmolar therapy for elevations in ICP

CO_2 35–45 mm Hg O_2 saturation >90%

Maintain normal glucose

Maintain euvolemia Serum sodium 140–145

Chemical DVT prophylaxis after 24 h

Goal Hemoglobin ≥7 g/dL

Fig. 1. Initial management of TBI. Initial means of managing TBI in the ICU. DVT, deep vein thrombosis; GCS, Glasgow coma scale score; TBI, traumatic brain injury. (Created with BioRender.com.)

controversial. The 2013 AANS/CNS guidelines recommend against their use, but the AO Spine guidelines from 2017 state high dose methylprednisolone should be given for 24 hours and within the first 8 hours of SCI.[61,62]

Stroke

Cerebrovascular accident (CVA) or stroke, defined as an acute focal injury of the CNS by a vascular cause, is the second leading cause of death and the third leading cause of disability worldwide among adults, with most of this burden falling on RLS.[63,64] Globally most strokes are ischemic, but in many RLS, they are primarily hemorrhagic.[65] Despite a decrease in stroke-associated disability-adjusted life years (DALY) in RRS, there has been an increase in RLS.[66] The most common risk factors for stroke are elevated systolic blood pressure, high body mass index, high fasting glucose, ambient particulate matter pollution, and smoking tobacco.[66]

Management of stroke relies on accurate and timely delineation of ischemic versus hemorrhagic etiology to determine candidacy for thrombolytic therapy. With a median availability of CT scanners of 6.1% among 10 RLS, a number of clinical prediction models have been created to attempt to address this gap.[67] Runchey and McGee evaluated prospective studies from 1966 to 2010 to determine which clinical characteristics might aid in separating stroke types. They discovered while certain clinical characteristics could suggest the presence of hemorrhage, none were strong enough to take the place of imaging.[68]

Tissue plasminogen activator (t-PA) administration within 3 hours of symptoms onset in acute ischemic stroke was established as the standard of care in 1995.[69]

This, along with mechanical thrombectomy, have proven to be first-line treatments for acute ischemic stroke in RRS.[70,71] Unfortunately, these are costly therapies that are challenging to provide in RLS, and rely on imaging modalities that may not be available.[72] A systematic review found that only 64 of 214 countries (30%) reported use of IV t-PA even though it is on the World Health Organization List of Essential Medicines.[73,74] LMICs had a reported use of 3% and 19%, respectively. A review by Khatib and colleagues found low use of evidence-based practices in the care of patients with stroke.[75] Fourteen of those study sites reported availability of t-PA, but only 3% of patients received this therapy. Barriers to its use are diagnostic certainty, the familiarity of using t-PA, and cost to the patient.

Outcomes are variable. One systematic review of more than 64,000 patients from RLS found in-hospital mortality ranged from 1% in Mexico to 45% in Nigeria, while the overall in-hospital mortality was 14%.[75] A retrospective cohort study conducted in Sierra Leonne noted an overall mortality rate of 35%.[76] A systematic review of stroke mortality in sub-Saharan Africa was high compared with that in RRS and believed by the authors of that study to result from weak health care systems and vascular risk factors.[77]

Rehabilitation is essential in improving outcomes, yet access to rehabilitation facilities and staff remain out of reach in many resource-constrained settings.[65] Chimatiro and colleagues found not only were services lacking, but there was a prolonged time between stroke onset to the initiation of rehabilitation.[72] Attempting to fill this gap on a more local level, home-based rehabilitation has been used with variable success. Task-sharing with family members and community health workers in India and South Africa has not substantially improved outcomes and has led to low satisfaction and unmet demands, highlighting the need for more support for families and more specific training of community health workers in proper rehabilitation techniques.[17,78]

The burden of stroke will likely only grow in RLS; thus it is critical to address this from a multi-faceted approach. Improvement in emergency medical services with decreasing time to arrival at care centers, increasing access to imaging, reducing the cost of thrombolytics, and growing multi-disciplinary teams are but a few areas that can potentially improve outcomes. Further, data registries, quality improvement initiatives, and local trials will increase awareness and provide relevant, context-specific solutions.

Central Nervous System Infection

CNS infections remain a significant etiology of morbidity and mortality. Depending on the geographic region, climate, and vaccination, they are due to different varieties of bacteria, viruses, fungi, and parasites.[79] Though difficult to accurately measure, the combined incidence and burden of these infections is highest in the World Health Organization (WHO) Africa, South-East Asia, and Western Pacific Regions.[80] Africa was identified as having highest incidence of bacterial meningitis and neurocysticercosis (NC) while Southeast Asia had the highest incidence of intracranial abscesses. Referring specifically to bacterial meningitis, RLS account for 98% of the nearly 5.6 million DALYs attributed to meningitis globally.[81]

Many CNS infections present with the triad of headache, fever, and meningismus, but these findings alone cannot discern between pathogenic etiologies. Therefore, one must have in mind a differential diagnosis when presented with a patient, young or old, complaining of headache and fever (**Table 1**). Most CNS infections are diagnosed through a combination of high index of suspicion, imaging, and lumbar puncture (LP), as physical examination maneuvers used to diagnose bacterial meningitis have an unacceptably low sensitivity.[79,82] Additionally, CT imaging is not routinely

Table 1
Differential diagnosis of individuals presenting with fever and headache

Pathogen	Clinical Manifestations	Diagnosis	Treatment	Complications
Bacteria				

Streptococcal Pneumoniae
Neisseria Meningitidis
Haemophilus Influenza
Listeria Monocytogenes
	• Headache
	• Fever
	• meningismus
		• LP
		  ○ Cell count
		  ○ Glucose
		  ○ Protein
		  ○ Culture if available
			• Third generation cephalosporin[a]
			• PLUS Vancomycin
			• PLUS Ampicillin if > 65 y of age
				• Hearing loss
				• Vison loss
				• Cognitive impairment
				• Infarcts
				• seizures

Mycobacterium Tuberculosis		• LP
		  ○ Cell count
		  ○ Glucose
		  ○ Protein
		  ○ AFB stain
		  ○ Genexpert if available
			• Anti-TB regimen
			• PLUS Glucocorticoids
				• Hydrocephalus
				• Coma
				• Death

Virus				
HIV Herpes simplex Rabies	• Fever • Encephalopathy	• LP as above ○ HSV PCR	• Acyclovir	• Seizures • Mesotemporal sclerosis
Fungus				
Cryptococcal Meningitis	• Headache • Confusion	• Cryptococcal antigen from CSF • India ink stain of CSF	• Amphotericin • PLUS Flucytosine or Fluconazole[b]	• Hydrocephalus
Parasite				
Cerebral Malaria	• Fever • Encephalopathy • Coma	• Thin and thick smear • Low threshold for considering diagnosis	• Artesunate OR Arthemether	• Coma • Epilepsy • Neurocognitive deficits
Neurocysticercosis	• Seizures	• Revised Del Brutto criteria	• Glucocorticoids • Anti-epileptics	• Epilepsy

Common, but not all inclusive list of infectious etiologies of meningitis and encephalitis.
AFB, acid fast bacilli; CSF, cerebrospinal fluid; HIV, human immunodeficiency virus; HSV, herpes simplex virus; LP, lumbar puncture; TB, tuberculosis.
[a] Based upon local antimicrobial sensitivities if available.
[b] Flucytosine not routinely available in RLS, therefore, fluconazole is indicated.

available in the resource-constrained setting, thereby making it difficult to follow guidelines that recommend imaging before LP.[83] This recommendation is not without debate, as there are 2 studies that discovered postmortem brainstem herniation in 1% of patients with meningococcal meningitis that underwent LP without imaging and a same 1% rate of herniation in a similar cohort of patients who did not undergo LP.[84,85] Despite microscopy and cerebrospinal fluid (CSF) culture being the gold standard for diagnosis, studies from RLS have proven difficult to achieve this due to lack of tools, laboratory personnel, or experienced clinicians to perform the LP.[86] When resources are available, CSF analysis itself makes it difficult to discern between bacteria, virus, or malaria as the culprit.

A novel approach of using colorimetric urine dipsticks to screen for meningitis has been undertaken. Several studies have attempted to use the leukocyte esterase tab to identify individuals with suspected bacterial meningitis for the purposes of not missing a deadly diagnosis and for triaging to higher centers of care.[87–89] However, none of these studies have shown high enough discrimination and calibration, but have begged the question: could CSF specific colorimetric strips be effective?

Bacterial Meningitis

The pathogens differ based on age, but common organisms are group B *Streptococcus, Neisseria meningitidis,* and *Haemophilus influenzae.*[79] According to the WHO, *N. meningitidis* is the main pathogen responsible for epidemic bacterial meningitis.[90] Other common pathogens are the gram negatives *Escherichia coli, Klebsiella pneumoniae,* and *Acinetobacter.* Prompt therapy with antimicrobials is the standard of care as a delay in the administration of therapy has been shown to have a negative impact on outcomes.[91] This should ideally be directed by local resistance patterns. There is growing evidence, and therefore concern, for antimicrobial resistance in RLS.[92–95]

Complications from bacterial meningitis are associated with long-term neurologic and cognitive impairment. In the neonatal period, these are not only impairments of hearing, vision, and motor function, but cerebral palsy and epilepsy.[96] Other complications include herniation, cerebral infarct, and intractable seizures.[97]

Neurocysticercosis

Neurocysticercosis (NC) was the most reported disease in publications of CNS infections and most prominently found in RLS with an incidence of 650 cases/100,000 people.[80,98] Caused by the larval form of the cestode, *Taenia solium,* the infection begins by the ingestion of food or water contaminated with the eggs.[98] NC is considered endemic in parts of sub-Saharan Africa, Asia, and Latin America.[99,100] While exact numbers are difficult to come by, in areas where NC is considered to be endemic, 30% of cases of epilepsy are due to the infection.

NC is capable of causing a variety of symptoms and signs depending on the number, size, stage, and location of the infection.[101] With highest affinity for the nervous system, the most devastating manifestations of epilepsy occur here due to single or multiple cysticerci. The cysticerci can occur in the brain parenchyma or ventricles, with ventricular disease potentially causing arachnoiditis, vasculitis, and even communicating hydrocephalus.[101] A group of experts simplified diagnostic criteria according to 2 principles: neuroimaging studies are essential for diagnosis, and all other information provides for indirect evidence favoring the diagnosis.[102] Management of NC involves 3 main classes of medications – antihelminth, antiepileptics (AEDs), anti-inflammatory (steroids). The overall treatment of NC is outside the scope of this critical care review, but it is important to note that for adolescent and adult patients with new-onset seizures and resultant epilepsy, a diagnosis of NC must be considered.

Cryptococcal Meningitis

Cryptococcal meningitis (CM) is the leading cause of meningitis in areas with a high prevalence of HIV infection and is the second leading cause of death among patients with HIV infection.[103] Despite the expansion and availability of antiretroviral therapy (ART), the prevalence of CM is unchanged in RLS.[104] CM is a subacute meningoen-cephalitis acquired by inhalation that can cause pulmonary symptoms, but due to its neurotropism, most of the presenting signs and symptoms are neurologic in nature.[105,106] It is well understood that individuals with HIV are at risk of CM infection. However, there are several conditions that place HIV-negative persons at risk for CM as well. These include prolonged steroid use, most commonly in the setting of the treatment of an autoimmune disease, sarcoidosis, and idiopathic CD4$^+$ lymphopenia.[105]

Patients often present with neurologic symptoms with headache and altered sensorium, and progression of disease can lead to increased ICP due to congestion and blockage of arachnoid granulations by dead organisms or shed cryptococcal polysaccharides.[104,105] This cellular debris decreases the reabsorption of CSF, resulting in rising pressure and hydrocephalus.

A prompt LP is both of diagnostic and therapeutic value. The opening pressure is often very high (>35 cm H_2O) and daily LPs may be required until the pressure is reduced below 25 cm H_2O. This practice has been shown to reduce mortality irrespective of initial opening pressure.[107] India Ink staining and CSF cryptococcal antigen (CrAg) are recommended for the rapid and accurate diagnosis of CM. Other notable findings in the CSF include elevated white blood cell count with lymphocyte predominance, elevated CSF protein, and low CSF glucose.[108,109] In the absence of CSF CrAg, a serum CrAg can be used to diagnose presumptive CM in those individuals with HIV. Antifungal therapies for CM have not changed much since the initial 1997 Mycoses Study Group trial and remain based on the three-step induction, consolidation, and maintenance approach.[107] The induction phase with intravenous flucytosine and amphotericin has proven itself to be difficult for the resource-constrained setting. Despite strong evidence supporting the use of flucytosine, an integral part of induction therapy for CM, availability, scarcity of in-country registration, and high cost have precluded flucytosine's use, leaving it out of reach for many.[110–113]

Adjunctive corticosteroids are not recommended in the treatment of CM. This is based on results from a multinational randomized controlled trial that was stopped early due to corticosteroids causing harm compared with the placebo group.[114]

Complications from CM itself as well as those due to the administration of amphotericin should be noted. Major complications of CM include hydrocephalus and immune reconstitution inflammatory syndrome (IRIS).[105,115] Adverse reactions to the administration of amphotericin include acute kidney injury, hypokalemia, and hypomagnesemia. The side effect of renal insufficiency has been one reason for the hesitancy to use amphotericin in the resource limited context due to the inability to measure serum drug levels. Recommendations to prevent this include generous administration of isotonic intravenous fluids before drug administration and careful attention to and repletion of electrolytes.[110,115,116]

Tuberculous Meningitis

Until the COVID-19 pandemic, tuberculosis (TB), an airborne disease caused by *Mycobacterium tuberculosis,* was the leading cause of death from a single infectious agent.[117] In 2020 there were an estimated 5.8 million new cases of TB worldwide. Tuberculous meningitis (TM) is an extra-pulmonary manifestation of TB and disproportionately affects children and those with HIV.[118,119] Accurate estimates of TM vary by location and are difficult to determine as cases are frequently unreported or even undiagnosed.

Pathogenesis involves hematogenous spread of *M. tuberculosis* to the brain followed by granuloma rupture and bacterial inoculation into the subarachnoid space. The resulting intracerebral inflammation is thought to contribute to the poor prognosis.[120]

The most well-documented risk factor for TM among adults is coinfection with HIV; these individuals have an increased risk of all-cause mortality compared with HIV-negative cohorts.[121,122] Age has also been described as a risk factor in that children are at increased risk for TM. Additionally, 1 in 5 infected children dies while only one in 3 survives without a significant disability.

Diagnosing TM clinically is difficult due to the nonspecific symptoms. Laboratory identification of TM using CSF (preferably large volume) can be difficult, prompting the WHO to recommend nucleic acid amplification for more rapid and accurate detection. The classic symptoms and signs of meningitis can appear, but as the infection progresses, more severe manifestations such as focal deficits, cranial nerve deficit, and coma can dominate. As with other CNS infections, LP is crucial in making the correct diagnosis. However, the low numbers of acid-fast bacilli in the CSF and the time required to find them make the utilization of microscopy cumbersome. This can be improved on by increasing the volume of CSF obtained for cytologic investigation.[123]

Since 2013 the WHO has recommended the use of nucleic acid amplification via GeneXpert for the rapid detection of TB.[124] This recommendation is based on a series of studies performed in settings of high TB burden and is a strong recommendation despite sensitivity varying between 51% and 100%. Given the easy and rapid use of this test, more than 23 million test cartridges have been procured for nearly 7,000 machines located in 130 countries.[125]

Therapy consists of a four-drug anti-tuberculous regimen with the addition of glucocorticoids.[126] Following up on this, a Cochrane review of 9 trials supported this initial study of showing the reduction in mortality for patients treated with corticosteroids.[127] Early detection and prompt therapy are essential to avoid complications, which often require surgical intervention. These include elevated ICP, ischemia, hydrocephalus, hyponatremia, and seizures, each contributing to poor outcome.[118,119] Management of elevated ICP, as well as the dearth of neurosurgeons in RLS, have been described elsewhere in this article.

Cerebral Malaria

Malaria is a parasitic disease caused by protozoans of the *Plasmodium* genus and there are 4 distinct species that are pathogenic to humans: *Plasmodium falciparum*, *P. vivax*, *P. ovale*, and *P. malariae*. *P falciparum* is considered the most dangerous and is responsible for most of the malaria infection mortalities.[128] From 2000 to 2019 there was a steady decline in malaria case incidence and deaths, but most of the cases occurred in the WHO African Region with a significant proportion of deaths from malaria occurring in children under age 5.[129] In 2020 there was an estimated 241,000 cases and 29 of the 85 countries where malaria is endemic accounted for nearly 96% of global malaria cases and deaths with most of these deaths occurring in children under 5 years of age.[129] Cerebral malaria is the most severe form of infection and has high rates of morbidity, including neurologic deficits such as new epilepsy, and mortality.[130] Cerebral malaria also carries the highest mortality rate as well as the greatest postinfectious sequelae in survivors.[131] The case fatality rate is around 15%.[132] Presentation, sequelae, and mortality rates are different between pediatric and adult populations. These differences are thought to be due to cellular maturity and host responses.[133,134] Clinically, it is hallmarked by impaired consciousness and coma. Other symptoms include diurnal fever, diffuse encephalopathy, seizures, and focal neurologic signs.[132] Diagnosis can prove difficult, especially among patients from regions with high rates of asymptomatic parasitemia. Practitioners have leveraged noninvasive measures of diagnosis such as fundoscopy, which has high sensitivity and specificity. However, this method is limited by large variability in the comfort of performing this examination as well as with the availability of ophthalmoscopes.[135]

Early and effective treatment is a key component in the fight against this disease. Treatment of severe and cerebral malaria has been the artemisinin derivatives, artesunate, and artemether, as the completion of 2 randomized controlled trials (RCTs) showed substantially reduced mortality in both adults and children.[136,137] However, as with all antimicrobial agents, resistance is an emerging issue. The extent to just how resistant *Plasmodium* is becoming has proven difficult to determine, as some studies suggest treatment failure by deviations from local protocols, as opposed to organism resistance.[129]

Given the rise in resistance and the further understanding of the host response to infection, the search for adjunctive therapies has been the topic of research for more than 30 years.[138] These have focused on modulating the immune response and clearing parasitemia. Systemic glucocorticoids and intravenous immunoglobulin were shown to be deleterious and are not recommended for the treatment of cerebral malaria.[139,140] Despite several case reports to suggest benefit, to date there have not been sufficient powered RCTs to suggest a benefit to exchange transfusion in patients with cerebral malaria.[141]

Seizures and Status Epilepticus

Seizures and epilepsy are widely prevalent, representing one of the most common neurologic disorders worldwide. Acute seizures have an estimated prevalence of 29 to 39 per 100,000 per year and the most common causes are TBI, cerebrovascular disease, drug withdrawal, infection, and metabolic insults. There is a bimodal distribution with the highest incidence peaks in the young and old.[142] The incidence of epilepsy is higher in RLS, and within RRS, the lower socioeconomic class has a higher incidence.[143] Status epilepticus (SE), the most severe form of an acute seizure, is associated with increased mortality. Due to inconsistent access to electroencephalography (EEG) in RLS to help diagnose nonconvulsive status epipleticus, our focus in this article will be on convulsive SE.[142] The true burden of disease in RLS is difficult to know due to a wide variety in reporting patterns, likely resulting in underreporting.

Challenges in treating acute seizures and SE consist of poor prehospital care and infrastructure, inconsistent access to antiepileptic drugs (AEDs), and lack of diagnostic services (eg, EEG, imaging studies) and skilled staff (eg, neurologists).[143,144] Surgical options for seizure management are few due to the small number of neurosurgeons and limited availability of specialized equipment.[145,146] Further, many RLS have the added complexity of cultural stigma associated with seizures and strong reliance on traditional medicine in some communities.[147] In general, first-line AEDs for SE are benzodiazepines with more variation on choice and availability of second-line agents. Laboratory testing, including evaluation for infections and electrolyte derangements, should be carried out where able.[148] Access to EEG, advanced imaging, and subspecialists is almost exclusively in tertiary referral centers within RLS.[144,149]

Despite many hurdles, clinicians in RLS have innovated methods to care for critically ill patients with seizures and SE. An example is the early initiation of enteral AEDs in Iran as part of the SE treatment algorithm when ICU beds or alternative drugs are not available.[150] Pediatric clinicians in South Africa without consistent access to levetiracetam and limited capacity to provide continuous infusions have demonstrated good effect at abating SE with intermittent doses of phenobarbital, thereby reducing ICU admissions and complications.[151] Allopathic practitioners have been welcomed to collaborate with traditional healers in Cape Town to bridge treatment gaps and augment cultural competency.[152]

Outcomes in RLS are highly variable. In-hospital mortality from SE in RLS is higher than in RRS with mortality ranging from 14.3% to 26.7% compared with 3.45% reported in a large US cohort.[152–157] In survivors, the development of neurologic sequelae, such as cognitive impairments or new focal deficits, was reported as ranging from 12% to 35.5% in RLS compared with 3.4% in a US cohort.[156,158–162]

It is estimated that around a quarter of patients with seizures in RLS represent potentially preventable conditions, including birth asphyxia, infections, and TBI.[158] Primary prevention strategies, including vaccination campaigns, expanded prenatal and birth care, and public health measures aimed at reducing road traffic accident injuries will have a deep impact on the burden of SE, particularly in children.[163] Interventions based on partnerships with RRS that have been piloted include low-cost educational programs in seizure management to enrich frontline health care providers and the establishment of telemedicine services.[164–166] These interventions, coupled with the expansion of prehospital services and increased access to diagnostics and therapeutics, can have a lasting impact on outcomes of SE in RLS.

Birth Asphyxia

The WHO defines birth asphyxia as "the failure to establish breathing at birth," a broad, nonspecific term that is gradually being replaced with more precise terminology beyond the scope of this review.[167] In survivors, it can lead to neonatal encephalopathy (NE), a syndrome characterized by abnormal neurologic function in the first days of life, which can result in significant disability, further burdening families and health care systems.[168,169] Up to 60% of cases of NE in RLS are due to intrapartum hypoxia.[170] In 2010, intrapartum hypoxia caused more than 500,000 deaths, more than 1 million new cases of NE, and more than 400,000 survivors with a significant neurologic disability; more than 95% of the deaths and disability occurred in LMICs.[168] Global stakeholders have prioritized the reduction of neonatal mortality due to lack of respiratory effort and developed targeted programming, such as the Helping Babies Breathe program.[171] These interventions have led to improved outcomes. Overall, neonatal mortality has reduced from 22.15 per 1000 live births in 2010 to 17 per 1000 live births in 2020. However, the burden still remains asymmetrically high in Africa, the Middle East, and South and Southeast Asia, which contained 90% of all deaths from "birth asphyxia" in 2017.[172] These statistics likely underrepresent the true burden of disease due to the lack of vital registration in many RLS.[173]

In RLS, the current management of intrapartum hypoxia has focused on reversing neonatal respiratory depression to prevent the development of NE. Protocols have been implemented to equip community birth attendants to use partographs, increase awareness of when to refer for emergency obstetric services, and once the baby is born, to perform interventions such as drying, stimulating, and assisted ventilation with success.[174–176] Management of NE due to intrapartum hypoxia in RRS relies on rapid transport of affected neonates to highly resourced tertiary referral centers to urgently receive therapeutic hypothermia with advanced hemodynamic and neurologic monitoring in a neonatal ICU. Many of these babies are intubated, mechanically ventilated, while receiving other advanced treatments and interventions. This is challenging to reproduce in RLS for many reasons. Despite these hurdles, there are centers that have successfully instituted therapeutic hypothermia with innovative, low-cost devices.[177,178] Outcomes data are mixed with several potential confounding factors such as the method of cooling, staff knowledge about neonatal resuscitation, or equipment used, further highlighting the need for RLS-specific guidelines.[179–183]

Substantial investment in primary prevention via the establishment of regular prenatal care and expansion in available resources and skilled staff to support pregnant women and newborns will dramatically reduce the incidence of NE and neonatal respiratory depression.[184] Indeed, several RLS have seen a reduction in incidence after successful implementation of public health measures.[185,186] Educational programs and exchange partnerships with RRS could facilitate these campaigns to effectively scale up interventions, as has been demonstrated with the Helping Babies Survive program sponsored by the WHO, the American Academy of Pediatrics, and the Laerdal Foundation. For more advanced management of NE, generation of data registries, expansion of neonatology services, and bilateral education exchanges are imperative to the care of newborns with critical neurologic illness in RLS.

Next Steps

Neurocritical care is a growing subspecialty within the field of critical care medicine and this expansion is a direct result of a steadily increasing burden of NCIs on a global scale. Unfortunately, this rapid growth is not commensurate with where cases of NCI occur.

In RLS, not only are cases of NCI becoming more prevalent, but the overall epidemiology is also changing. Historically, infectious etiologies such as bacterial meningitis and cerebral malaria made up the bulk of admissions of patients with a neurologic condition requiring intensive care. However, given rapid globalization and longer life expectancy, many noncommunicable diseases have overtaken these as the primary pathologies of NCI.

To effectively care for this growing patient population, there must be a multifaceted approach with the engagement of multiple stakeholders. At the hospital level, clinicians and caregivers in RLS must be able to recognize and address NCI. Capacity building in the space of human resources would result in specialized training for nurses and midlevel clinicians with skills to meet the unique needs of this cohort of patients. Other members of the multidisciplinary team should include physiotherapists, occupational therapists, speech therapists, respiratory therapists, pharmacists, and nutritionists. Utilization of these team members may mean the genesis of the position as many may not be available in the resource-constrained context, but each has shown to be beneficial in improving outcomes for patients with neurocritical conditions.[72]

Other areas of needed growth are training programs for general surgeons, nonsurgeon physicians, and nonphysicians to be able to address neurologic emergencies from the field to the hospital across the continuum of care. This has been accomplished in similar settings and should be replicated, building on what worked and what needs to be improved on.[187–189] Further, there is a desperate need to improve access to neurosurgical services throughout the continent. At present there are only 76 training programs across the African continent with an abysmal 0.03 neurosurgeons available per 100,000 patients across LICs; only 41% of African countries have at least one neurosurgical training program.[13,190] This incredibly low number is mirrored by the number of neurologists in LICs (0.03 per 100,000 patients).

Research focused on these settings can help standardize care and improve outcomes by focusing on measures of proven benefit and ignoring practices that do not. A more in-depth focus on local resources and capabilities will improve the generalizability of the results and be less likely to waste precious resources. Additionally, research regarding management and outcomes, such as patient registries, can be used for benchmarking and quality improvement initiatives, ultimately helping individual facilities and regions make decisions based on objective data.

Finally, emergency medical services are another spoke of the NCC wheel that needs attention. This will require a concerted effort among policymakers, public health officials, hospitals, and stakeholders to improve outcomes by decreasing the time to medical presentation.

Neurocritical illness has long been present in the RLS. However, there has been a seismic epidemiologic shift as most countries are enjoying a longer life expectancy. While this is an accomplishment in and of itself we must recognize that, older populations are at risk for more noncommunicable forms of neurocritical disease. This will shift the burden of disease from the young to those of middle and older ages, and further tax an already stressed health care ecosystem in most RLS. Without preparation and appropriate recognition of these illnesses becoming more prevalent, there may be tremendous downstream societal effects. The time to take action is now, starting with investing in systemic change by engaging public health officials, policymakers, and large nongovernmental organizations. Capacity-building efforts take time to have effect, and in the meantime, creative solutions to address treatment gaps, such as specialized training for nonsurgeons and modified care protocols, will need to be used to improve outcomes for patients requiring NCC. It truly does take a "village" and growing the village of trained caregivers can improve the care and outcomes of those presenting to RLS with NCI.

DISCLOSURE

The authors have no commercial or financial disclosures.

CLINICS CARE POINTS

- TBI is a common problem in the resource constrained setting. The best management is prevention of secondary injury followed by a focus on rehabilitative services, if available.
- Neurocysticercosis is one of the most common causes of new onset seizures in the resource constrained setting and should be considered upon presentation.
- Despite cerebrovascular events becoming more common in the resource constrained setting, the prevalence of therapeutic interventions is lagging behind.

REFERENCES

1. Wijdicks EFM. The history of neurocritical care. Handb Clin Neurol 2017; 140:3–14.
2. Groeger JS, Guntupalli KK, Strosberg M, et al. Descriptive analysis of critical care units in the United States: patient characteristics and intensive care unit utilization. Crit Care Med 1993;21(2):279–91.
3. Lilly CM, Swami S, Liu X, et al. Five-year trends of critical care practice and outcomes. Chest 2017;152(4):723–35.
4. Fink EL, Kochanek PM, Tasker RC, et al. International survey of critically ill children with acute neurologic insults: the prevalence of acute critical neurological

disease in children: a global epidemiological assessment study. Pediatr Crit Care Med 2017;18(4):330–42.

5. Brown MW, Foy KE, Chanda C, et al. Neurologic illness in Zambia : a neurointensivist ' s experience. J Neurol Sci 2018;385:140–3.

6. Zimmerman JE, Kramer AA, Knaus WA. Changes in hospital mortality for United States intensive care unit admissions from 1988 to 2012. Crit Care 2013;17(2). https://doi.org/10.1186/cc12695.

7. Chin JH, Vora N. The global burden of neurologic diseases. Neurology 2015; 83(4):349–51.

8. The top 10 causes of death. World Health Organization; 2020. Available at: https://www.who.int/news-room/fact-sheets/detail/the-top-10-causes-of-death. Accessed April 8, 2022.

9. Wong JC, Linn KA, Shinohara RT, et al. Traumatic brain injury in Africa in 2050: a modeling study. Eur J Neurol 2016;23(2):382–6.

10. JI S, RH M, Colleen B, et al. Worldwide organization of neurocritical care: results from the PRINCE study Part 1. Neurocrit Care 2020;32(1):172–9.

11. Rao CPV, Suarez JI, Martin RH, et al. Global survey of outcomes of neurocritical care patients: analysis of the PRINCE study Part 2. Neurocrit Care 2020;32: 88–103.

12. Shrestha GS, Lamsal R. Neurocritical care in resource-limited settings. J Neurosurg Anesthesiol 2020;32(4):285–6.

13. Shrestha GS, Goffi A, Aryal D. Delivering neurocritical care in resource-challenged environments. Curr Opin Crit Care 2016;22(2):100–5.

14. Mateen FJ. Neurocritical care in developing countries. Neurocrit Care 2011; 15(3):593–8.

15. Injuries and violence. World Health Organization; 2021. Available at: https://www.who.int/news-room/fact-sheets/detail/injuries-and-violence.   Accessed April 8, 2022.

16. Puvanachandra Prasanthi, Hyder AA. The burden of traumatic brain injury in Asia : a call for research. Pak J Neurol Sci 2009;4(1):27–32.

17. Hyder AA, Wunderlich CA, Puvanachandra P, et al. The impact of traumatic brain injuries: a global perspective. NeuroRehabilitation 2007;22(5):341–53.

18. Puvanachandra P, Hyder AA. Traumatic brain injury in Latin America and the Caribbean: a call for research. Salud Publica Mex 2008;50(SUPPL. 1):13–6.

19. de Silva MJ, Roberts I, Perel P, et al. Patient outcome after traumatic brain injury in high-, middle- and low-income countries: analysis of data on 8927 patients in 46 countries. Int J Epidemiol 2009;38(2):452–8.

20. Kumar R, Lim J, Mekary RA, et al. Traumatic spinal injury: global epidemiology and worldwide volume. World Neurosurg 2018;113(May):e345–63.

21. Elf K, Nilsson P, Enblad P. Outcome after traumatic brain injury improved by an organized secondary insult program and standardized neurointensive care. Crit Care Med 2002;30(9):2129–34.

22. O'Lynnger TM, Shannon CN, Le TM, et al. Standardizing ICU management of pediatric traumatic brain injury is associated with improved outcomes at discharge. J Neurosurg Pediatr 2016;17(1):19–26.

23. Kiragu AW, Dunlop SJ, Mwarumba N, et al. Pediatric trauma care in low resource settings: challenges, opportunities, and solutions. Front Pediatr 2018;6:1–14.

24. Punchak M, Mukhpadhyay S, Sachdev S, et al. Neurosurgical care: availability and access in low-income and middle-income countries. World Neurosurg 2018;112:e240–54.

25. Kochanek PM, Tasker RC, Carney N, et al. Guidelines for the Management of Pediatric Severe Traumatic Brain Injury, Third Edition: Update of the Brain Trauma Foundation Guidelines [published correction appears in Pediatr Crit Care Med. 2019 Apr;20(4):404]. Pediatr Crit Care Med. 2019;20(3S Suppl 1):S1–S82. doi:10.1097/PCC.0000000000001735.

26. Carney N, Totten AM, O'Reilly C, et al. Guidelines for the management of severe traumatic brain injury, 4th edition. Neurosurgery 2017;80(1):6–15.

27. Wooldridge G, Hansmann A, Aziz O, et al. Survey of resources available to implement severe pediatric traumatic brain injury management guidelines in low and middle-income countries. Child's Nerv Syst 2020;36(11):2647–55.

28. Barkley AS, Spece LJ, Barros LM, et al. A mixed-methods needs assessment of traumatic brain injury care in a low- and middle-income country setting: building neurocritical care capacity at two major hospitals in Cambodia. J Neurosurg 2021;134(1):244–50.

29. Callese TE, Richards CT, Shaw P, et al. Trauma system development in low- and middle-income countries: a review. J Surg Res 2015;193(1):300–7.

30. Patel A, Vieira MMC, Abraham J, et al. Quality of the development of traumatic brain injury clinical practice guidelines: a systematic review. PLoS One 2016; 11(9):1–17.

31. Debenham S, Fuller M, Stewart M, et al. Where there is No EMS: lay providers in emergency medical services care-EMS as a public health priority. Prehosp Disaster Med 2017;32(6):593–5.

32. Chesnut RM, Temkin N, Carney N, et al. A trial of intracranial-pressure monitoring in traumatic brain injury. N Engl J Med 2012;367(26):2471–81.

33. Chesnut RM, Temkin N, Videtta W, et al. Consensus-based management protocol (CREVICE protocol) for the treatment of severe traumatic brain injury based on imaging and clinical examination for use when intracranial pressure monitoring is not employed. J Neurotrauma 2020;37:1291–9.

34. Ramesh A, Fezeu F, Fidele B, et al. Challenges and solutions for traumatic brain injury management in a resource-limited environment: example of a public referral hospital in Rwanda. Cureus 2014;6(5):1–7.

35. Staton CA, Msilanga D, Kiwango G, et al. A prospective registry evaluating the epidemiology and clinical care of traumatic brain injury patients presenting to a regional referral hospital in Moshi, Tanzania: challenges and the way forward. Int J Inj Contr Saf Promot 2017;24(1):69–77.

36. Kesinger MR, Nagy LR, Sequeira DJ, et al. A standardized trauma care protocol decreased in-hospital mortality of patients with severe traumatic brain injury at a teaching hospital in a middle-income country. Injury 2014;45(9):1350–4.

37. Sahoo SS, Agrawal D. Correlation of optic nerve sheath diameter with intracranial pressure monitoring in patients with severe traumatic brain injury. Indian J Neurotrauma 2013;10(1):9–12.

38. Gupta S, Khajanchi M, Kumar V, et al. Third delay in traumatic brain injury: time to management as a predictor of mortality. J Neurosurg 2020;132(January): 289–95.

39. Kuo BJ, Vaca SD, Vissoci JRN, et al. A prospective neurosurgical registry evaluating the clinical care of traumatic brain injury patients presenting to Mulago National Referral Hospital in Uganda. PLoS One 2017;12(10):1–16.

40. Elahi C, Rocha TAH, da Silva NC, et al. An evaluation of outcomes in patients with traumatic brain injury at a referral hospital in Tanzania: evidence from a survival analysis. Neurosurg Focus 2019;47(5):1–9.

41. Choi JH, Park PJ, Din V, et al. Epidemiology and clinical management of traumatic spine injuries at a major government hospital in Cambodia. Asian Spine J 2017;11(6):908–16.
42. Abio A, Bovet P, Valentin B, et al. Changes in mortality related to traumatic brain injuries in the Seychelles from 1989 to 2018. Front Neurol 2021;12:1–8.
43. Magogo J, Lazaro A, Mango M, et al. Operative treatment of traumatic spinal injuries in Tanzania: surgical management, neurologic outcomes, and time to surgery. Glob Spine J 2021;11(1):89–98.
44. Krebs E, Gerardo CJ, Park LP, et al. Mortality-associated characteristics of patients with traumatic brain injury at the university teaching hospital of Kigali, Rwanda. World Neurosurg 2017;102:571–82.
45. Chhabra HS, Sharma S, Arora M. Challenges in comprehensive management of spinal cord injury in India and in the Asian spinal cord network region: findings of a survey of experts, patients and consumers. Spinal Cord 2018;56:71–7.
46. FIENS. Available at: https://fiens.org/partners/. Accessed April 9, 2022.
47. Corley J, Lepard JR, Barthelemy E, et al. Essential neurological workforce needed to address neurotrauma in low- and middle-income countries. World Neurosurg 2019;123:295–9.
48. Lepard JR, Ammar A, Shlobin NA, et al. An assessment of global neurotrauma prevention and care delivery: the provider. World Neurosurgery2 2021; 156(December):e183–91. Available at: http://kiss.kstudy.com/journal/thesis_name.asp?tname=kiss2002&key=3183676.
49. Galea MD. Telemedicine in rehabilitation. Phys Med Rehabil Clin N Am 2019; 30(2):473–83.
50. Tyagi N, Amar Goel S, Alexander M. Improving quality of life after spinal cord injury in India with telehealth. Spinal Cord Ser Cases 2019;5(1). https://doi.org/10.1038/s41394-019-0212-x.
51. Dhakal R, Baniya M, Solomon RM, et al. TEleRehabilitation Nepal (TERN) to improve quality of life of people with spinal cord injury and acquired brain injury. A proof-of-concept study 2021. https://doi.org/10.1101/2021.06.21.21257001. medrxiv. Published online.
52. Upadhyayula PS, Yue JK, Yang J, et al. The current state of rural neurosurgical practice: an international perspective. J Neurosci Rural Pract 2018;9(1):123–31.
53. Brouwer MC, van de Beek D, Thomas S, et al. Bacterial Meningitis 1 Dilemmas in the diagnosis of acute community-acquired bacterial meningitis. Lancet 2012; 380:1684–92.
54. Jahns FP, Miroz JP, Messerer M, et al. Quantitative pupillometry for the monitoring of intracranial hypertension in patients with severe traumatic brain injury. Crit Care 2019;23(1):1–9.
55. Robba C, Santori G, Czosnyka M, et al. Optic nerve sheath diameter measured sonographically as non-invasive estimator of intracranial pressure: a systematic review and meta-analysis. Intensive Care Med 2018;44(8):1284–94.
56. Rasulo FA, Bertuetti R, Robba C, et al. The accuracy of transcranial Doppler in excluding intracranial hypertension following acute brain injury: a multicenter prospective pilot study. Crit Care 2017;21(1):1–8.
57. Eckert MJ, Martin MJ. Trauma : spinal cord injury. Surg Clin 2017;97:1031–45. https://doi.org/10.1038/s41393-018-0155-2%0A10.1007/s12028-018-0537-5%0A10.1016/j.mporth.2016.07.006%0A10.1016/j.bpa.2015.11.003%0A10.1016/j.mpaic.2017.05.010%0A10.1. Available at:.
58. Eli I, Lerner DP, Zoher G. Acute traumatic spinal cord injury. Neurol Clin 2021; 39(2021):471–88.

59. Karsy M, Hawryluk G. Modern medical management of spinal cord injury. Curr Neurol Neurosci Rep 2019;19(9):1–7.

60. Menacho ST, Floyd C. Current practices and goals for mean arterial pressure and spinal cord perfusion pressure in acute traumatic spinal cord injury: defining the gaps in knowledge. J Spinal Cord Med 2021;44(3):350–6.

61. Walters BC, Hadley MN, Hurlbert RJ, et al. Guidelines for the management of acute cervical spine and spinal cord injuries: 2013 update. Neurosurgery 2013;60(SUPPL. 1):82–91.

62. Fehlings MG, Wilson JR, Tetreault LA, et al. A clinical practice guideline for the management of patients with acute spinal cord injury: recommendations on the use of methylprednisolone sodium succinate. Glob Spine J 2017; 7(3_supplement):203S–11S.

63. Campbell BCV, Khatri P. Stroke *Lancet* 2020;396:129–42.

64. Krishnamurthi RV, Ikeda T, Feigin VL. Global, regional and country-specific burden of ischaemic stroke, intracerebral haemorrhage and subarachnoid hae-morrhage: a systematic analysis of the global burden of disease study 2017. Neuroepidemiology 2020;54(2):171–9.

65. Kisa A, Kisa S, Collaborators GBD, et al. Global, regional, and national burden of stroke and its risk factors, 1990–2019: a systematic analysis for the Global Burden of Disease Study 2019. Lancet Neurol 2021;20(October):26.

66. Feigin VL, Brainin M, Norrving B, et al. World stroke organization (WSO): global stroke fact sheet 2022. Int J Stroke 2022;17(1):18–29.

67. Yadav H, Shah D, Sayed S, et al. Availability of essential diagnostics in ten low-income and middle-income countries: results from national health facility sur-veys. Lancet Glob Heal 2021;9(11):e1553–60.

68. Runchey S, McGee S. Does this patient have a hemorrhagic stroke? Clinical findings distinguishing hemorrhagic stroke from ischemic stroke. JAMA - J Am Med Assoc 2010;303(22):2280–6.

69. The National Institute of Nerulogical Disorders and Stroke rt-PA Stroke Study Group. Recombinant tissue plasminogen activator for acute ischemic stroke. N Engl J Med 1995;333(24).

70. Nogueira RG, Jadhav AP, Haussen DC, et al, TGJ. Thrombectomy 6 to 24 hours after STroke with a mismatch between deficit and infarct. N Engl J Med 2018; 378(1):11–21.

71. Albers G, Marks M, Kemp S, et al. Thrombectomy for stroke at 6 to 16 hours with selection by perfusion imaging. N Engl J Med 2018;378(8):708–18.

72. Chimatiro GL, Rhoda AJ. Scoping review of acute stroke care management and rehabilitation in low and middle-income countries. BMC Health Serv Res 2019;19(1).

73. Berkowitz AL, Mittal MK, Mclane HC, et al. Worldwide reported use of IV tissue plasminogen activator for acute ischemic stroke. Int J Stroke 2014;9(3):349–55.

74. World Health Organization. Model list of essential medicines, 21st list, 2019. 2019. Available at: http://apps.who.int/iris/.

75. Khatib R, Arevalo YA, Berendsen MA, et al. Presentation, evaluation, manage-ment, and outcomes of acute stroke in low- and middle-income countries: a sys-tematic review and meta-analysis. Neuroepidemiology 2018;51(1–2):104–12.

76. Russell JBW, Charles E, Conteh V, et al. Risk factors, clinical outcomes and pre-dictors of stroke mortality in Sierra Leoneans: a retrospective hospital cohort study. Ann Med Surg 2020;60(November):293–300.

77. Adoukonou T, Kossi O, Fotso Mefo P, et al. Stroke case fatality in sub-Saharan Africa: systematic review and meta-analysis. Int J Stroke 2021;16(8):902–16.

78. Scheffler E, Mash R. Surviving a stroke in South Africa: outcomes of home-based care in a low-resource rural setting. Top Stroke Rehabil 2019;26(6): 423–34.
79. Wall EC, Chan JM, Gil E, et al. Acute bacterial meningitis. Curr Opin Neurol 2021;35(3):386–95.
80. Robertson FC, Lepard JR, Mekary RA, et al. Epidemiology of central nervous system infectious diseases: a meta-analysis and systematic review with implications for neurosurgeons worldwide. J Neurosurg 2019;130(4):1107–26.
81. McIntyre PB, O'Brien KL, Greenwood B, et al. Effect of vaccines on bacterial meningitis worldwide. Lancet 2012;380:1703–11.
82. Thomas KE, Hasbun R, Jekel J, et al. The diagnostic accuracy of kernig's sign, brudzinski's sign, and nuchal rigidity in adults with suspected meningitis. Clin Infect Dis 2002;35(1):46–52.
83. Tunkel AR, Hasbun R, Bhimraj A, et al. Infectious diseases society of America's clinical practice guidelines for healthcare-associated ventriculitis and meningitis. Clin Infect Dis 2017;64(6):e34–65.
84. Durand M, Calderwood S, Weber D, et al. Acute bacterial meningitis in adults. N Engl J Med 1993;328(1):21–6. Available at: http://content.nejm.org/cgi/content/abstract/329/14/977%5Cnhttp://www.nejm.org/doi/abs/10.1056/NEJM199309303291401.
85. Wylie PAL, Stevens D, Drake W, et al. Epidemiology and clinical management of meningococcal disease in west Gloucestershire: retrospective, population based study. Br Med J 1997;315(7111):774–9.
86. Gudina EK, Tesfaye M, Adane A, et al. Challenges of bacterial meningitis case management in low income settings: an experience from Ethiopia. Trop Med Int Heal 2016;21(7):870–8.
87. DeLozier JS, Auerbach PS. The leukocyte esterase test for detection of cerebrospinal fluid leukocytosis and bacterial meningitis. Ann Emerg Med 1989;18(11): 1191–8.
88. Bortcosh W, Siedner M, Carroll RW, et al. Utility of the urine reagent strip leucocyte esterase assay for the diagnosis of meningitis in resource-limited settings: meta- analysis. Trop Med Int Heal 2017;22(9):1072–80.
89. Bruce C, Mashimango L, Remi T, et al. Bedside colorimetric reagent dipstick in the diagnosis of meningitis in low – and middle – income countries : a prospective , international blinded comparison with laboratory analysis. Afr J Emerg Med 2022;12(3):161–4.
90. World Health Organization. Weekly epidemiological record. 2020. Available at: www.who.int/wer.
91. Eisen DP, Hamilton E, Bodilsen J, et al. Longer than 2 hours to antibiotics is associated with doubling of mortality in a multinational community - acquired bacterial meningitis cohort. Nat Sci Rep 2022;12(672):1–11.
92. Agata EMCD, Dupont-rouzeyrol M, Magal P, et al. The impact of different antibiotic regimens on the emergence of antimicrobial-resistant bacteria. PLoS One 2008;3(12):4–12.
93. Leopold SJ, van Leth F, Tarekegn H, et al. Antimicrobial drug resistance among clinically relevant bacterial isolates in sub-Saharan Africa: a systematic review. J Antimicrob Chemother 2014;69(9):2337–53.
94. Dailey PJ, Osborn J, Ashley EA, et al. Antimicrobial resistance among clinically relevant bacterial isolates in Accra: a retrospective study. BMC Res Notes 2015; 11(1):254.

95. Tadesse BT, Ashley EA, Ongarello S, et al. Antimicrobial resistance in Africa: a systematic review. BMC Infect Dis 2017;17(1):1–17.

96. John CC, Montano SM, Bangirana P, et al. Global research priorities for infections that affect the nervous system. Nature 2015;527(7578):S178–86.

97. Sharew A, Bodilsen J, Hansen BR, et al. The cause of death in bacterial meningitis. BMC Infect Dis 2020;20(182):1–9.

98. Gripper LB, Welburn SC. Neurocysticercosis infection and disease–A review. Acta Trop 2017;166:218–24.

99. Millogo A, Njamnshi AK, Kabwa-pierreluabeya M. Neurocysticercosis and epilepsy in sub-Saharan Africa. Brain Res Bull 2022;145(June 2018):30–8.

100. Coyle CM, Mahanty S, Zunt JR, et al. Neurocysticercosis: neglected but not forgotten. Plos Negl Trop Dis 2012;6(5):9–11.

101. Winkler AS. Neurocysticercosis in sub-Saharan Africa: a review of prevalence, clinical characteristics, diagnosis, and management. Pathog Glob Health 2012;106(5):261–74.

102. Del Brutto OH, Nash TE, White AC, et al. Revised diagnostic criteria for neurocysticercosis. J Neurol Sci 2017;372:202–10.

103. Rajasingham R, Smith RM, Park BJ, et al. Global burden of disease of HIV-associated cryptococcal meningitis: an updated analysis. Lancet Infect 2017; 17(8):873–81.

104. Wall EC, Everett D, Mukaka M, et al. Bacterial meningitis in malawian adults, adolescents, and children during the era of antiretroviral scale-up and haemophilus influenzae type B vaccination, 2000-2012. Clin Infect Dis 2014;58(10): 2000–12.

105. Williamson PR, Jarvis JN, Panackal AA, et al. Cryptococcal meningitis: epidemiology, immunology, diagnosis and therapy. Nat Rev Neurol 2016;13(1):13–24.

106. Alanio A, Vernel-Pauillac F, Sturny-Leclère A, et al. Cryptococcus neoformans host adaptation: toward biological evidence of dormancy. MBio 2015;6(2). https://doi.org/10.1128/mBio.02580-14.

107. Rolfes MA, Hullsiek KH, Rhein J, et al. The effect of therapeutic lumbar punctures on acute mortality from cryptococcal meningitis. Clin Infect Dis 2014; 59(11):1607–14.

108. Jarvis JN, Bicanic T, Loyse A, et al. Determinants of mortality in a combined cohort of 501 patients with HIV-associated cryptococcal meningitis: implications for improving outcomes. Clin Infect Dis 2014;58(5):736–45.

109. World Health Organization. Rapid advice diagnosis, prevention and management of cryptococcal disease in HIV-infected adults, adolescents and children. World Health Organization; 2011.

110. Loyse A, Burry J, Cohn J, et al. Leave no one behind: response to new evidence and guidelines for the management of cryptococcal meningitis in low-income and middle-income countries. Lancet Infect Dis 2019;19(4):e143–7.

111. Mfinanga S, Chanda D, Kivuyo SL, et al. Cryptococcal meningitis screening and community-based early adherence support in people with advanced HIV infection starting antiretroviral therapy in Tanzania and Zambia: an open-label, randomised controlled trial. Lancet 2015;385(9983):2173–82.

112. Molloy SF, Kanyama C, Heyderman RS, et al. Antifungal combinations for treatment of cryptococcal meningitis in Africa. N Engl J Med 2018;378(11):1004–17.

113. Organisation (WHO) World Health. World health organization model list of essential medicines. Ment Holist Heal Some Int Perspect 2019;21:119–34.

114. World Health Organization. Diagnosis, prevention and management of cryptococcal disease in HIV-infected adults , adolescents and children 2018.

115. Chen SCA, Korman TM, Slavin MA, et al. Antifungal therapy and management of complications of cryptococcosis due to Cryptococcus gattii. Clin Infect Dis 2013;57(4):543–51.

116. Loyse A, Thangaraj H, Easterbrook P, et al. Cryptococcal meningitis: improving access to essential antifungal medicines in resource-poor countries. Lancet Infect Dis 2013;13(7):629–37.

117. World Health Organization. Global tuberculosis report. 2021. Available at: https://www.who.int/publications-detail-redirect/9789240037021.

118. Donovan J, Figaji A, Imran D, et al. The neurocritical care of tuberculous meningitis. Lancet Neurol 2019;18(8):771–83.

119. Wilkinson RJ, Rohlwink U, Misra UK, et al. Tuberculous meningitis. Nat Rev Neurol 2017;13(10):581–98.

120. Van Laarhoven A, Dian S, Ruesen C, et al. Clinical parameters, routine inflammatory markers, and LTA4H genotype as predictors of mortality among 608 patients with tuberculous meningitis in Indonesia. J Infect Dis 2017;215(7):1029–39.

121. Marais S, Pepper DJ, Schutz C, et al. Presentation and outcome of tuberculous meningitis in a high HIV prevalence setting. PLoS One 2011;6(5). https://doi.org/10.1371/journal.pone.0020077.

122. Roy RB, Bakeera-Kitaka S, Chabala C, et al. Defeating paediatric tuberculous meningitis: applying the who "defeating meningitis by 2030: global roadmap. Microorganisms 2021;9(4):1–18.

123. Thwaites GE, Chau TTH, Farrar JJ. Improving the bacteriological diagnosis of tuberculous meningitis. J Clin Microbiol 2004;42(1):378–9.

124. World Health Organization. Automated real-time nucleic acid amplification technology for rapid and simultaneous detection of tuberculosis and rifampicin resistance: xpert MTB/RIF assay for the diagnosis of pulmonary and extrapulmonary TB in adults and children. 2013. Available at: https://apps.who.int/iris/handle/10665/112472.

125. Brown S, Leavy JE, Jancey J. Implementation of genexpert for tb testing in low- and middle-income countries: a systematic review. Glob Heal Sci Pract 2021;9(3):698–710.

126. Thwaites GE, Bang ND, Dung NH, et al. Dexamethasone for the treatment of tuberculous meningitis in adolescents and adults. N Engl J Med 2004;351:1741–51.

127. Prasad K, Singh MB, Ryan H. Corticosteroids for managing tuberculous meningitis. Cochrane Database Syst Rev 2016;2016(4). https://doi.org/10.1002/14651858.CD002244.pub4.

128. Luzolo AL, Ngoyi DM. Cerebral malaria. Brain Res Bull 2022;145(2019):53–8.

129. World Health Organization. World malaria report 2021. Vol 1. Available at: https://www.who.int/teams/global-malaria-programme/reports/world-malaria-report-2021, 2021. Accessed June 1, 2022.

130. Mishra SK, Newton CRJC. Diagnosis and management of the neurological complications of falciparum malaria. Nat Rev Neurol 2009;5(4):189–98.

131. Schiess N, Rueda AV, Cottier KE, et al. Pathophysiology and neurologic sequelae of cerebral malaria. Malar J 2020;19(266).

132. Birbeck GL, Molyneux ME, Kaplan PW, et al. Blantyre Malaria Project Epilepsy Study (BMPES) of neurological outcomes in retinopathy-positive paediatric cerebral malaria survivors: a prospective cohort study. Lancet Neurol 2010;9(12):1173–81.

133. Hawkes M, Elphinstone RE, Conroy AL, et al. Contrasting pediatric and adult cerebral malaria: the role of the endothelial barrier. Virulence 2013;4(6):543–55.

134. Gillrie MR, Lee K, Gowda DC, et al. Plasmodium falciparum histones induce endothelial proinflammatory response and barrier dysfunction. Am J Pathol 2012;180(3):1028–39.

135. Beare NAV, Taylor TE, Harding SP, et al. Malarial retinopathy: a newly established diagnostic sign in severe malaria. Am J Trop Med Hyg 2006;75(5):790–7.

136. White NJ. Artesunate versus quinine for treatment of severe falciparum malaria: a randomised trial. Lancet 2005;366(9487):717–25.

137. Dondorp AM, Fanello CI, Hendriksen IC, et al. Artesunate versus quinine in the treatment of severe falciparum malaria in African children (AQUAMAT): an open-label, randomised trial. Lancet 2010;376(9753):1647–57.

138. Varo R, Crowley VM, Sitoe A, et al. Adjunctive therapy for severe malaria: a review and critical appraisal. Malar J 2018;17(1):1–18.

139. Warrell DA, Looareesuwan S, Warrell MJ, et al. Dexamethasone proves deleterious in cerebral malaria. A double-blind trial in 100 comatose patients. N Engl J Med 1982;306(6):313–9.

140. Taylor TE, Molyneux ME, Wirima JJ, et al. Intravenous immunoglobulin in the treatment of paediatric cerebral malaria. Clin Exp Immunol 1992;90(3):357–62.

141. Riddle MS, Jackson JL, Sanders JW, et al. Exchange transfusion as an adjunct therapy in severe Plasmodium falciparum malaria: a meta-analysis. Clin Infect Dis 2002;34(9):1192–8.

142. Hauser WA, Beghi E. First seizure definitions and worldwide incidence and mortality. Epilepsia 2008;49(SUPPL. 1):8–12.

143. Fiest KM, Sauro KM, Wiebe S, et al. Prevalence and incidence of epilepsy: a systematic review and meta-analysis of international studies. Neurology 2017; 88:296–303.

144. Lee B, Mannan MA, Zhou D, et al. Treatment gap for convulsive status epilepticus in resource-poor countries. Epilepsia 2018;59:135–9.

145. Kissani N, Nafia S, El Khiat A, et al. Epilepsy surgery in Africa: state of the art and challenges. Epilepsy Behav 2021;118(2021). https://doi.org/10.1016/j.yebeh.2021.107910.

146. Dewan MC, Rattani A, Fieggen G, et al. Global neurosurgery: the current capacity and deficit in the provision of essential neurosurgical care. Executive summary of the global neurosurgery initiative at the program in global surgery and social change. J Neurosurg 2019;130(4):1055–64.

147. Baskind R, Birbeck G. Epilepsy care in Zambia: a study of traditional healers. Epilepsia 2005;46(7):1121–6.

148. Ciccone O, Mathews M, Birbeck GL. Management of acute seizures in children: a review with special consideration of care in resource-limited settings. Afr J Emerg Med 2017;7:S3–9.

149. Caraballo R, Tion C, Fejerman N. Seminar in Epileptology Management of epilepsy in resource-limited settings. Epileptic Disord 2015;17(171):13–8.

150. Asadi-Pooya AA, Jahromi MJ, Izadi S, et al. Treatment of refractory generalized convulsive status epilepticus with enteral topiramate in resource limited settings. Seizure 2015;24(C):114–7.

151. Burman RJ, Ackermann S, Shapson-Coe A, et al. A comparison of parenteral phenobarbital vs. Parenteral phenytoin as second-line management for pediatric convulsive status epilepticus in a resource-limited setting. Front Neurol 2019; 10:1–12.

152. Keikelame MJ, Swartz L. 'A thing full of stories': Traditional healers' explanations of epilepsy and perspectives on collaboration with biomedical health care in Cape Town. Transcult Psychiatry 2015;52(5):659–80.

153. Gams Massi D, Endougou Owona CD, Magnerou AM, et al. Convulsive status epilepticus in an emergency department in Cameroon. Epilepsy Behav Rep 2021;16. https://doi.org/10.1016/j.ebr.2021.100440.

154. Amare A, Zenebe G, Hammack J, et al. Status epilepticus: clinical presentation, cause, outcome, and predictors of death in 119 Ethiopian patients. Epilepsia 2008;49(4):600–7.

155. Tiamkao S, Pranbul S, Sawanyawisuth K, et al. A national database of incidence and treatment outcomes of status epilepticus in Thailand. Int J Neurosci 2014; 124(6):416–20.

156. Phabphal K, Geater A, Liimapichart K, et al. Adult tonic-clonic convulsive status epilepticus over the last 11 years in a resource-poor country: a tertiary referral centre study from southern Thailand. Epileptic Disord 2013;15(3):255–61.

157. Koubeissi M, Alshekhlee A. In-hospital mortality of generalized convulsive status epilepticus: a large us sample. Neurology 2007;69:886–93.

158. Tiamkao S, Pranboon S, Thepsuthammarat K, et al. Incidences and outcomes of status epilepticus: a 9-year longitudinal national study. Epilepsy Behav 2015; 49(2015):135–7.

159. Sadarangani M, Seaton C, Scott JAG, et al. Incidence and outcome of convulsive status epilepticus in Kenyan children: a cohort study. Lancet Neurol 2008; 7(2):145–50.

160. Cascino GD, Hesdorffer D, Logroscino G, et al. Morbidity of nonfebrile status epilepticus in Rochester, Minnesota, 1965-1984. Epilepsia 1998;39(8):829–32.

161. Shatirishvili T, Kipiani T, Lomidze G, et al. Short-term outcomes and major barriers in the management of convulsive status epilepticus in children: a study in Georgia. Epileptic Disord 2015;17(3):292–8.

162. Hassan H, Rajiv KR, Menon R, et al. An audit of the predictors of outcome in status epilepticus from a resource-poor country: a comparison with developed countries. Epileptic Disord 2016;18(2):163–72.

163. Cochran MF, Berkowitz AL. A global health delivery framework approach to epilepsy care in. J Neurol Sci 2015;358:263–5.

164. Skupski R, Toth A, McCurdy MT, et al. Utilizing anesthesiologists, emergency and critical care physicians with telemedicine monitoring to develop intubation and ventilation services in an intensive care unit in the austere medical environment: a case series. Expansion of the EP/CC GAS project. Open J Anesthesiol 2018;08(06):183–97.

165. Patel AA, Wibecan L, Tembo O, et al. Improving paediatric epilepsy management at the first level of care: a pilot education intervention for clinical officers in Zambia. BMJ Open 2019;9(7). https://doi.org/10.1136/bmjopen-2019-029322.

166. Carrizosa J, Braga P, Albuquerque M, et al. Epilepsy for primary health care: a cost-effective Latin American E-learning initiative * A report from the education commission of the international league against epilepsy international league against epilepsy. Epileptic Disord 2018;20(5):386–95.

167. Perinatal asphyxia. World health organization. Available at: https://www.who.int/teams/maternal-newborn-child-adolescent-health-and-ageing/newborn-health/perinatal-asphyxia. Accessed April 10, 2022.

168. Lee ACC, Kozuki N, Blencowe H, et al. Intrapartum-related neonatal encephalopathy incidence and impairment at regional and global levels for 2010 with trends from 1990. Pediatr Res 2013;74(SUPPL. 1):50–72.

169. Lawn JE, Lee ACC, Kinney M, et al. Two million intrapartum-related stillbirths and neonatal deaths: where, why, and what can be done? Int J Gynecol Obstet 2009;107(SUPPL):5–19.

170. Kurinczuk JJ, White-Koning M, Badawi N. Epidemiology of neonatal encephalopathy and hypoxic-ischaemic encephalopathy. Early Hum Dev 2010;86(6):329–38.

171. Pediatrics AA of. Helping babies survive. Accessed April 10, 2022. Available at: https://www.aap.org/en/aap-global/helping-babies-survive/.

172. Number of deaths in children aged <5 yearsw, by cause. World Health Organization. Available at: https://www.who.int/data/gho/data/indicators/indicator-details/GHO/number-of-deaths. Accessed April 10, 2022.

173. Ariff S, Lee ACC. Global burden, epidemiologic trends, and prevention of intrapartum-related deaths in low-resource settings. Clin Perinatol 2016;43(3):593–608.

174. Msemo G, Massawe A, Mmbando D, et al. Newborn mortality and fresh stillbirth rates in Tanzania after helping babies breathe training. Pediatrics 2013;131(2):353–60.

175. Carlo WA, Goudar SS, Jehan I, et al. Newborn-care training and perinatal mortality in developing countries. N Engl J Med 2010;362(7):614–23.

176. Bang AT, Bang RA, Baitule SB, et al. Management of birth asphyxia in home deliveries in rural: the effect of two types of birth attendants and of resuscitating with mouth-to-mouth, tube-mask or bag - Mask. J Perinatol 2005;25(SUPPL. 1). https://doi.org/10.1038/sj.jp.7211275.

177. Oliveira V, Kumutha JR, Narayanan E, et al. Hypothermia for encephalopathy in low-income and middle-income countries: feasibility of whole-body cooling using a low-cost servo-controlled device. BMJ Paediatr Open 2018;2(1):1–9.

178. Prashantha YN, Suman Rao PN, Nesargi S, et al. Therapeutic hypothermia for moderate and severe hypoxic ischaemic encephalopathy in newborns using low-cost devices–ice packs and phase changing material. Paediatr Int Child Health 2019;39(4):234–9.

179. Robvertson N, Nakakeeto M, Hagmann C, et al. Therapeutic hypothermia for birth asphyxia in low-resource settings : a pilot randomised. Lancet 2008;372(9641):801–3.

180. Thayyil S, Pant S, Montaldo P, et al. Hypothermia for moderate or severe neonatal encephalopathy in low-income and middle-income countries (HELIX): a randomised controlled trial in India , Sri Lanka , and Bangladesh. Lancet Glob Heal 2021;9:1273–85.

181. Montaldo P, Pauliah SS, Lally PJ, et al. Cooling in a low-resource environment: lost in translation. Semin Fetal Neonatal Med 2015;20(2):72–9.

182. Bharadwaj SK, Vishnu Bhat B. Therapeutic hypothermia using gel packs for term neonates with hypoxic ischaemic encephalopathy in resource-limited settings: a randomized controlled trial. J Trop Pediatr 2012;58(5):382–8.

183. Catherine RC, Ballambattu VB, Adhisivam B, et al. Effect of therapeutic hypothermia on the outcome in term neonates with hypoxic ischemic encephalopathy-A randomized controlled trial. J Trop Pediatr 2021;67(1). https://doi.org/10.1093/tropej/fmaa073.

184. Wall SN, Lee ACC, Niermeyer S, et al. Neonatal resuscitation in low-resource settings: what, who, and how to overcome challenges to scale up? Int J Gynecol Obstet 2009;107(SUPPL):47–64.

185. Lee AC, Cousens S, Darmstadt GL, et al. Care during labor and birth for the prevention of intrapartum-related neonatal deaths: a systematic review and Delphi estimation of mortality effect. BMC Public Health 2011;11(SUPPL. 3). https://doi.org/10.1186/1471-2458-11-S3-S10.

186. Wallander JL, Bann C, Chomba E, et al. Developmental trajectories of children with birth asphyxia through 36months of age in low/low-middle income countries. Early Hum Dev 2014;90(7):343–8.

187. Ellegala DB, Simpson L, Emanuel Mayegga AMO, et al. Neurosurgical capacity building in the developing world through focused training. J Neurosurg 2014; 121(6):1526–32.

188. Park BE. The African experience: a proposal to address the lack of access to neurosurgery in rural sub-Saharan Africa. World Neurosurg 2010;73(4):276–9.

189. Burton A. Training non-physicians as neurosurgeons in sub-Saharan Africa. Lancet Neurol 2017;16(9):684–5.

190. Dada OE, Karekezi C, Mbangtang CB, et al. State of neurosurgical education in Africa: a narrative review. World Neurosurg 2021;151:172–81.

Building Critical Care Capacity in a Low-Income Country

Arthur Kwizera, MD[a],*, Cornelius Sendagire, MD[a],
Yewande Kamuntu, PharmD[b], Meddy Rutayisire, MD[a],
Jane Nakibuuka, PhD[c], Patience A. Muwanguzi, PhD[d],
Anne Alenyo-Ngabirano, MD[e], Henry Kyobe-Bosa, MD[e,f,g],
Charles Olaro, MD[e]

KEYWORDS

- Intensive care units • Capacity building • Low-income country • Uganda • COVID

KEY POINTS

- Uganda, like many other other low income countries, has very limited critical care capacity.
- The COVID 19 pandemic spurred governtments efforts to improve critical care capacity not just for COVID but also for the post pandemic era.
- This paper describes the process of building a low income country's critical care capacity in the pandemic era.

INTRODUCTION

Among people with COVID-19 about 5% have critical disease with complications such as respiratory failure, acute respiratory distress syndrome (ARDS), severe sepsis and septic shock, thromboembolism, and/or multiorgan failure, including acute kidney injury and cardiac injury.[1,2] All these people required critical care, including admission to intensive care units (ICU), use of equipment to continuously monitor vital signs and

[a] Department of Anaesthesia and Critical Care, Makerere University, College of Health Sciences, Plot 1 Upper Mulago Hill Road, P O Box 2191, Kampala, Uganda; [b] Clinton Health Access Initiative, Plot 8a, Moyo Close, P O Box 2191, Kampala, Uganda; [c] Department of Medicine, Intensive Care Unit, Mulago National Referral Hospital, Plot 1 Upper Mulago Hill Road, P O Box 2191, Kampala, Uganda; [d] Department of Nursing, College of Health Sciences, Makerere University, Plot 1 Upper Mulago Hill Road, P O Box 2191, Kampala, Uganda; [e] Ministry of Health, Plot 6 Lourdel Road, P O Box 2191, Wandegeya, Kampala, Uganda; [f] Uganda Peoples Defense Forces, Chwa II Road, Mbuya , P O Box 2191, Kampala, Uganda; [g] Kellogg College, University of Oxford, 60-62 Banbury Road, Park Town, Oxford OX2 6PN, United Kingdom
* Corresponding author.
E-mail address: arthur.kwizera@mak.ac.ug

Crit Care Clin 38 (2022) 747–759
https://doi.org/10.1016/j.ccc.2022.07.003
0749-0704/22/© 2022 Elsevier Inc. All rights reserved.

support organs, as well as administration of specialized treatments. Similar to the rest of sub-Saharan Africa,[1] Uganda's limited ICU capacity was already well documented,[3] and the COVID-19 pandemic had already required numerous countries to expand their surge capacity to meet the needs of patients with severe and critical illness.[4–6] In anticipation of increased ICU admissions, understanding that medical oxygen was a critical need for the management of cases of COVID-19, the government of Uganda decided to strengthen critical care health care services at regional referral hospitals by establishing numerous ICU around the nation, to avoid overwhelming the new ICU at national referral hospital at Mulago. It was also recognized that the national medical oxygen scale-up implementation plans needed updating.

General Response

In anticipation of the COVID-19 pandemic, the Ugandan Ministry of Health activated the Incident Management System through the National Task Force (NTF) and District Task Forces for coordination of the COVID-19 response and preparedness.[7] The NTF is multisectoral and multidisciplinary in nature, comprising of key ministries, agencies, and departments as well as partners and relevant stakeholders, and works through its subcommittees. The NTF assigned an Incident Management Commander as the overall team lead of the response that had 9 pillars: Surveillance, Case management, Laboratory, Risk Communication, Logistics, SIRI (Strategic Information Research and Innovations), Community Engagement, Vaccination, and Continuity of Essential Health Services.

Critical Care Planning Committee

In April 2020, the national critical care subcommittee was drawn from ICU clinicians, Ministry of Health senior management, biomedical engineers, and development partners under the Continuation of Essential health services pillar.

Conceptual Framework Underpinning This Exercise

We modified the approach used by Arabi and colleagues,[8] which drew on concepts from a capacity building model by Hawe and colleagues.[9] This model has within its framework key strategies we considered important to guide our exercise. These strategies were organizational development, workforce development, resource allocation, leadership,

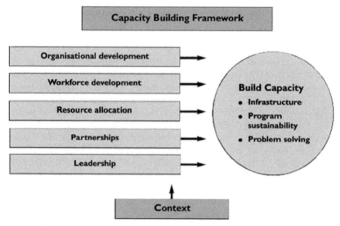

Fig. 1. Conceptual framework underpinning this exercise.

and partnership. We initially focused on building the capacity around 3 domains: infrastructure, human resources, and sustainability (instead of problem solving) (**Fig. 1**).

Therefore, the response was divided into 2 assignments: (1) needs assessment, (2) interventions.

Summary of Uganda's Healthcare System

According to the ministry of health,[10] the number of health facilities (public, private, and private not for profit) in Uganda now totals 6937. The data also show that 45.16% (3133) of health facilities are government owned, 14.44% (1002) are private and not for profit (PNFP), whereas the remaining 40.29% (2795) are private for profit and 0.10% (7) community-owned facilities.

The government and PNFPs are mostly higher levels of health facilities, whereas the private for profit facilities majorly consists of lower levels (Health Center II [HC IIs] and clinics).

Uganda's health facilities are stratified into 7 levels based on the services they provide and the catchment area they are intended to serve. The lowest level health facilities are designated as HC I followed by HC II to HC IV as level 2 to level 4 health facilities with ability to provide more health services: General Hospital (GH), Regional Referral Hospital, and National Referral Hospitals as the topmost level facilities in this structure.

Referrals for patient care follow this level of stratification. In addition, the country now has 5 Specialized Hospitals, which include Mulago National Specialized Hospital, Mulago Specialized Women and Neonatal Hospital, Regional Pediatric Surgical Hospital in Entebbe, Uganda Heart Institute, and Uganda Cancer Institute.

The country also has 4 National Referral Hospitals, namely Mulago National Referral Hospital, Kawempe National Referral Hospital, Kiruddu National Referral Hospital, and Butabika National Referral Hospital. There are 16 Regional Referral Hospitals and 62 GHs in the country.

Intensive care services start at the regional referral hospital level, where the scheme of service for the anesthesiologist begins.

Assessment of Human Resource for Critical Care Provision

The assessment was carried out using telephonic surveys as well as site visits. A structured questionnaire was used to determine the number of acute care providers.

As many African countries, physician-anaesthesia providers play a leading role in management of critical illness[11]; however, this health workforce is still a key bottleneck for the appropriate provision of critical care health services, with key challenges such as inadequate numbers of anesthesiologists, limited skills, retention, motivation, and service delivery.[12] According to the Ministry of Health, only one-quarter of the anesthesia human resource required in Uganda as of 2020 had been met to match the Health Sector Development Plan 2020 (eg, Uganda has less than 30 registered public sector anesthesiologists compared with the 359 required).[13] Likewise in the nursing sector, there were 171 ICU nurses, of whom only13 had formal training in critical care nursing (and yet the country needed about 2400 ICU/ high dependency unit [HDU] nurses).[3] At the national referral hospital ICU, there is a modular critical care training initiative, leading to a World Federation of Critical Care Nurses–accredited competency certificate.

Several reasons leading to the critical shortage of this cadre were highlighted in this assessment: production of critical care professionals does not adequately match health service needs and demands. The number of physician and nonphysician anesthetists graduating each year is meager and cannot fill the ever-widening gaps. There was only one critical care nurses' program at the time, and it graduated a handful of nurses per year.

As a means of temporarily closing the gap (task shifting), the government developed the anesthetic officer training program. However, their training focused on perioperative medicine and not critical care.

Later an improved program, the Bachelor of Science (BSc) in anesthesia, was developed and launched. However, the program is still in its nascent stages and is slowly picking momentum.

We noted low staff retention and motivation mainly stemming from a lack of paths for career development as well as low pay. Inadequate remuneration further undermines efforts at recruitment, retention, and effective service provision.

It was also noted that in the current staffing structure, there is no unifying body or cadre to provide the much-needed visionary leadership, setting, and monitoring of standards, co-ordination with regulatory bodies, health policy formulation and analysis, and creation of a sense of mission in critical care services in Uganda.

Assessment of Infrastructure for Critical Care Services

Data from a recent (2019) study of the country's ICU capacity revealed only 12 functional ICUs, most of which were in the central region. There were 55 ICU beds making up a ratio of 1.3 ICU beds per million population.[3] The ICU beds comprised 1.5% of the total bed capacity of the studied hospitals. Most of the ICUs were mixed (paediatric-adults), anaesthesia-led were 9 and 5 operated in a closed model. An additional assignment to update this information was proposed, to inform planning.

The assignment was split into 2 components. (1) the national survey and (2) the quantification exercise. Because this was a public health emergency response with no patients involved, there was no need for ethical approvals required from regulatory bodies.

The national survey was conducted by teams of biomedical engineers and technicians based at 16 regional referral hospitals. Each health subdistrict is served by the regional referral hospital. Data were gathered by site inspections and through researcher administered questionnaires. The findings confirmed the study findings.

Assessment of Oxygen Capacity

A previous quantification for the national oxygen plan had assumed that at least 124,348 m^3 per month would be needed as of to fulfill the oxygen need of all public facilities from HC IV, GH, regional referral hospitals, and the national referral hospitals. Admittedly, this was made on the back of inadequate data and best estimates.

We assessed 16 referral hospitals around the country. The national referral hospital at Mulago was assessed in 2 sections, that is Upper Mulago National Referral Hospital and Lower Mulago National Referral Hospital because the 2 have had independent oxygen supplies for some years now.

The study team conducted this assessment during physical visits to the hospitals over a period of 3 months/weeks. We obtained information on sources of oxygen, functionality of the oxygen sources, backup sources of power, human resource attending to hospital oxygen needs, and presence of a HDU or ICUs within the facility.

The sources of oxygen identified at the various hospitals included Pressure Swing Adsorption oxygen plants, oxygen concentrators, and oxygen cylinders.

Of the 16 regional referral hospitals assessed, all used oxygen cylinders and oxygen concentrators in different parts of the hospitals, and 17 hospitals had oxygen plants.

All hospitals reported unstable power supply for their oxygen service, with black outs occurring every week. Only one hospital had a back-up power source specifically for their oxygen plant. All hospitals reported having generators for backup power supply for GH activities.

All hospitals had staff assigned to the oxygen plants/supply. However, 2 hospitals had 1 staff to run these activities for the entire week, 3 had 2 staff, and the rest had 3 or more staff. Moroto and Fort portal had the highest number of staff (7) for this purpose.

We determined that the regional referral hospitals' pressure swing adsorption plants could only produce 120,000 L of oxygen in an 8-hour work shift; this is equivalent to 17 cylinders of the J size, which were the most common cylinders available.

Interventions

Human resources

A multidisciplinary team that included ICU-based anaesthesiologists and physicians, biomedical engineers, and human resources administrative staff was set up to develop a human resource for critical care plan. Continuous stakeholder engagements were made, and a strategy evolved. This strategy had short-, medium-, and long-term goals. Short-term goals included short courses in critical care nursing, oxygen therapy, and infection prevention for patient management during the COVID-19 pandemic; this was done by in-service training of existing health workers. The association of Anaesthesiologists of Uganda with support from development partners and in conjunction with the ministry did this by training dedicated ICU staff at the regional referral hospitals; this was supplemented by recruitment of health workers on short-term contracts for the pandemic response. The medium- and long-term goals focus on identifying and increasing the presence of critical care specialists at the regional referral hospitals; this is being done by development of a 4-year collegiate training program (based on the College of Anaesthesiologists of East, Central, and Southern Africa (CANECSA) anaesthesiology and critical care curriculum) that would target and retain medical officers at the regional referral hospitals; this is intended to supplement the current Master of Medicine Specialist programs at the 2 national universities (Makerere and Mbarara) that are inadequate to cater for national needs.[13] In addition, the Ministry of Health through its existing collaboration with National Health Service Health Education England has developed a government-to-government program to develop specialty training in key areas of the health sector including Critical Care. The Strengthening Workforce Capacity through global Learning in Critical Care (SCALE-Critical Care) is expected to develop human resource capacity to deliver intensive care at facility level as well as drive health system improvement. The program will further create opportunities for virtual learning and global placements to UK professionals and trainees to learn from a clinically rich environment in Uganda. The overall goal of the program is to increase critical care capacity through workforce development between Uganda and the UK by developing distant learning in critical care between training institutions in Uganda and the UK; enabling Ugandan Health workers benefit from the Medical Training Initiative Scheme and other training and scholarship pathways in the UK for critical care; and increasing Global Placement of UK professionals to support Critical Care training, practice, and research in Uganda. In addition, a pulmonary critical care fellowship is in the later stages of development.

Regarding critical care nursing, capacity building began with the Ministry of Health's recognition of critical care nursing as a nursing subspecialty, followed by inclusion of dedicated salaried posts in critical care nursing in the health service commission at the regional and national referral hospital levels. Before the COVID-19 pandemic, the only recognized critical care nursing training program was a master's in nursing (Critical Care Nursing) offered at one university in the country. The Ministry of Health further provided 25 scholarships for Masters in Critical Care Nursing and 400 slots for an In-service Certificate in Intensive Care Nursing taught at Mbarara University of Science and Technology. In addition, 2 other universities are now offering postgraduate studies in critical care nursing. There is also continuous engagement at a multisectoral level, to retain and remunerate the various cadres that have successfully completed these courses/programs.

Infrastructure

The quantification exercise was conducted through a series of meetings in which clinical data from the regional referral hospitals were used to determine ICU bed capacity per hospital and in line with human resources as well as budgetary allocations.

Clinical scenarios were created to aid in planning. In all scenarios COVID-19 and non-COVID-19 care was considered. In addition, the costing exercise took into consideration all supplies and consumables expended during treatment of a critically ill patient, regardless of age.

Reference was made to the national oxygen plan National Scale up of Medical Oxygen Implementation Plan (2018–2022)[14] to enable the team to leverage the exercise on existing infrastructure.

As a result, the decision was to construct/renovate and equip 10-bed ICUs at all regional referral hospitals. To provide guidance and recommendations for the planning or renovation of intensive care units, the committee of the health infrastructure division was composed of biomedical engineers, and critical care clinicians used various evidence-based resources with context in consideration.[15–17] The planned units were to be open semipartitioned general ICUs staffed by a mix of both critical care– and noncritical care–trained nurses. The highest form of organ support therapy to be provided was cardiorespiratory in terms of mechanical ventilation and use of vasopressors. Specifications for major ICU equipment (such as mechanical ventilators, high-flow oxygen devices, fluid infusion, medical furniture, patient monitors) were designed according to the National Equipment Guidelines,[18] and in addition, local biomedical limitations were put into consideration. For example, the lack of medical air meant that ventilators had to have their own source of driving gas (turbine or other electronically driven pneumatics). Floor plans for the units considered patient flow/monitoring as well as possible future poor staffing ratios. Later, some ICUs had isolation units ($\pm$ negative pressure), added as extensions (**Fig. 2**). In addition, an update of planned ICUs from other public sectors was created (**Fig. 3**).

Oxygen Quantification

The committee came up with 2 clinical scenarios borne out of the national response plan (**Fig. 4**); this was based on assumptions modeled by the scientific advisory committee that at worst case scenario ~180,000 total cases to be registered up to the period 20th August of 2020 with the proportion of cases needing oxygen at 15% severe (27,000) and 5% critical (9000). We assumed the ratio of adults to pediatric cases would be 9:1 and each of the 16 treatment centers to manage 2250 severe and critical care cases.

Firstly, illness severity was graded according to oxygen demand (determined by the average flow rate) on a scale 1 to 4 as follows: 1 = 3 L/min by nasal prongs; 2 = 8 L/min by simple Hudson or venturi face mask; 3 = 12 to 15 L/min by nonrebreather mask; 4 = 20 to 60 L/min by CPAP/NIV/IMV/HFNC.

Being that at the time there were no functional ICUs at most hospitals, demand was expected from the repurposed 30-bed COVID isolation wards and from ongoing

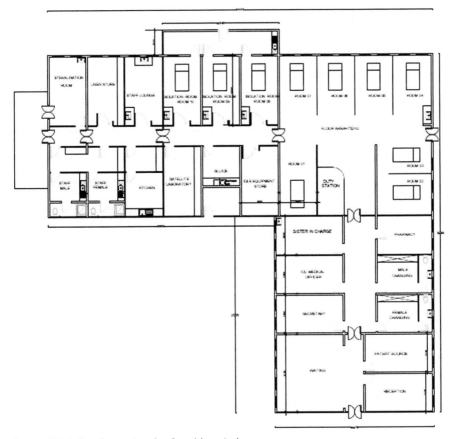

Fig. 2. ICU design for regional referral hospitals.

hospital care (operating theaters, labor wards, emergency department); this created the basis for the first scenario (see **Fig. 4**).

The second scenario took into consideration the new 10-bed ICU infrastructure that was being planned and added this to all aspects of scenario 1 (see **Fig. 4**).

It was therefore predicted that at surge, in scenario 1, the 30 dedicated COVID beds would have 20 level one patients; 8 level two; and 2 level three patients. The 20 non-COVID beds (includes surgical and ward patients) 10 level one patients and 10 level two patients.

In scenario 2, the 30 dedicated COVID beds would have 20 level one patients, 8 level two, and 2 level three patients. The 20 non-COVID beds (includes surgical and ward patients) 10 level one patients and 10 level two patients. In addition, there would be 10 ICU patients, 7 on mechanical ventilation and 3 on high-flow nasal cannula, all at level four status.

Following the aforementioned process, it was calculated that each regional referral would need to generate 374,400 L of oxygen per day for scenario 1 and 728,640 L of oxygen per day for scenario 2 (see **Fig. 4**).

In addition, it was determined that prepositioning a buffer supply of 275 cylinders was needed to ensure sufficient oxygen buffer supply of 5 days for scenario 1. It was also determined that these 275 cylinders would be depleted within 6 days, and

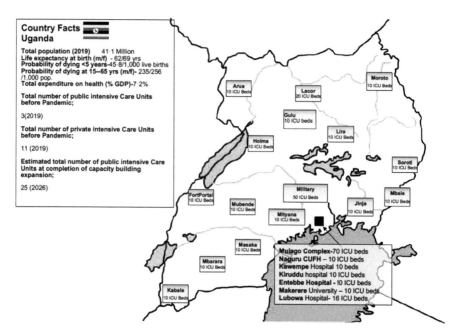

Fig. 3. Distribution of planned and built public intensive care units across the country.

therefore, the number of cylinders required across all 15 regional referral hospitals to be 4125 (**Fig. 5**).

For scenario 2, it was determined that prepositioning a buffer supply of 536 cylinders was needed to ensure sufficient oxygen buffer supply of 5 days for scenario 1. It was also determined that these cylinders would be depleted within 6 days, and therefore, the number of cylinders required across all 15 regional referral hospitals to be 8036 (**Fig. 6**).

scenario	# COVID ICU beds	#COVID beds	# non-COVID patients requiring oxygen	oxygen level 1	# cylinders	oxygen level 2	# cylinders	oxygen level 3	# cylinders	oxygen level 4 (HFNC)	# cylinders	oxygen level 4 (MV)	# cylinders	TOTAL # cylinders	TOTAL oxygen volume (L)
1	30	0	20	30	19.1	18	30.5	2	5.5	0	0.0	0	0.0	55.1	374,400
2	30	10	20	30	19.1	18	30.5	2	5.5	3	25.4	7	26.7	107.2	728,640

Scenario 1
- 50 total beds:
  - **30 dedicated COVID beds** → level 1 = 20; level 2 = 8; level 3 = 2
  - **20 non-COVID beds** (includes surgical and ward patients) → level 1 = 10; level 2 = 10

Scenario 2
- 60 total beds:
  - **30 dedicated COVID beds** → level 1 = 20; level 2 = 8; level 3 = 2
  - **20 non-COVID beds** (includes surgical and ward patients) → level 1 = 10; level 2 = 10
  - **10 ICU beds** → level 4 (HFNC) = 3; level 4 (MV) = 7

Fig. 4. Oxygen demand for 2 different COVID-19 scenarios with and without dedicated ICU beds (6800L).

Scenario 1 (@6800L)										
# days buffer supply (initial)	5									
Day	1	2	3	4	5	6	7	8	9	10
# cylinders (in use)	55.1	55.1	55.1	55.1	55.1	55.1	55.1	55.1	55.1	55.1
#cylinders (starting buffer)	275.3	237.9	200.5	163.1	125.6	88.2	50.8	13.4	-24.0	-61.4
#cylinders (daily production)	17.6	17.6	17.6	17.6	17.6	17.6	17.6	17.6	17.6	17.6
# cylinders (new buffer)	292.9	255.5	218.1	180.7	143.3	105.9	68.5	31.1	-6.4	-43.8
# days buffer supply (actual)	5.3	4.6	4.0	3.3	2.6	1.9	1.2	0.6	-0.1	-0.8

- With a buffer supply of 5 days:
  - ~275 cylinders would need to be prepositioned
  - supply would be depleted within 6 days
- Number of cylinders required across all 15 regional referral hospitals → 4125.0
- Increasing the buffer supply would proportionally increase the time to depletion of stock
- RRH without cases can continue to increase buffer stocks as part of a national supply that can be mobilized for surge hot spots

Fig. 5. Prepositioning a buffer supply of cylinders to ensure sufficient oxygen supply for a finite period (Scenario 1).

Challenges

Introduction or scale-up of a relatively new specialty in a low-resource setting is conflicted by competition with limited resources. Making significant additions to the national drug/consumables' procurement process required frequent engagement with key stakeholders; this was quite difficult to do in the middle of a budget cycle and a pandemic.

Global consensus on appropriate nurse-to-patient ratio in resource-limited ICUs has not yet been achieved.[4,16] Some HIC data were used to inform some of the planning for recruitment and retention, although ultimately the number of nurses who received training was decided by whichever resources were available.

We have experienced underutilization of procured equipment because of the continued of lack of human resources. In addition, the demand for critical capacity still far outstrips the pace of training. For example, technicians were expected to carry out their day jobs (maintaining hospital equipment) while also running the plants. There is no night shift, so the plants were run at half capacity. There were no backup generators, and power cuts shut off the supply.

Scenario 2 (@6800L)										
# days buffer supply (initial)	5									
Day	1	2	3	4	5	6	7	8	9	10
# cylinders (in use)	107.2	107.2	107.2	107.2	107.2	107.2	107.2	107.2	107.2	107.2
#cylinders (starting buffer)	535.8	446.3	356.8	267.2	177.7	88.2	-1.3	-90.8	-180.3	-269.8
#cylinders (daily production)	17.6	17.6	17.6	17.6	17.6	17.6	17.6	17.6	17.6	17.6
# cylinders (new buffer)	553.4	463.9	374.4	284.9	195.4	105.9	16.4	-73.1	-162.6	-252.1
# days buffer supply (actual)	5.2	4.3	3.5	2.7	1.8	1.0	0.2	-0.7	-1.5	-2.4

- With a buffer supply of 5 days:
  - ~536 cylinders would need to be prepositioned
  - supply would be depleted within 5 days
- Number of cylinders required across all 15 regional referral hospitals → 8036.5
- Increasing the buffer supply would proportionally increase the time to depletion of stock
- RRH without cases can continue to increase buffer stocks as part of a national supply that can be mobilized for surge hot spots

Fig. 6. Prepositioning a buffer supply of cylinders to ensure sufficient oxygen supply for a finite period (Scenario 2).

There was frequent burnout among key people in this process. The already few critical care human resources also participated in COVID case management, as well as other sector responses. Many fell ill and had to isolate themselves, with a few needing hospitalization; this had a significant impact on the capacity building process and has been observed globally.[19]

There is a lack of contextual evidence to drive practice guideline development, and this has limited the development process to "best practice" protocols or using guidelines that have taken into consideration diversity of resources. In addition, we also noted that there was poor or no implementation of recommendations from locally conducted done research.

Future Considerations

Building up a national ICU system from scratch is a laborious and expensive undertaking, more so when done in a resource-limited setting. This is an ongoing project, which is likely to undergo significant evolution, as lessons are learned and there is an improvement in resource allocation for critical care. The most important hurdle will be improving the quality and quantity of the human resource.

The care for the critically ill patient in Africa places significant strain on an already constrained health care system, which means that significant focus should go to capacity building in recognition and treatment of life-threatening acute illness. Early interventions reduce organ dysfunction progression and lessen the strain on limited resources[20]; this is what the bulk of our short-term training courses are focused on.

By using the "chain of survival" model enables the concept of "task sharing" to be appropriately adopted, with every cadre having an important role from "bystander" recognition of critical illness to the intensivist in the ICU along a referral continuum. Other acute care professions with relatively similar skillsets can be positioned along this continuum. This brings in the importance of strengthening prehospital care and emergency unit professionals' capacity to fill the gaps in this continuum. One such program that seems to embrace this is the Essential Emergency and Critical Care (EECC).[21] EECC is defined as the care that should be provided to all critically ill patients of all ages in all hospitals in the world. It is distinguished by 3 principles: first, priority to those with the most urgent clinical need, including both early identification and timely care; second, provision of the life-saving treatments that support and stabilize failing vital organ functions; and third, a focus on effective care of low cost and low complexity. We are considering a clinical trial in our setting for this.

One such example is one where a staffing model allows accredited critical care personnel (critical care trained anesthesiologists, emergency, and internal medicine physicians) to oversee nonaccredited staff and for outside specialists to contribute to areas in which they excel, such as nonphysician anesthesiologists and emergency care physicians managing airways; this has been alluded to in a white paper.[16] Uganda has already laid the foundation for this framework. And the next steps would be to harmonize this process.

Embracing point of care medicine in the "chain of survival" would minimize delays, reduce cost of care, and prevent congestion at diagnostic departments. The COVID pandemic highlighted the importance of lung ultrasound in helping improve management while maintaining infection control and prevention, and this is one of many ways in which critical care will never be the same.[5]

Conducting critical care research in low- and middle-income countries (LMICs) is hampered by lack of skills and funding. The lack of context-specific research impairs treatment guideline development. Even when research is done, data collected during clinical studies are based on specific research questions of a time-limited value.

In high-income countries ongoing patient registries provide a continual evaluation of service provision, epidemiology, and quality of care by providing real-time access to data.[22] In Uganda we are establishing a national perioperative and ICU registry, which is hoped to provide a platform for shared learning as well as embed clinical research. It will strengthen our understanding of the burden of surgical and critically ill patients in Uganda and allow us to continually improve the quality of patient care in the country.

Evidence suggests that treatment by trained critical care providers improves survival in critically ill patients.[23] In LMICs, many critically ill patients lack access to this cadre. A telemedicine technology–based approach where experienced critical care–trained providers can monitor and treat patients from a centralized location can help address this issue. This has the potential improving the overall quality of care. Although published studies of ICU telemedicine show mixed results,[24] studies that consider context are associated with improvements in adherence to simple evidence-based daily care processes and survival outcomes.[25,26]

As in some LMICs, Ugandan ICU patients' treatment costs are often not fully covered by the health/insurance systems; this implies that patients and their families incur high out-of-pocket expenses. Indeed, this was the experience at the height of the COVID pandemic. The possible solution to ensuring a minimum critical package lies in the ongoing setup of the national health insurance and ministry of health cost-sharing schemes and regional and national referral hospitals. An intentional and well-thought-out stand-alone critical care financing policy/package would ensure equitable access for most of the people who would otherwise find the costs prohibitive.

SUMMARY

This paper highlights a systematic, multisectoral approach to build ICU (critical care) capacity in a low-income, low-resource setting for COVID and beyond. We share on-going challenges, important lessons learned so far, and perspectives for the future.

CLINICS CARE POINTS

- The critical care or intensive care unit is an important place in the healthcare system for supportive management of patients with acute organ dysfunction.
- Availability of well-resourced critical care facilities is associated with a reduction in all cause morbidity and mortality.
- Low-income countries have severely limited and under resourced critical care capacity. The COVID pandemic left many countries severely exposed.
- Building national critical care capacity in a low-income country is a continuous resource consuming multidisciplinary process.

AUTHOR CONTRIBUTIONS

A. Kwizera conceptualized the article. All authors made substantial contributions to the writing of the manuscript article as well as to the process described in the article.

Funding sources: no funding was used for this effort.

ACKNOWLEDGMENTS

The authors would like to thank the ministry of health and all stakeholder in the government of Uganda for their role in this effort.

DISCLOSURE

The authors have no conflicts of interest to declare with regard to this article.

REFERENCES

1. African C-CCOSI. Patient care and clinical outcomes for patients with COVID-19 infection admitted to African high-care or intensive care units (ACCCOS): a multi-centre, prospective, observational cohort study. Lancet 2021;397(10288): 1885–94. https://doi.org/10.1016/S0140-6736(21)00441-4 [published Online First: 2021/05/24].
2. Estenssoro E, Loudet CI, Rios FG, et al. Clinical characteristics and outcomes of invasively ventilated patients with COVID-19 in Argentina (SATICOVID): a prospective, multicentre cohort study. Lancet Respir Med 2021;9(9):989–98. https://doi.org/10.1016/S2213-2600(21)00229-0 [published Online First: 2021/07/06].
3. Atumanya P, Sendagire C, Wabule A, et al. Assessment of the current capacity of intensive care units in Uganda; A descriptive study. J Crit Care 2020;55:95–9. https://doi.org/10.1016/j.jcrc.2019.10.019 [published Online First: 2019/11/13].
4. Kodama C, Kuniyoshi G, Abubakar A. Lessons learned during COVID-19: building critical care/ICU capacity for resource limited countries with complex emergencies in the World Health Organization Eastern Mediterranean Region. J Glob Health 2021;11:03088. https://doi.org/10.7189/jogh.11.03088 [published Online First: 2021/07/31].
5. Arabi YM, Azoulay E, Al-Dorzi HM, et al. How the COVID-19 pandemic will change the future of critical care. Intensive Care Med 2021;47(3):282–91. https://doi.org/10.1007/s00134-021-06352-y [published Online First: 2021/02/23].
6. Caresia CE. Management of critically ill COVID-19 patients: challenges and affordable solutions. Pan Afr Med J 2021;38:270.
7. Ministry of Health U. Uganda COVID19 Response and preparedness plan. 2020.
8. Arabi YM, Taher S, Berenholtz SM, et al. Building capacity for quality and safety in critical care: a roundtable discussion from the second international patient safety conference in April 9-11, 2013, Riyadh, Saudi Arabia. Ann Thorac Med 2013;8(4): 183–5. https://doi.org/10.4103/1817-1737.118480 [published Online First: 2013/11/20].
9. Hawe P, Lloyd B, King L, et al. Indicators to help with capacity building in health promotion. NSW Health Department; 2000.
10. Ministry of Health U. Uganda's healthcare provider network. 2021.
11. Metogo JAM, Tochie JN, Etoundi PO, et al. Anaesthesiologist-intensivist phycisians at the core of the management of critically ill COVID-19 patients in Africa: persistent challenges, some resolved dilemma and future perspective. Pan Afr Med J 2020;37(Suppl 1):44. https://doi.org/10.11604/pamj.supp.2020.37.44. 25234 [published Online First: 2021/02/09].
12. Lipnick MS, Bulamba F, Ttendo S, et al. The need for a global perspective on task-sharing in anesthesia. Anesth Analg 2017;125(3):1049–52. https://doi.org/10.1213/ANE.0000000000001988 [published Online First: 2017/04/30].

13. F Bulamba RB, Kimbugwe J, Ochieng JP, et al. Development of the anaesthesia workforce and organisation of the speciality in Uganda: a mixed-methods case study. South Afr J Anaesth Analg 2022. https://doi.org/10.36303/SAJAA.2022. 28.3.2646.

14. Ministry of Health U. National Scale up of Medical Oxygen Implementation Plan. 2018-2022. 2018.

15. Papali A, Adhikari NKJ, Diaz JV, et al. Infrastructure and organization of adult intensive care units in resource-limited settings. In: Dondorp AM, Dunser MW, Schultz MJ, editors. Sepsis management in resource-limited settings. Cham: CH); 2019. p. 31–68.

16. Losonczy LI, Papali A, Kivlehan S, et al. White paper on early critical care services in low resource settings. Ann Glob Health 2021;87(1):105. https://doi.org/10.5334/aogh.3377 [published Online First: 2021/11/18].

17. Valentin A, Ferdinande P, Improvement EWGoQ. Recommendations on basic requirements for intensive care units: structural and organizational aspects. Intensive Care Med 2011;37(10):1575–87. https://doi.org/10.1007/s00134-011-2300-7 [published Online First: 2011/09/16].

18. Ministry of Health U. National Medical Equipment Policy. 2009.

19. Mehta S, Machado F, Kwizera A, et al. COVID-19: a heavy toll on health-care workers. Lancet Respir Med 2021;9(3):226–8. https://doi.org/10.1016/S2213-2600(21)00068-0 [published Online First: 2021/02/09].

20. Turner HC, Hao NV, Yacoub S, et al. Achieving affordable critical care in low-income and middle-income countries. BMJ Glob Health 2019;4(3):e001675. https://doi.org/10.1136/bmjgh-2019-001675.

21. Schell CO, Khalid K, Wharton-Smith A, et al. Essential Emergency and Critical Care: a consensus among global clinical experts. BMJ Glob Health 2021;6(9). https://doi.org/10.1136/bmjgh-2021-006585 [published Online First: 2021/09/23].

22. Haniffa R. Linking of global intensive care c. Future perspectives for clinical quality registries in critical care. J Crit Care 2021;63:279. https://doi.org/10.1016/j.jcrc.2020.12.004 [published Online First: 2020/12/15].

23. Diaz JV, Riviello ED, Papali A, et al. Global critical care: moving forward in resource-limited settings. Ann Glob Health 2019;85(1):3.

24. Kahn JM, Rak KJ, Kuza CC, et al. Determinants of intensive care unit telemedicine effectiveness. An ethnographic study. Am J Respir Crit Care Med 2019; 199(8):970–9. https://doi.org/10.1164/rccm.201802-0259OC [published Online First: 2018/10/24].

25. Kovacevic P, Dragic S, Kovacevic T, et al. Impact of weekly case-based tele-education on quality of care in a limited resource medical intensive care unit. Crit Care 2019;23(1):220. https://doi.org/10.1186/s13054-019-2494-6 [published Online First: 2019/06/16].

26. Flurin L, Tekin A, Bogojevic M, et al. International virtual simulation education in critical care during COVID-19 pandemic: preliminary description of the virtual checklist for early recognition and treatment of acute illness and iNjury program. Simul Healthc 2022;17(3):205–7 [published Online First: 2022/04/20].

Critical Care Pandemic Preparation: Considerations and Lessons Learned from COVID-19

Mervyn Mer, MD, MMed, PhD[a,*], Diptesh Aryal, MD[b],
Nathan D. Nielsen, MD, MSc[c,d], Ary Serpa Neto, MD, MSc, PhD[e,f,g,h],
Bhavna Seth, MD, MHS[i], Madiha Raees, MD[j],
Martin W. Dünser, MD[k], Kristina E. Rudd, MD, MPH[l]

KEYWORDS

- COVID-19 • Pandemics • Global health • Critical care

KEY POINTS

- Pandemics are inevitable occurrences.
- Advance planning, clear lines of communication, and consistent messaging are essential.
- Critical care services and staff are an integral and vital component of all pandemic preparation, planning, and health care delivery.

Continued

[a] Department of Medicine, Divisions of Critical Care and Pulmonology, Charlotte Maxeke Johannesburg Academic Hospital and Faculty of Health Sciences, University of the Witwatersrand, 7 York Road, Parktown 2193, Johannesburg, South Africa; [b] Nepal Intensive Care Research Foundation, Basbari Road, Kathmandu 44606, Nepal; [c] Division of Pulmonary, Critical Care, and Sleep Medicine, Department of Medicine, University of New Mexico School of Medicine, Albuquerque, NM 87131, USA; [d] Section of Transfusion Medicine and Therapeutic Pathology, Department of Pathology, University of New Mexico School of Medicine, Albuquerque, NM 87131, USA; [e] Australian and New Zealand Intensive Care Research Centre (ANZIC-RC), School of Public Health and Preventive Medicine, Monash University, Level 3 553 St Kilda Rd, Melbourne, Victoria 3004, Australia; [f] Department of Critical Care, University of Melbourne, Parkville, Victoria 3010, Australia; [g] Department of Intensive Care, Austin Health, 145 Studley Road, Heidelberg, Victoria 3084, Australia; [h] Department of Critical Care Medicine, Hospital Israelita Albert Einstein, Avenue Albert Einstein 627/701, Sao Paulo, Brazil; [i] Division of Pulmonary and Critical Care Medicine, Department of Medicine, Johns Hopkins School of Medicine, 1830 East Monument Street, 5th Floor, Baltimore, MD 21205, USA; [j] Division of Critical Care Medicine, Department of Anesthesia and Critical Care Medicine, Children's Hospital of Philadelphia, 3401 Civic Center Blvd, Wood Building 6107, Philadelphia, PA 19104, USA; [k] Department of Anesthesiology and Intensive Care Medicine, Kepler University Hospital and Johannes Kepler University Linz, Krankenhausstrasse 9, 4020 Linz, Austria; [l] Clinical Research, Investigation, and Systems Modelling of Acute Illness (CRISMA) Center, Department of Critical Care Medicine, University of Pittsburgh, 3520 Fifth Avenue, Suite 100, Pittsburgh, PA 15206, USA
* Corresponding author.
E-mail address: mervyn.mer@wits.ac.za

Crit Care Clin 38 (2022) 761–774
https://doi.org/10.1016/j.ccc.2022.07.002
0749-0704/22/© 2022 Elsevier Inc. All rights reserved.
criticalcare.theclinics.com

Continued

- The 6 "S's" (staff, stuff, space, systems, support, sustainability) are crucial elements that need to be adequately addressed in pandemic management.
- We need to learn from past mistakes to optimize for the future.

INTRODUCTION

Pandemics and large-scale outbreaks of infectious disease present huge challenges to health care systems and in particular to policymakers, public health authorities, clinicians and all health care workers (HCWs). Large numbers of afflicted patients are likely to overwhelm hospital systems, including, importantly, critical care services. The recent COVID-19 pandemic has resulted in an unprecedented number of patients who have required hospital and intensive care unit (ICU) admission, and underscored the relevance and importance of critical care as a discipline. Critical care units are a vital and integral component of pandemic preparedness providing care to seriously ill patients, many of whom may require organ support. Safe and effective critical care has the potential to improve outcomes, motivate individuals to seek timely medical attention, and attenuate the devastating sequelae of a severe pandemic. To achieve this, suitable planning and preparation are essential. Various excellent publications, guidelines, and suggested approaches to ICU pandemic preparedness and organization have been published in recent years.[1–12] This article discusses the key principles and strategies that can be used to better prepare critical care services during a pandemic. Many of the lessons learned pertaining to critical care have emanated from recent experiences with the COVID-19 pandemic.

History

More human beings have died from infectious diseases than as a consequence of any other entity. The emergence and spread of infectious disease with pandemic potential have occurred regularly throughout history.[13] Conditions such as plague, cholera, influenza, severe acute respiratory syndrome coronavirus (SARS-CoV), Middle East respiratory syndrome coronavirus (MERS-CoV), Ebola virus disease, and most recently, coronavirus disease 2019 (COVID-19) have infected vast numbers of individuals and resulted in millions of deaths.[14,15] They have also highlighted the capacity of certain pathogens for rapid transmission and spread, as well as the risks posed to HCWs. The polio scourge of 1952 marked the start of intensive care medicine and the use of mechanical ventilation outside the operating theater, a pivotal step that has saved many lives and revolutionized medicine.[16–18]

Terminology

Various terms and definitions are relevant to clarify and understand to better inform and assist in optimizing decisions by those involved in pandemic planning. These include the terms "outbreak," "epidemic," "pandemic," "critical care," and "intensive care unit."

Outbreaks refer to local increases in disease incidence that may place a significant burden on a health care facility or health care facilities in a particular region. Epidemics are similar to outbreaks but generally involve larger geographic areas and have a greater potential impact on health care services. A pandemic relates to an epidemic that affects multiple areas and regions of the world.[19]

Critical illness is defined as a state of ill health in which vital organ dysfunction is present and whereby a high risk of imminent death exists. It is the most severe form of acute illness due to any underlying disorder and results in millions of deaths globally annually.[20–22] Improving the way health care manages critical illness has the potential to save countless lives.[23–25]

An intensive care unit (ICU) is an organized system for the provision of care to critically ill patients that provides intensive and specialized medical and nursing care, an enhanced capacity for monitoring, and multiple modalities of physiologic organ support to sustain life during a period of life-threatening organ system insufficiency. Although an ICU may be based on a designated and defined area of a hospital, its activities often extend beyond the walls of the physical space to include the emergency department, hospital ward, and follow-up clinic. Various levels of ICU capacity and capability are recognized. These definitions and descriptions can inform health care decision-makers in planning and measuring capacity and provide clinicians and patients with a benchmark to evaluate the level of resources available for clinical care.[24] An understanding of these terms has important implications for optimal pandemic preparation and planning.

Key Elements Involved in Planning and Principles of Intensive Care Unit Processes: the "S's"

Several key elements are discussed which are relevant to ameliorate surge capacity and address important aspects pertinent to pandemics with respect to critical care service planning. The COVID-19 pandemic, in particular, and many of the important lessons learned from it and other pandemics, epidemics, and outbreaks, have helped to inform a better understanding of what is required. These elements are best considered as the "S's"[26,27] (**Fig. 1**).

Staff

In pandemic conditions, all elements of the health care system are placed under additional and often overwhelming stress, and this includes health care personnel. The

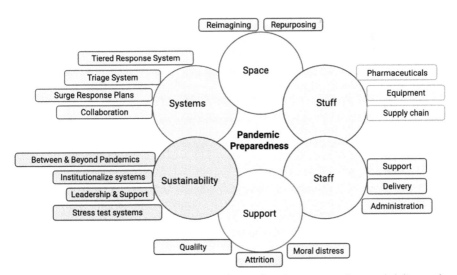

Fig. 1. Key components for critical care pandemic planning, preparation, and delivery: the six S's.

demands generated by a sharp rise in patient numbers and additional challenges posed by the pandemic illness place substantive stress on HCWs who may already be functioning in less than ideal conditions at baseline. Several important considerations must be taken into account when appraising the *staff* element: (I) essential health care staffing incorporates far more than nurses and physicians; (2) different considerations apply to the allocation of different types of health care staff; (3) HCWs are not readily exchangeable and often are not able to move freely across regional or national borders; (4) HCWs are among the individuals at highest risk during pandemic conditions while simultaneously being among the most difficult to replace should they fall ill.

Modern health care is far more complex than just the workings of physicians and nurses—a hospital providing critical care services requires the contributions of allied health professionals and other professionals (such as pharmacists, dieticians, physiotherapists, occupational therapists, respiratory therapists, social workers, chaplaincy staff) and infrastructure staff (including physical plant engineers, environmental engineers, medical device maintenance, housekeepers, food services, laundry services, mortuary services, and security personnel among others). As patient numbers increase rapidly, the additional workload and demands placed on all these roles increase and expanded staffing (and staffing "backup") plans are as essential to hospital functioning as those for physicians or nurses.

When it comes to direct patient care, another set of considerations apply—due to the nature of their work and required "hands on time," ideal nurse-to-patient ratios as may be the norm, may no longer be possible. This may be compounded as patient admission numbers rise by insufficient available skilled nurses—simply put, too many patients, not enough nurses. Similar elements pertain to the number of available physicians and critical care trained specialists. This has the potential to impact on the quality and personalization of care, increase errors, and enhance the risk of staff burnout. Hospital administrators and planners must be cognizant of these hugely relevant facts and plan accordingly. It is important to recognize that while it may be necessary to "do more with less," it is just as relevant to ensure that "less is not done for more."[27,28]

Not all HCWs possess the same skill set—specifically, not all physicians or nurses have the skills, experience, or psychological makeup to function at a satisfactory level in the critical care setting, especially as mortality rates begin to climb. Critical care specialists in medicine, nursing, and allied health professions are trained to deal with emergencies and acutely ill patients and situations, and while other professionals may be redeployed from other locations and pressed into service, they may not function at the same level as those trained formally in critical care. Some may not be able to function in this arena at all. Another challenge is that the health care workforce is not a freely mobile one—matters of licensure, credentialing, and even immigration status can limit the movement of HCWs from a location under less stress to a location that is in need. As pandemic waves strike regions and nations at differing times, initiatives to facilitate the mobility of the health care workforce to areas in crisis are essential to reduce the stress on personnel on the ground. In view of many of these elements, as well as experience gleaned from the COVID-19 pandemic, critical care staff have been referred to as a "scarce resource."[27]

A final consideration in the *staff* element is the acknowledgment of the risks that HCWs face in pandemic conditions. In every pandemic, among the most vulnerable are front-line HCWs and any death among this group may impact adversely on the collective psyche of these professionals, adding an additional set of fears and stressors to a workforce already under duress. Each individual lost to either convalescence or death generates a trickle-down effect on their colleagues—be it additional shifts to be covered or more patients to be seen. Hospitals that cannot adequately protect their staff in pandemic conditions are at progressive risk for collapse due to simple attrition, and administrators must appreciate their staff as the finite, precious resource that they are.

Stuff

This aspect pertains to the supply requirements necessary to deal with a pandemic and relates to relevant consumables, including pharmaceuticals, as well as to appropriate equipment required to support patients. This includes reliable and sufficient oxygen supply, safe blood products for transfusion, or giving sets for intravenous fluids and medications. A major challenge during the COVID-19 pandemic was the increased demand for personal protective equipment (PPE), resulting in critical shortages for HCWs. Among some reasons, the lack of information visibility combined with the inability to precisely track product movement within the supply chain, are the most important. Recent studies provided innovative initiatives to deal with these problems, such as blockchain-based solutions.[29]

Other *stuff* to be accounted for in pandemic preparation is dependent on the nature of the infection that results. A pathogen such as SARS-CoV-2 that predominantly causes respiratory failure led to a demand for mechanical ventilators; other pathogens may generate a similar demand in dialysis machines or blood purification technologies; still others in intravenous fluids, antibiotics, or immune-system modulating therapies. A fully functioning supply chain should be able to rapidly adapt to the unique medical challenges posed by rampant pathogen spread and be able to ensure an equitable and timely distribution of such life support materials.

Case study 1: oxygen supply in Nepal

The number of severely ill patients requiring supplemental oxygen therapy in Nepal was significant during the peak of the pandemic waves. There were insufficient supplies and skilled personnel in the system for delivering health care services. Hundreds of patients were already on oxygen in ICUs; most of them were on mechanical ventilation and receiving oxygen through high-flow oxygen delivery devices. Unfortunately, the hospital oxygen supply was disrupted on several occasions. The country lacked sufficient oxygen plants. The government instituted a quota system in which hospitals were given a set amount of oxygen cylinders each day. Families were even required to carry their own oxygen cylinders to some hospitals. The hospitals were forced to refer patients to other facilities due to overcrowding and a substantial reduction in oxygen supplies. The predicament was not unique to Nepal; several low- and middle-income countries had to deal with it as well.

A tiered approach to health care delivery and the creation of a well-structured referral system would have resulted in more efficient use of available resources, especially oxygen. Patients who needed organ support, such as mechanical ventilators and high-flow oxygen cannulas, could have been pooled together at tertiary hospitals. Meanwhile, the noncritically ill patients may have been managed by the district hospitals. The construction of oxygen plants and oxygen concentrator banks is a critical intervention that needs to be undertaken as preparedness for the pandemic. Capacity planning based on anticipated demand and securing a reliable supply chain mechanism are critical.

Space

Traditionally, the practice of critical care has occurred in a designated and defined space within a hospital. The COVID-19 pandemic has resulted in a global reimagining of the critical care *space*—both within and without the traditional ICU setting. Within the ICU, nontraditional spaces (closets, treatment rooms, offices, hallways) have been transformed into patient "rooms"; room capacities have been expanded beyond previously prescribed limits. Non-ICU wards have been transformed into ICU-like treatment environments following the requisite reengineering; critical care has even become "portable," delivered in non-ICU locales until limited ICU space becomes available.

In the most extreme cases, ICU "spaces" have been created even outside of hospital walls—critical care has been provided in tents, in parking garages, and in open spaces. Redefining and reevaluating critical care services, including whereby it can be delivered, is part of a flexible response that is required in pandemic circumstances. This reflects the important principle that critical care is defined primarily by the teams and underlying principles of the care delivered, rather than the physical space in which it takes place.

Systems

The COVID-19 pandemic has clearly demonstrated that the proper organization of health care *systems* translates directly into improved health care delivery on the front lines. Properly structured organizational responses, particularly those with tiered responses based on the number and trajectory of hospitalizations, improve the efficiency of patient distribution and the maintenance of equitable access to care. Additionally, the presence of strong pandemic response systems can reduce anxiety and confusion among frontline HCWs, who all too often feel in the dark about rapidly changing administrative priorities and decision-making.

Of particular importance in this regard is the need for well-defined, properly structured triage systems for when the demand for care resources, and in particular critical care, outstrips all available supply. During a pandemic, decisions may have to be made as to who receives certain resources and who does not. Resource allocation schema, sometimes also referred to as "crisis standards of care," should be laid out in advance, clearly codified and accessible, be made as transparent as feasible, and based on objective criteria whenever possible.[30] It is also essential that these schema include community perspectives and be equitable, ensuring that consideration is given to ensure that the most vulnerable and systemically marginalized members of a community are not further excluded. Decisions regarding allocations should include objective, detached administrators. The psychological trauma experienced by physicians forced into making such immediate life-or-death decisions cannot be understated, and all steps to ameliorate and assist in these difficult decisions should be taken.

In a similar vein, close collaborations between physicians and nonphysicians are essential in ensuring that a health care *system,* whatever the scale, can operate as efficiently as possible during a pandemic. The skills of non-HCWs such as administrators, logisticians, ethicists, lawyers, and government leaders are as important for framing an adaptive response to a pandemic as are those of clinicians. Lines of communication between these various professionals working to address the challenges of a pandemic must be open and readily available. Transparency in decision-making processes and clear, consistent messaging are essential. Adaptability is absolutely necessary, as is the ability to learn from immediate and past mistakes. Critical care never takes place in a vacuum, and a *System* that can be as flexible and inventive as the practitioners operating within it can save even more lives, albeit under the most challenging of circumstances.

Support

Burnout is a major risk for every person in the health care arena, irrespective of role, during a pandemic.[31–40] The reasons for this complex burnout and moral distress are wide-ranging and its presence and downstream effects need to be acknowledged within any institutional plan for pandemic response. Burnout not only directly increases attrition within the already strained health care work force but it also contributes to poor health care outcomes and clinical errors.[41,42]

The importance of appropriate *support* for all the members of the critical care team cannot be sufficiently emphasized, and these support mechanisms should be made available both during and after the pandemic response. A wide range of activities and resources should be provided, ranging from small on-the-job "morale boosts," to professional psychological counseling. It is important to acknowledge that every individual HCW on the pandemic frontlines will cope with the stresses in a different manner and that a "one size fits all" approach to supporting them will never be effectual. Additionally, putting the onus on frontline workers to "take care of themselves" or build resilience is rarely helpful—persons at the limits of their reserves may see this as yet another demand on their time and energy, another task to accomplish, another potential avenue for failure. Effective institutional *support* strategies for strained HCWs involve tangible steps to make the workday easier, such as limiting paperwork or documentation requirements, resources that are accessible at the workplace or during convenient times, and interventions that actively reach out and attempt to identify struggling individuals rather than empty encouragements of "self-care." For many persons, the psychological trauma of delivering critical care during pandemic conditions will not be a short-term struggle, and institutions should make resources for their staff available for months to years after a pandemic resolves.

Sustainability

All of the above need to be *sustained* during the time of a pandemic, and *sustainability* beyond pandemics offers the possibility of enhancing and improving health care for many citizens. It also ensures delivery of the best possible care for critically ill patients while reducing the risk to HCWs.

Special and Specific Considerations

Interaction with government and policymakers

Consistent, fact-based messaging from political leadership, ideally grounded in data and science, is critical. This helps the general public make informed choices regarding safety measures and preventative behaviors, and can also improve HCW morale. Leaders that involve scientists, physicians, or public health experts in the crafting of messaging, and who are seen as listening to evidence and reason, immediately gain credibility and respect from the health care community. Well-grounded messaging to the public also has the potential to prevent the further spread of the pandemic and thus reduce the pressure on the health care system overall.

Early preparation

"Failing to prepare is preparing to fail." Early preparation cannot be overemphasized. A tragic reality of the COVID-19 pandemic is that despite early warnings of potential danger and spread at the outset, most of the nations of the world were not properly prepared, politically, structurally, or medically, for a scourge as persistent, aggressive, and easily transmitted as SARS-CoV-2. Five actions are recommended by the WHO during a pandemic[43]: (1) planning and coordination (to provide leadership and coordination across different sectors); (2) situation monitoring and assessment (to collect, interpret, and disseminate information on the risk of a pandemic before it occurs and, once underway, to monitor pandemic activity and characteristics); (3) reducing the spread of disease (through "social distance" measures); (4) continuity of health care provision (for patients with other diseases than the pandemic one); and (5) communication (to provide and exchange relevant information with the public, partners, and stakeholders). Preparedness on every level, both prompt and efficient, from national to the individual hospital unit, is pivotal in better preparation for inevitable future pandemics.[44]

Involvement of nonintensive care unit staff

Because there may be a paucity of adequately trained critical care staff in a pandemic, the pool of physicians, nurses, and ancillary health care staff may by necessity need to be expanded. Creative measures such as novel restructuring of critical care teams may need to be initiated, for instance, critical care trained practitioners supervising small teams of noncritical care trained practitioners rather than practicing direct patient care. In such circumstances, standard credentialing, scope-of-practice and medico-legal rules need to be adjusted accordingly, and both the new supervisors and those supervised informed of the new processes and protocols as well as being reassured that their licensure is protected.

Other creative measures to rapidly increase critical care human resource "capacity" may be required, and include condensed training programs or online training programs created by professional societies or other organizations tailored to specific pandemic-induced demands. These initiatives are complex, however, and will involve not only trained critical care clinician-educators, but also professional societies, licensing authorities, and governmental regulatory agencies.

Case study 2: the pandemic of misinformation

In January 2020, the first verified case of COVID19 was reported in Nepal. Over the next few months, the number of cases, as well as the hospitalization rate, continued to grow. While the disease was being researched extensively mostly in high-income countries, the HCWs in resource-limited settings like Nepal tried treatments most of which were not backed up by scientific evidence. Health care professionals struggled to provide the standard of care in the absence of timely protocols. The treatment was driven by clinical judgments based on insufficient information. Most of the time, the results of preprint scientific research were misinterpreted. Nothing, however, seemed to work. The panic that ensued in the initial stages of the pandemic was entirely due to misinformation.

The impact would have been mitigated if efforts had been made to publish evidence on therapeutics in a timely manner. Looking back, we can see that most of the drugs used back then were either ineffective or even hazardous in some situations. Implementing research with the goal of generating newer evidence could have been beneficial. Clinical trials using locally available and affordable drugs during the initial stages of the pandemic could have had a timely and favorable impact on the course of the pandemic.

Therapeutic protocols

Protocols play an important role in assisting with a standard accepted approach to the management of patients. They may serve as very useful resources in all settings, but particularly where noncritical care trained practitioners are involved in critical care practice, and where critical care is provided outside of traditional critical care settings. Protocols may include sets of instructions, flow charts, checklists, and guidance statements. It is essential, however, that these clinical protocols be practical, easy to follow, situation-relevant, and reflect the resources available at the individual facility. They must also be evidence- or best practice-based whenever possible, and be properly vetted by practitioners with the relevant expertise and knowledge of local conditions, resources, and epidemiology. Furthermore, these protocols must above all be *adaptable*—in pandemics, local conditions may change rapidly, resources may shift, and knowledge regarding the pathogen involved may evolve rapidly. Rigid protocols that cannot adapt to changing circumstances or scientific understanding may become more of a hindrance and a source of waste, inefficiency, and suboptimal care than no protocols at all. Thus, in the development and adoption of such protocols, there should be planned periodic updates, as well as mechanisms for rapidly implementing changes, should circumstances demand.

Clinical trials

Clinical research undertaken during a pandemic has the potential to positively impact on the pandemic course. Current and future pandemics cannot be overcome without scientific knowledge, and credible knowledge cannot be generated without properly conducted clinical trials. One major challenge during a pandemic is to design clinical trials that can mitigate concerns related to time to complete traditional clinical trials, and quickly identify effective or harmful interventions. Careful consideration is required to optimize the trial design to achieve this, and several novel trial designs are available and could be considered. These include adaptive sequential designs, response-adaptive randomization, historical and dynamic borrowing, multistage multiarm trials, shared controls, and strategies that aim to "pick the winner" to identify early which treatments are effective.[45]

Health care facilities and institutions, including importantly, critical care units, can contribute significantly to providing valuable information, imparting a better understanding and supplying pertinent details and facts regarding incidence, case presentation, risks, infection and prevention control aspects, resource elements, management aspects, and outcome. This information is key to informing clinical, including critical care, as well as broader public health decision making.[46] Research performed during a pandemic should conform to the same vigorous scientific and ethical standards expected during nonpandemic times. All conducted research should have the goal of promoting knowledge and enhancing health, be scientifically and methodologically sound, and whereby benefits to communities and the individuals supersede any harm. Ethics and study protocols should ideally be expedited by oversight bodies in order for potentially meaningful and relevant research to take place during a pandemic. Appropriate and ethically correct consent procedures must always be adhered to. Similarly, submitted research must be subjected to the same diligent and meticulous review processes that are present in nonpandemic periods.[47,48]

Team work and support

Communication with staff is a vital and essential component of fostering good teamwork—engaging, polite, constructive, and inclusive with all parties and at all times.[41] This approach will often address and overcome many significant challenges including fear, panic, and anxiety. Regular staff debriefings or communication sessions are important to provide positive feedback, encouragement, and support, and to acknowledge the input from each team member. It is also important that team members are reassured that when resources are stretched, it may not be possible to treat patients to the high standards usually demanded under normal conditions and that doing everything possible in these circumstances is suitably appropriate. Psychological support for personnel is imperative and must be available for all medical, nursing and allied teams, as the risk of burnout poses a real possibility and staff wellbeing is crucial for continued efficiency, productivity, and effective functionality of critical care units. Elements pertaining to staff burnout have been alluded to previously.

Family interaction

Pandemics bring with them real challenges in many instances regarding family–patient interactions related to safety concerns. Consequently, direct patient–family interactions are often not feasible. This frequently creates anxiety and loneliness for both the patient and their family. Regardless of the huge demands that may be experienced in an excessively busy ICU, time must be set aside to communicate with families on a regular basis and to keep them suitably updated on their loved one's condition and progress. Telephonic discussion, text messages, and video calls are simple ways of achieving this and go a long way to both creating rapport, as well as to ameliorating family concerns and apprehension. These modalities should be considered as a basic minimum in terms of communication and information sharing. In the sad event of a terminal patient, a dignified video call can often assist families in not feeling that their loved one has died alone, and many have expressed that it has helped enormously in finding closure.

Futility

It is important to appreciate that there is a need to determine futility, particularly in the face of limited resources. Appropriate selection of patients to ICU should be based on unit capacity and patient profile. Triage elements have been previously alluded to, and as a general principle, patients should not be admitted to the ICU or submitted to organ support interventions if they are going to die regardless of the efforts on the part of ICU staff. This is not only a futile and unkind step for the patient and their family but also impacts on wider society, restricting the availability of such services for those who could genuinely benefit. Moreover, the high mortality rates associated with admitted cases whereby further care is futile may also impact negatively on the morale of ICU personnel. Formalized criteria for ICU admission and the use of life-support therapies, at all times, including during pandemics, assist enormously in determining that only patients who are likely to benefit are included.

Impact on patients not affected by the pandemic

It should always be borne in mind that patients not afflicted by the pandemic but who require ICU services should not be forgotten. Where possible, such patients should be afforded ICU care and provisions for this patient cohort should be part of the planning efforts. Failure to do so may have deleterious consequences and result in unnecessary unfavorable patient outcomes. This has been a neglected issue and frequent oversight during pandemics. The impact of not addressing nonpandemic patient needs may be seen for years to come. The cancellation of routine procedures, the fear of going to hospital and health care facilities during a pandemic and possibly contracting disease, loss of patients to follow-up and missing treatments, and delayed presentations are all factors that must be considered during pandemics. The COVID-19 pandemic has highlighted and brought all of these aspects to the fore. Psychological issues as a consequence of lockdowns, social isolation, fear, and loneliness among those not affected are also important additional considerations.

Challenges in resource-limited settings

Health care infrastructures vary widely around the world. Fragile health care systems exist in many low- and middle-income country (LMIC) settings and in several domains, these are severely resource constrained. Critical care facilities in some regions are grossly lacking, and this may be further compounded by challenges in oxygen supplies, water safety, electricity, trained personnel and staffing, medical equipment, protective equipment, support services, and transportation. Notwithstanding these elements, excellent quality care is feasible and possible with adherence to sound practices and basic clinical principles.[27] This approach should always be strived for, even under extremely difficult circumstances, to ensure that patient care and dignity are never compromised. Telemedicine has a potentially very useful role to play and this benefit can in fact extend to all global regions, whether resource-limited or not.

Follow-up clinics
Long-term sequelae in survivors of pandemics are not infrequent occurrence, and appropriate follow-up services and rehabilitation programs should be initiated for these patients to allow for further ongoing management, support, and care to enhance recovery. Where appropriate, vaccine education and rollout are additional very important aspects to address.

CLINICS CARE POINTS

- Pandemics are inevitable occurrences.
- Critical Care services and staff are an integral and vital component of all pandemic preparation, planning and health care delivery.
- The 6 "S's" (staff, stuff, space, systems, support, sustainability) are crucial elements that need to be adequately addressed in pandemic preparation.
- Effective communication with staff and families of patients is essential.
- Burnout is a major risk for every person in the health care arena, irrespective of role during a pandemic.
- Psychological support for personnel is imperative.
- Patients not afflicted by the pandemic but who also require Critical Care services should not be forgotten and should be incorporated into planning efforts.
- Despite many challenges that may prevail in resource-limited settings, delivery of sound care is possible.
- Clinical research conducted during a pandemic has the potential to positively impact on the pandemic course.
- Research performed during a pandemic should conform to the same vigorous scientific and ethical standards expected during nonpandemic times.
- Appropriate follow-up services and rehabilitation programmes should be initiated for pandemic survivors.
- Where appropriate, vaccine education and rollout are important aspects to address.

FUTURE AND SUMMARY

Pandemics place unprecedented strains on health care systems, with resultant increases in morbidity, mortality, and human suffering, including among HCWs.[27] These events are inevitable, but can also be powerful drivers of technological, structural, and care delivery innovations. Critical care is an integral component of all pandemic preparation, planning and health care delivery.[27] The COVID-19 pandemic has emphasized and highlighted the relevance, importance, and need for critical care services and staff, and that appropriate planning for such services is vital. Reflection and introspection at all organizational levels, and based on cumulative experiences, will assist in further optimizing this indispensable service moving forward.

REFERENCES

1. Gomersall CD, Loo S, Joynt GM, et al. Pandemic preparedness. Curr Opin Crit Care 2007;13:742–7.
2. Sprung CL, Zimmerman JL, Joynt GM, et al. Recommendations for intensive care unit and hospital preparations for an influenza epidemic or mass disaster: summary report of the European Society of Intensive Care Medicine's Task Force for intensive care unit triage during an influenza epidemic or mass disaster. Intensive Care Med 2010;36:428–43.
3. Wurmb T, Scholtes K, Kolibay F, et al. Hospital preparedness for mass critical during SARS-CoV-2 pandemic. Crit Care 2020;24:386.
4. Society of Critical Care Medicine. Configuring ICUs in the COVID-19 era. Available at: https://www.sccm.org. Rapid Resource Center.
5. Goh KJ, Wong J, Tien J-CC, et al. Preparing your intensive care unit for the COVID-19 pandemic: practical considerations and strategies. Crit Care 2020;24:215.
6. Griffen KM, Karas MG, Ivascu NS, et al. Hospital preparedness for COVID-19: a practical guide from a critical care perspective. Am J Respir Crit Care Med 2020;(11):1337–44.
7. Maves R, Downar J, Dichter JR, et al. Triage of scarce critical care resources in COVID-19. An implementation guide for regional allocation. An expert panel report of the task force for mass critical care and the American college of chest physicians. CHEST 2020;158(1):212–25.
8. Kain T, Fowler R. Preparing intensive care for the next pandemic influenza. Crit Care 2019;23:337.
9. Aziz S, Arabi YM, Alhazzani W, et al. Managing ICU surge during the COVID-19 crisis: rapid guideline. Intensive Care Med 2020;46:1303–25.
10. Thomas T, Laher AE, Mahomed A, et al. Challenges around COVID-19 at a tertiary-level healthcare facility in South Africa and strategies implemented for improvement. S Afr Med J 2020;110(9):964–7.
11. Barbash IJ, Kahn JM. Fostering hospital resilience – lessons from COVID-19. JAMA 2021;326(8):693–4.
12. Dichter JR, Devereaux AV, Sprung CL, et al. Mass critical care surge response during COVID-19. Implementation of contingency strategies – a prelimininary report of findings from the task force for mass critical care. CHEST 2022;161(2):429–47.
13. Humermovic D. Brief history of pandemics (pandemics throughout history). Pages 7-35. In: Huremovic D, editor. Psychiatry of pandemics. Switzerland AG: Springer Nature; 2019. https://doi.org/10.1007/978-3-030-15346-5.
14. Piret J, Boivin G. Pandemics throughout history. Front Microbiol 2021;11:631736.
15. Christian M, Lapinsky SE, Stewart TE. Critical care pandemic preparedness primer. Intensive Care Med 2007;2007:999–1010.
16. Lassen HC. A preliminary report on the 1952 epidemic of poliomyelitis in Copenhagen with special reference to the treatment of acute respiratory insufficiency. Lancet 1953;1(6749):37–41.
17. Reisner-Senelar L. The birth of intensive care medicine: Bjorn Ibsen's records. Intensive Care Med 2011;37(7):1084–6.
18. Wunsch H. The outbreak that invented intensive care. Nature 2020. https://doi.org/10.1038/d41586-020-01019-Y.
19. Kelly H. The classic definition of a pandemic is not elusive. Bull World Health Organ 2011;89:539–40.

20. Adhikari NK, Fowler RA, Bhagwanjee S, et al. Critical care and the global burden of critical illness in adults. Lancet 2010;376(9749):1339–46.

21. Rudd KE, Johnson SC, Agesa KM, et al. Global, regional and national sepsis incidence and mortality, 1990-2017: analysis for the Global Burden of Disease Study. Lancet 2020;395(10219):200–11.

22. Razzak J, Usmani MF, Bhutta ZA. Global, regional and national burden of emergency medical diseases using specific emergency disease indicators: analysis of the 2015 Global Burden of Disease Study. BMJ Glob Health 2019;4(2):e000733.

23. Weil MH, Tang W. From intensive care to critical care medicine: a historical perspective. Am J Respir Crit Care Med 2011;183(11):1451–3.

24. Marshall JC, Bosco L, Adhikari NK, et al. What is an intensive care unit? a report of the task force of the world federation of societies of intensive and critical care medicine. J Crit Care 2017;37:270–6.

25. Schell CO, Beane A, Kayambankadzanya RK, et al. Global critical care: add essentials to the roadmap. Ann Glob Health 2019;85(10):97.

26. Seda G, Parrish JS. Augmenting critical care capacity in a disaster. Crit Care Clin 2019;35:563–73.

27. Mer M, Nielsen ND. Pandemics and critical care. In: Pandemics and health care: principles, processes and practice. Cape Town, South Africa: Juta and Company (Pty) Ltd; 2021. p. 339–54.

28. Mer M - Personal quotation. From talk delivered at the 3rd World Sepsis Congress held on 21 April 2021 as well as from talk delivered at Critical Care Society of Southern Africa Symposium 8 May 2021.

29. Omar IA, Debe M, Jayaraman R, et al. Blockchain-based supply chain traceability for COVID-19 personal protective equipment. Comput Ind Eng 2022;167:107995.

30. Piscitello G, Kapania EM, Miller WD, et al. Variation in ventilator allocation guidelines by us state during the coronavirus disease 2019 pandemic. a systematic review. JAMA Netw Open 2020;3(6):e2012606.

31. Stocchetti N, Segre G, Zanier ER, et al. Burnout in intensive care unit workers during the second wave of the COVID-19 pandemic: a single center cross-sectional Italian study. Int J Environ Res Public Health 2021;18:6102.

32. Azoulay E, De Waele J, Ferrer R, et al. Symptoms of burnout in intensive care unit specialists facing the COVID-19 outbreak. Ann Intensive Care 2020;10:110.

33. Khasne RW, Dhakulkar BS, Mahajan HC, et al. Burnout among healthcare workers during COVID-19 pandemic in India: results of a questionnaire. Indian J Crit Care Med 2020;28(8):664–71.

34. Kerlin MP, McPeake J, Mikkelson ME. Burnout and joy in the profession of critical care medicine. Crit Care 2020;24:98.

35. Luo M, Guo L, Yu M, et al. The psychological and mental impact of coronavirus disease 2019 (COVID-19) on medical staff and general public – a systematic review and meta-analysis. Psychiatry Res 2020;291:113190.

36. Chidiebere Okechukwu E, Tibaldi L, La Torre G. The impact of COVID-19 pandemic on mental health of Nurses. Clin Ter 2020;171(5):e399–400.

37. Buselli R, Corsi M, Baldanzi S, et al. Professional quality of life and mental health outcomes among health care workers exposed to sars-cov-2 (Covid-19). Int J Environ Res Public Health 2020;17(17):6180.

38. Greenberg N, Weston D, Hall C, et al. Mental health of staff working in intensive care during Covid-19. Occup Med (Lond) 2021;71(2):62–7.

39. Kok N, van Gurp J, Teerenstra S, et al. Coronavirus disease 2019 immediately increases burnout symptoms in ICU professionals: a longitudinal cohort study. Crit Care Med 2021;49(3):419–27.

40. Gardiner E, Baumgart A, Tong A, et al. Perspectives of patients, family members, health professionals and the public on the impact of COVID-19 on mental health. J Ment Health 2022. https://doi.org/10.1080/09638237.2021.2022637.

41. Reader T, Cuthbertson BH, Decruyenaere J. Burnout in the ICU: potential consequences for staff and patient well-being. Intensive Care Med 2008;34(1):4–6.

42. Garrouste-Orgeas M, Flaatten H, Moreno R. Understanding medical errors and adverse events in ICU patients. Intensive Care Med 2016;42:107–9.

43. WHO Global Influenza Programme & World Health Organization. Pandemic influenza preparedness and response: a WHO guidance document. World Health Organization; 2009. Available at. https://apps.who.int/iris/handle/10665/44123.

44. Mer M. Lessons I have learnt from COVID-19. Wits J Clin Med 2020;2(3):217–20.

45. Serpa Neto A, Hodgson C. Will evidence-based medicine survive the COVID-19 pandemic? Ann Am Thorac Soc 2020;17(9):1060–1.

46. Fineberg H. Pandemic preparedness and response – lessons from the H1N1 influenza of 2009. N Engl J Med 2014;370:1335–42.

47. Tong A, Elliot JH, Azevido LC, et al. Core outcome set for trials in people with coronavirus disease 2019. Crit Care Med 2020;48(11):1622–35.

48. Yeoh K-W, Shah K. Research ethics during a pandemic (COVID-19). Int Health 2021;13(4):374–5.

Bleeding, Hemorrhagic Shock, and the Global Blood Supply

Isabella Faria, MD[a,b,1], Neil Thivalapill, MS[c], Jennifer Makin, MD[d],
Juan Carlos Puyana, MD[e,f], Nakul Raykar, MD, MPH[a,g],*

KEYWORDS

• Hemorrhage • Hemorrhagic shock • Blood transfusion • Global health • Critical care

KEY POINTS

• Bleeding is responsible for high mortality and morbidity worldwide, and safe blood is a scarce resource, especially in low- and middle-income countries.

• Timely recognition and addressing the "lethal diamond" – coagulopathy, hypothermia, acidosis, and hypocalcemia – is key to better outcomes in treating hemorrhagic shock.- Traumatic injury, obstetric hemorrhage, and upper gastrointestinal bleed are the leading causes of severe bleeding requiring transfusion.

• While hemorrhagic shock requires urgent blood for transfusion, a 114 million unit shortfall makes transfusion scarce or impossible in much of the world. Blood scarcity is a complex, multifactorial issue in low-resource environments encompassing donor supply, availability, and management; processing and testing of blood; and administration and post-transfusion monitoring.

[a] Program in Global Surgery and Social Change, Harvard Medical School, 641 Hungtington Avenue, Boston, MA 02115, USA; [b] Faculdade de Medicina da Universidade Federal de Minas Gerais, 190 Avenida Professor Alfredo Balena, Belo Horizonte, MG 31130450, Brazil; [c] Institute for Public Health and Medicine, Northwestern University Feinberg School of Medicine, 420 East Superior Street, Chicago IL 60611, USA; [d] Department of Obstetrics, Gynecology and Reproductive Science, The University of Pittsburgh Medical Center Magee – Women's Hospital, 300 Halket Street, Pittsburgh, PA 15213, USA; [e] Critical Care Medicine, and Clinical Translational Science, Pittsburgh, PA 15213, USA; [f] University of Pittsburgh, UPMC Presbyterian, F1263, 200 Lothrop Street, Pittsburgh, PA 15213, USA; [g] Division of Trauma & Emergency Surgery, Center for Surgery and Public Health, Brigham and Women's Hospital, 75 Francis Street, Boston, MA 02215, USA
[1] Present address: 641 Hungtington Avenue, Boston, MA 02115.
* Corresponding author. Division of Trauma & Emergency Surgery, Center for Surgery and Public Health, Brigham and Women's Hospital, 75 Francis Street, Boston, MA 02215.
E-mail address: nraykar@bwh.harvard.edu
Twitter: @nakulraykar (N.R.)

Crit Care Clin 38 (2022) 775–793
https://doi.org/10.1016/j.ccc.2022.06.013
0749-0704/22/© 2022 Elsevier Inc. All rights reserved.
criticalcare.theclinics.com

INTRODUCTION

Hemorrhage is responsible for at least 40% of deaths after trauma and 27% of maternal deaths worldwide.[1,2] Patients with hemorrhagic shock are among the most acutely ill that are treated in medicine; attentive critical care and transfusion of blood products are requisites to avoid death resulting from acidosis, coagulopathy, hypothermia, hypocalcemia, and multisystem organ failure. And although the availability of safe blood for transfusion is central to the management of severe bleeding, safe blood is a scarce resource, especially in low- and middle-income countries (LMICs).[3] In this review, the authors provide a brief overview of bleeding, hemorrhage, and hemorrhagic shock; describe its epidemiology as well as the key diagnostic and management approaches to the major causes of hemorrhagic shock in the global context; and provide an overview of the current barriers to transfusion and emerging solutions in many of the world's poorest areas.

Definitions

Bleeding is the loss of blood components from the cardiovascular system. There are several types of bleeding, ranging from location, rate, and duration. The Oxford dictionary defines hemorrhage as "severe loss of blood from a damaged blood vessel inside a person's body."[4] What precisely separates bleeding from hemorrhage is less defined, but brisk bleeding is known as hemorrhage. And when hemorrhage progresses unchecked, it leads to inadequate oxygen delivery for cellular metabolism and thereby tissue hypoxia; this state is known as hemorrhagic shock. **Table 1** provides detailed definitions for various classifications of bleeding.

Recognizing Hemorrhagic Shock

Although unchecked hemorrhage can quickly progress to hemorrhagic shock and death within a matter of minutes, the initial signs of hemorrhagic shock can be subtle and may not show until the patient has lost an extensive amount of blood. **Table 2** outlines the widely accepted classes of hemorrhagic shock, which are based on the traditional classifications based on volume of blood lost.[5] Newer studies suggest that the rate of blood loss is as important a factor as the total blood loss.[6]

Nonetheless, alterations in mental status or increases in respiratory rate, slight agitation, or increased anxiety might be some of the only signs of early hemorrhagic shock in otherwise young and healthy patients. Pale, ashy, or cyanotic skin and a capillary refill time more than 2 seconds can be direct evidence of inadequate tissue perfusion.[7] A fast central pulse and a weak or absent peripheral pulse suggest hypotension. The Advanced Trauma Life Support manual has famously taught that the presence of a peripheral pulse suggests a systolic blood pressure (SBP) of at least 80 mm Hg, and a central pulse typically correlates with an SBP of 60 mm Hg.[5] There is some debate as to the exact blood pressures required to generate a palpable pulse, but the radial pulse will disappear before a femoral pulse that will disappear before a carotid pulse.[8] Hence, as the carotid pulse is often the easiest location to palpate a central pulse, its presence should not lower concern for severe hemorrhagic shock although its absence does correlate strongly with severe hemorrhagic shock. Finally, hypotension itself may be a late finding in healthy young adults, and the provider should not rule out severe bleeding in the setting of normal blood pressure.

Pathophysiology of Hemorrhagic Shock and the Lethal Triad

A complex combination of processes on the cellular and tissue level leads to the well-known "lethal triad" of coagulopathy, hypothermia, and acidosis in severe

Table 1
Types of bleeding by blood components and duration

	Type of Bleeding
By location of bleeding:	
Internal	Happens when blood leaked from blood vessels is contained within the body, usually in a cavity.
External	Happens when blood leaked from blood vessels exits through an open injury in the skin.
By type of blood:	
Capillary	Very slow blood loss. Most common, the least dangerous, easy to control by applying pressure.
Venous	Flowing, darker red blood (lower O2). Steady but not as strong as arterial flow.
Arterial	Pulsatile, bright red blood (more O2). Usually from lacerations, punctures, amputations. Arterial blood is lost at an increased speed compared with others, so it is usually the most dangerous.
By frequency:	
Acute	Happens when there is abrupt blood loss in a short time span, which results in reduction of circulating blood. Sharp circulating volume loss causes immediate body responses to compensate for new hypoxic state.
Chronic	Happens due to a gradual and continuing blood loss over a longer period of time. Usually, circulating blood volume is maintained. In the early stages, patients present with mild iron deficiency anemia, and the body compensates for the blood loss.
Acute-on-chronic	Acute transformation of a chronic condition managed as acute. Usually occurs in overlap with acute bleeding (eg, hematemesis or chronic GI bleeding). This is usually seen in patients with portal hypertensive lesions.

Table 2
Classification of hemorrhage by severity

Class	
Class I (Mild)	Blood volume loss of up to 15% with heart rate minimally elevated or normal but no change in BP, pulse pressure, and respiratory rate
Class II (Moderate)	Blood volume loss between 15% and 30% with HR (100–120), RR,[20–24] decreased pulse pressure with a normal or minimally changed systolic blood pressure. Skin may be cool to touch, and moist, capillary refill may be delayed.
Class III (Severe)	Blood volume loss between 30% and 40%, significant decreases in blood pressure ± mental status changes. SBP < 90 and drop in BP >20%–30% from presentation are of particular concern. Assume this is due to bleeding until proved otherwise. Heart rate ≥ 120 and "thready" with elevated RR and decreased urine output.
Class IV (Severe)	Blood volume loss >40%, significant decreases in blood pressure ± mental status changes. Hypotensive (SBP < 90), narrowed pulse pressure (≤25 mm Hg), and HR > 120. Skin will be cold and pale, and capillary refill will be delayed.

Data from American College of Surgeons. Committee on Trauma. Advanced Trauma Life Support: Student Course Manual (Tenth Edition). American College of Surgeons; 2018.

hemorrhagic shock and worsens outcomes.[9] Because blood delivers oxygen to tissues, hemorrhage leads to diminished oxygen delivery. The resulting transition to anaerobic metabolism leads to an accumulation of lactic acid, free radicals, and other inflammatory molecules.

Concomitantly, although the coagulation cascade activates at the local site of blood loss to promote fibrin formation, blood clotting, and limiting blood loss, systemic inflammatory markers activate endothelium in other parts of the body into a fibrinolytic state.[10] In states of injury and bleeding, this is a protective physiologic response that allows for a prothrombotic state at the site of injury while protecting against unnecessary clot formation in other regions of the body. In severe hemorrhage, this typically careful balance between local fibrin formation and systemic fibrinolysis is dysregulated, and a profound coagulopathy ensues.

Finally, to complete the triad, blood loss results in massive dissipation of heat. With lower body temperatures comes diminished function of critical enzymes, including those central to the clotting cascade; this further potentiates blood loss and the triad of coagulopathy, acidemia, and even more hypothermia.

There is increasing consensus that the "lethal triad" should be modified into the "lethal diamond" to account for the important role of calcium in this process and prompt providers to take note (**Fig. 1**).[11] Calcium plays a central role in the coagulation cascade, its presence is essential for cardiac contractility and vascular tone, and hypothermia can worsen hypocalcemia by affecting the hepatic processing of citrate. Further, necessary transfusion can exacerbate hypocalcemia, perpetuating the cycle.

On a more macro level, severe hypovolemia from hemorrhage leads to decreased perfusion of critical body tissues, leading to multisystem organ failure. In the most extreme, irreversible circumstance, reduced perfusion of the brain and heart leads to death from brain anoxia and nonperfusing cardiac arrhythmias. In less severe but often equally debilitating circumstances, multisystem organ failure ensues from hypoperfusion of the kidneys, liver, intestine, and extremities.

The Key Role of Critical Care: Rewarming and Appropriate Resuscitation

The role of high-quality critical care in the treatment of hemorrhagic shock is obvious. High-quality warming is central to addressing the lethal diamond. Forced air and convection warming devices are highly effective in maintaining an appropriate patient temperature and ubiquitous in the high-income country setting.[12] Many different techniques exist, some better than others, including the use of warming blankets and warmed fluids, and techniques can be tailored to the local context.[13]

Although appropriate resuscitation is essential to breaking the deadly downward spiral of hemorrhagic shock, inappropriate resuscitation can potentiate it. Remarkably, for decades, crystalloid administration was the first step in the resuscitation of hemorrhage-related hypovolemia. The adverse impact of this approach on severe hemorrhage has only been fully recognized over the past decade: (1) crystalloid temporarily enhances circulating volume at the expense of diluting blood's oxygen-carrying capacity, clotting factors, and platelets, worsening blood loss and coagulopathy; (2) cold, acidic crystalloid solutions further bicarbonate losses and lower body temperature, furthering acidemia- and hypothermia-related enzyme dysfunction; and (3) crystalloid solution is only transiently retained in the intravascular space, worsening interstitial edema in multiple body organs and compartments.[14]

Similar to replacement of lost blood volume with crystalloid, replacement with packed red blood cells (PRBC) alone is also inadequate. A PRBC resuscitation strategy, although improved over crystalloid, also can potentiate coagulopathy instead of breaking the cycle.[15] As over a decade of evidence has now shown, resuscitation with

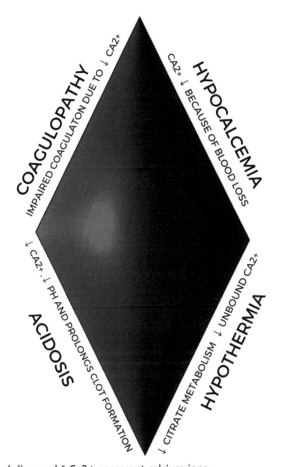

Fig. 1. The "lethal diamond." Ca2+ represent calcium ions.

blood products must be carefully "balanced," replacing all the components of blood that are lost with severe hemorrhage.

Evidence-backed consensus now supports an equal ratio of platelets and plasma relative to blood products administered during resuscitation or a target ratio of 1:1:1.[16] Even though science is evolving, whole blood is likely the preferred transfusion fluid for severe hemorrhagic shock. Although a 1:1:1 ratio of PRBC to plasma and platelets approximates the composition of whole blood, it does not achieve it.[17] Whole blood has a higher concentration of red blood cells, platelets, and clotting factors compared with its 1:1:1 approximation.

HEMORRHAGE IN TRAUMA
Epidemiology

Trauma is one of the 10 leading causes of death and disability in the world and is the lead cause of death for the young.[18,19] Accidental injury constitutes the highest proportion of global injury burden, responsible for more than 5 million deaths per year, almost equal to 9% of global annual mortality.[20] Road traffic injury itself kills 1.3 million and injures 50 million annually.[21] Ninety percent of these deaths occur in LMICs, and the risk of death in a road traffic collision is more than 3 times higher in LMICs than in high-income countries (HICs).[21] Violence and self-inflicted injuries account for 16% of injury-related mortality worldwide but are the leading cause of death among 15- to 44-year-olds.[22]

In the context of this massive global injury burden, its notable that up to 29% of all injury-related deaths are considered preventable, and uncontrolled bleeding accounts for 64% of these preventable deaths.[23] And although most of the hemorrhage-related deaths (56%) occur before arrival to definitive care,[24] hemorrhage accounts for the largest proportion of mortality within the first hour in emergency services care. Half of hospital deaths within the first 24 hours and 80% of operating room deaths after major trauma are due to bleeding.[24]

Initial Evaluation

As famously stated by the "Advanced Trauma Life Support" program, the top 3 causes for hypotension in trauma are "bleeding, bleeding, and bleeding."[5]

Two quick calculations can help serve as decision aids and either raise or lower the clinician's suspicion for bleeding: (1) the Shock Index and (2) the Assessment of Blood Consumption (ABC) Score. The Shock Index is simply a ratio of the patient's heart rate to the SBP.[25] A ratio of less than 0.7 is considered typically normal, but ratios at 0.9 and higher should elicit concern for hemorrhage.

The ABC score was designed to predict the need for a massive blood transfusion and consists of 4 easy-to-calculate components: tachycardia, hypotension, presence of penetrating trauma mechanism, and a bedside ultrasound positive for intrabdominal free fluid. Presence of 2 or more of these is considered a high likelihood of requiring a transfusion.[26]

Diagnosis

The "primary" and "secondary" surveys are focused evaluations incorporating physical examination, vital signs, and bedside imaging to identify emergent physiologic and anatomic threats to life. Identifying bleeding is a core objective.

External bleeding can lead to blood loss in the field before hospital arrival and, although usually easy to identify, can be hidden by hair, clothing, and in areas not immediately obvious to the examiner. As such, manual palpation and visual exploration of every surface—palpating the scalp underneath hair, turning patients on their side to visualize the back—are key elements of the initial evaluation to identify external bleeding.

Hemodynamically significant internal bleeding can occur in almost any closed body cavity and can be less obvious. Identifying where the patient is bleeding is critical, as it will guide management. The chest, abdomen, pelvis, and extremities can harbor significant quantities of blood. Bleeding in the abdomen is approached very differently than bleeding in the extremity, chest, or pelvis. Assessing for chest trauma, "softness" of the abdomen, and extremity compartments and checking the pelvis for stability are important to raise the examiner's suspicion for potential hemorrhage at these sites. The thigh compartment, for example—especially in the obese with lots of soft tissue—can easily harbor more than a liter of blood.

Imaging adjuncts are often necessary to diagnose or rule out internal bleeding. The extended Focused Assessment for Sonography in Trauma is a bedside ultrasound examination that can be performed as part of the trauma evaluation. It works to identify free fluid in the abdominal, chest, and pericardial spaces. Although a negative FAST examination does not rule out bleeding, a positive one is highly predictive. FAST can have lower sensitivity (68%) in patients with blunt abdominal injury, and a reference test such as computed tomography (CT) should be performed next. On the other hand, the FAST specificity is very high (95%) for the presence of internal hemorrhage.[27] The hazard ratio increases by 1.5 for every 10 minutes increase in time to the operating room after a positive FAST examination.[28] Chest and pelvis radiographs can help quickly assess whether there is fluid in the chest or pelvic fracture, respectively, allowing the clinician to either adjust their level of concern for bleeding in these areas. CT scan is often the next line of imaging but does not have a role in management of patients with severe hemorrhage and hemodynamic instability. Surgery should not be delayed if there is an indication of emergent laparotomy, as patients with bleeding can rapidly decompensate while obtaining diagnostic imaging and are typically in a setting (the radiology suite) that makes them less accessible for immediate intervention, if needed. Similarly, the CT imaging should not be performed if it delays transferring the patient to another center for definitive care.[5]

Management

Rapid bleeding should be addressed with rapid urgency. External hemorrhage should be controlled on initial evaluation. High-quality compression should be to areas that can be compressed (the scalp, most parts of the skin). When this is inadequate in the extremities, a tourniquet can effectively control exsanguination from an extremity. Deeper wounds in noncompressible areas such as the anatomic junctions of the neck, upper chest, and groins may benefit from packing to exert intrinsic compression.

When internal bleeding is suspected as the cause of hemorrhagic shock, operative management is typically required. The initial evaluation and diagnostic workup will guide which body cavity is of focus. Anterolateral thoracotomy can provide broad exposure to identify and control bleeding in the chest. Midline laparotomy provides rapid entrance and exposure to the abdominal cavity. When hemorrhage is from the pelvis, a lower midline incision can facilitate entrance to the preperitoneal space, which can be packed as a temporizing measure.

OBSTETRIC HEMORRHAGE
Epidemiology

Obstetric hemorrhage is the leading direct cause of maternal death worldwide, and postpartum hemorrhage accounts for approximately 25% of all cases.[29–31] In 2017, approximately 295,0000 women died from preventable causes related to pregnancy and childbirth. Maternal mortality is defined as the death of a woman during pregnancy and within 42 days following termination of pregnancy regardless of the cause, duration, or site of the pregnancy.[32]

The main categories of obstetric hemorrhage include vaginal bleeding in early pregnancy (less than 20 weeks); antepartum hemorrhage (AH) or vaginal bleeding after 20 weeks; and postpartum hemorrhage (PPH), massive blood loss after delivery, defined as greater than 1000 mL or bleeding associated with signs/symptoms of hypovolemia within 24 hours of birthing regardless of delivery route.[33] **Table 3** presents the main causes and incidence of obstetric hemorrhage.

In the United States, 11.4% of all pregnancy-related mortality was due to obstetric hemorrhage,[34] but 94% of all maternal deaths occur in LMICs.[35] And among all maternal deaths related to obstetric hemorrhage, PPH is responsible for more than three-fourths of them and, with an increasing global incidence of 3% to 10% of all deliveries, was one of the top 5 causes of maternal mortality in both LMICs and HICs.[29] The risk of death from PPH is much higher in LMICs, although, for a multitude of reasons, some of which relate to blood transfusion availability as well as health

Table 3
Classification of obstetric hemorrhage by incidence rates and specific cause

Classification of Obstetric Blood Loss	Incidence of Bleeding	Specific Cause of Hemorrhage
Vaginal bleeding in early pregnancy	20%–40% of all pregnancies[42,87]	Ectopic pregnancy Abnormal implantation: cesarean scar/cervical pregnancy Miscarriage Unsafe abortion Cervical/vaginal/uterine pathology Molar pregnancy/choriocarcinoma
Antepartum hemorrhage	2%–6% of all pregnancies[37–39]	Placenta previa Placental abruption Placenta accreta spectrum Uterine rupture Vasa previa Amniotic fluid embolism
Postpartum hemorrhage	5%–18% of all pregnancies[88–90]	Uterine atony Retained placenta Cervical/vaginal lacerations Coagulopathy/disseminated intravascular coagulopathy Uterine inversion

infrastructure and workforce.[30] Mortality has been noted to be 2- to 3-fold higher in northern Africa, for example, compared with the 16.3% in HICs.[29] Further, mortality is likely inadequate to measure the true impact—17.6% of postpartum hemorrhage episodes result in severe maternal outcomes as measured by death or a "near miss" of resultant organ-system dysfunction.[36]

Initial Evaluation

For AH in early pregnancy, the history and extent of bleeding should be determined. A detailed history will solicit symptoms that indicate significant blood loss, including passage of blood clots or blood soaking through their clothes, lightheadedness, significant cramping, and passing of tissue. A physical examination should include an examination of any tissue and abdominal and pelvic examination. Uterine size (an estimate of gestational age) and the presence of midline or lateralized tenderness should be determined. A speculum examination should determine the amount of bleeding; the appearance of the cervix; presence of cervical dilation; or any signs of laceration/injury, masses, or infection. Laboratory studies should include a complete blood count, a qualitative or preferably quantitative human chorionic gonadotropin level, and blood grouping. A transvaginal and transabdominal ultrasound should assess the uterus, adnexa, the presence of masses, fetus and fetal heart rate, and free fluid. For second and third trimesters AH, evaluation consists of assessing the extent of bleeding, presence of pain, hemodynamic stability, assessment of fetal viability, and well-being (fetal nonstress test, ultrasound, biophysical profile). An abdominal examination should assess for uterine size and tenderness. A speculum examination should assess the cervical os for the presence of amniotic fluid, bleeding, or fetal membranes/parts/placental tissue. Ultrasound should confirm the location of the placenta, amniotic fluid, fetal gestational age, and estimated fetal weight.[37–39]

In PPH, all blood loss should be quantified. The patient should be monitored for hemodynamic stability and oxygenation. On examination, look for significant vaginal or cervical lacerations, even in patients who underwent cesarean delivery, as cervical dilation and descent can cause lacerations. Repeat examination even if performed at birth time. Assess the uterus for tone, retained placenta, abnormal placentation (placenta accreta spectrum), and uterine inversion. If the patient presents with anal pain out of proportion, a rectal examination should be performed to look for vaginal hematoma. A FAST examination can be performed to evaluate the abdomen, and uterine tone should also be assessed during this examination.[33,40]

Delayed response to change in vitals after delivery is a common factor of preventable maternal death.[41] Assume progressively increasing heart rate and decreasing blood pressure are due to blood loss/hypovolemia until these causes are positively excluded. Some patients may only present mild signs of shock such as mild tachycardia and mild hypotension. If the patient is potentially unstable, moving them to an operating room is the safest option in case further action is needed. Deterioration of maternal vital signs out of proportion to vaginal bleeding suggests intraperitoneal or retroperitoneal bleeding (eg, ruptured uterus, hepatic rupture due to preeclampsia, expanding vaginal hematoma).

Diagnosis

Vaginal bleeding in early pregnancy could represent a threatened abortion, incomplete abortion, or complete abortion. All patients with early pregnancy bleeding and pain should be assumed to have an ectopic pregnancy until proved otherwise. A pregnancy should be seen within the uterus by transvaginal ultrasound once the human chorionic gonadotropin (HCG) level is greater than 2000 to 3500 IU. A decreasing beta-HCG is consistent with failed pregnancy.[42–44]

For second and third trimester bleeding, patients should be assessed for placental location and placental abruption. Placenta previa generally is painless, and a placental abruption typically presents with vaginal bleeding, uterine tenderness, and uterine contractions with or without abnormalities on fetal heart rate. Ultrasound has low sensitivity for placental separation. Ultrasound evaluation of uterine rupture would show free fluid in the abdomen with possible extravasation of the fetus. Management depends on gestational age, cause and severity of bleeding, and maternal and fetal status.[45,46]

In PPH, timelines in its recognition, determination of cause, and initiating treatment are critical. Although challenging in the obstetric setting, careful quantification of blood loss is recommended.[47] In most cases, a vaginal and bimanual examination can determine the cause of postpartum hemorrhage. Patients should be assessed for coagulopathy with thromboelastography when available or use a simple red top tube to assess for clotting ability. FAST can be used to assess shock signs with no vaginal bleeding associated. However, because sensitivity is low, a negative result should not rule out internal bleeding.[48,49]

Management

Ruling out life-threatening vaginal bleeding is the first step in working up first-trimester acute hemorrhage. Miscarriages can be managed expectantly, medically, or surgically with manual vacuum aspiration or suction dilation and curettage.[50] Surgical evacuation is indicated in patients who are actively bleeding and unstable. A ruptured ectopic pregnancy with evidence of intraabdominal bleeding mandates surgical management and gynecologic consultation when available. Laparoscopy or laparotomy must not be delayed in unstable patients with suspected ectopic pregnancy. In all cases of hemorrhage, management involves supportive care with intravenous fluids, checking blood levels, and transfusing as indicated.[42–44]

For second and third trimester bleeding, rapid obstetric consultation should be obtained in case cesarean delivery is needed. In hemodynamically unstable patients and in patients with cardiac arrest displacing the uterus to the patient's left side significantly improves cardiac output. Substantial changes in vital signs may not occur until more than 20% of total blood volume has been lost due to the hypervolemia and normal physiology of pregnancy. Fetal heart rate monitoring, when appropriate based on viability (>20 weeks gestation), is essential for determining the condition of the fetus. RhD-negative women with abdominal or pelvic trauma or with vaginal bleeding should receive anti-D immune globulin, per standard protocols.

Treatment goals for PPH are to restore circulatory volume, maintain tissue oxygenation, reverse or prevent coagulopathy, and eliminate the obstetric cause. Uterine atony is the most common cause of PPH. In this case the patient should have her bladder emptied and fundal and bimanual uterine massage should be attempted (misoprostol, oxytocin/carbetocin, methergine, hemabate, tranexamic acid). If the atony is persistent, uterine tamponade methods should be attempted such as an intrauterine balloon (condom balloon or Bakri), gauze packing, or suction compression (Jada). Some patients may require an operation where uterine-sparing surgery can be attempted with ligation of the hypogastric, the B-Lynch suture, O'Leary suture, or placement of a uterine artery embolization by interventional radiology. Ultimately, a peripartum hysterectomy may be necessary to control blood loss.[33,51–53]

Retained products of conception are more common after a vaginal birth but can happen after any delivery. If the first 2 fail, the procedure is performed manually, with forceps, curettage, or a suction catheter. An unstable patient should be examined for uterine rupture, a rare complication that can happen even with vaginal births when there is instrumental delivery or induced labor. Persistent pain and vaginal bleeding after drugs should serve as an alert for this complication, and the management is usually hysterectomy. Blood might accumulate in the retroperitoneum or inside the uterine cavity and not be seen after the wound is closed. If the patient presents with laceration, a repair should be made.[51] A uterine inversion should be identified before placental separation and manually replaced. In rare cases muscle relaxing agents or surgical intervention is necessary.[54]

Blood loss should always be measured. It can be done by weighing pads soaked with blood subtracting the weight of a dry pad.[50] In case of blood loss exceeding 1.5 L, the physician should ask for complete blood count, type and crossmatch, coagulation studies, thromboelastographic examinations, and proceed with blood transfusion. Consider autologous transfusion early, either in vaginal or cesarean delivery. Blood can be collected after delivery of the placenta, and an effort should be made to avoid contamination with fecal material or amniotic fluid.[55] For PPH, an aggressive transfusion approach can be used, and there is no current specific guideline. An approach used by the Stanford University Medical Center is the use of an initial package consisting of 6 units RBCs, 4 units fresh frozen plasma, and 1 apheresis platelet unit and a hemoglobin target of greater than 7 g/dL.[56]

In general, management of all of these conditions is the same across low and high-resource settings. Challenges within low-resource settings include delays in access to care, with patients presenting in late stages of hemorrhagic shock.[57] There are often challenges in access to medications, anesthetists, specialist health care providers such as obstetricians and gynecologists, blood for transfusion, and diagnostic tests including blood work and imaging.[58,59] Important adaptations in a low-resource setting might include transferring to higher level of care, use of ketamine for anesthesia, reliance on affordable temperature stable medications such as misoprostol and tranexamic acid, task shifting to allow nurses and mid-levels perform manual vacuum aspiration, uterine tamponade with a condom balloon, and autologous blood transfusions using devices such as the hemafuse.[60–62]

UPPER GASTROINTESTINAL BLEEDING
Epidemiology

Upper gastrointestinal bleeding (UGIB) is a common source of hemorrhage that occurs in the proximal gastrointestinal tract. Hospitalization rates for UGIB are 6 times higher than lower GI bleeding and result in substantial morbidity, mortality, and medical expense.[63–65] The mortality varies from 5% in the United States to 30% in Sub-Saharan Africa,[66] with the higher rates attributed to delay in diagnosis, treatment, and inadequate infrastructure, including access to blood.[67]

Multiple conditions can lead to a UGIB, and these vary in prevalence across the world. For example, the 2 major causes of severe bleeding from UGIB are peptic ulcer disease and esophagogastric varices. Peptic ulcers are typically the most common cause of hemorrhage in the upper GI tract, and gastric ulcers are the most common. The proportion of UGIB due to peptic ulcers ranges as high as 30% to 65% in some studies from Egypt, Brazil, and India. Varices occur due to portal hypertension, which is another major cause of UGIB. In many African studies, esophageal varices were found to be the main cause of UGIB.[67,68] Some of these variations may be related to the prevalence of infections such as hepatitis B, hepatitis C, and schistosomiasis that are endemic in many parts of the world, particularly LMICs, and can result in cirrhosis.[67] Most patients with cirrhosis develop varices, with an annual hemorrhage rate of 5% to 15%[69] and a mortality rate around 20% with active bleeding.[67,69] **Table 4** outlines common causes of UGIB and prevalence from studies across the world.

Initial Evaluation

Most commonly, patients with UGIB present with hematemesis, which is vomiting of blood and/or melena, which are black, tarry stools, the result of blood that has traveled through the GI tract. It is worth noting that part of the patients might present with hematochezia, or bloody bowel movements, even though this sign is more common in LGIB. Patients with variceal cause usually present more to care with active bleeding compared with nonvariceal causes, such as ulcerations and erosive lesions.[70]

The goal of the initial evaluation is to assess the severity of the bleed, identify potential sources of the bleed, and determine other conditions present that may affect management. Rectal examination can help assess stool color (melena vs hematochezia vs brown). A nasogastric tube may provide evidence of upper GI bleeding when the presenting sign is melena or hematochezia. History is a key component—up to 60% of patients with a history of a previous UGIB are bleeding from the same lesion.[71]

Diagnosis

Endoscopy is often diagnostic and therapeutic. Although endoscopy should be performed as soon as possible, preferably within 24 hours of UGIB, its performance at any point can decrease patient mortality.[67] Nonetheless, there is scant availability of endoscopy in many of the world's rural settings.[72] As such, many GI bleeds remain unexplained after clinical and/or endoscopic evaluation (where available) and are often called "undetermined" or "obscure GI bleeding." Advances in diagnostic imaging have steadily decreased the prevalence of obscure GI bleeding but most settings across the world lack access to these diagnostics.[73,74] A CT angiogram has high sensitivity and specificity for bleed location and can further guide therapeutic options when available.

Management

As in all cases of hemorrhagic shock, the key management principles are to stop the bleeding and replace lost blood volume. In the process of doing this, special attention should be given to airway status, monitoring of vital signs and cardiac rhythm, urine output, and nasogastric output. All patients with suspected or known severe bleeding should be started on high-dose proton pump inhibitors.[75] For patients with known or suspected esophagogastric variceal bleeding, the goal of therapy is to control acute hemorrhage and to prevent its recurrence.[76] These patients should receive somatostatin or analogues such as octreotide to decrease portal pressure and prophylactic antibiotics covering gram negatives.[69]

Judicious blood transfusion is important with a hemoglobin target of 7 to 9 g/d. A transfusion target of 9 to 11 g/dL in patients with cirrhosis is associated with increased mortality, possibly due to an increased hepatic venous pressure gradient, which can lead to increased variceal bleeding.[77]

Stopping the bleeding requires first making a diagnosis and localizing the bleed. Gastroenterologists and interventional radiologists, where available, play a critical role, as therapies are more directed and less morbid than surgical exploration. Emergency surgery for UGIB may be indicated in low-resource settings when there is limited capacity for nonsurgical treatment.[72] Endoscopy offers many advantages including diagnosis and therapy with thermal coagulation, hemostatic clips, and injection therapy.[75] For variceal hemorrhage, esophageal balloon tamponade can be used as a temporizing measure before definitive therapy.[69] Esophageal banding and scleral therapy are the first line of treatment.[67,78] Although transjugular intrahepatic portosystemic shunting (TIPS) is often the fallback for severe variceal bleeding, its availability across the world is limited. Surgical shunts, although effective at stopping bleeding, have high mortality rates and have largely been supplanted by TIPS, where available.

Table 4	
Most common causes of upper gastrointestinal bleeding worldwide	
Most Common Causes	**Prevalence (%)**
Gastric and/or duodenal ulcers	6–65
Esophagogastric varices	12.8–56.3
Severe or erosive gastritis/duodenitis	2.5–12.9
Severe or erosive esophagitis	0.3–14.7
Mass lesions	1.7–8
Angiodysplasia	0.5–4.7
Mallory-Weiss syndrome	1–5
Unknown source	1–38

Unknown source is * defined by normal findings at the time of endoscopy after episode of bleeding and unknown causes for active bleeding.
Data from Refs.[67,68,70,74,91–93]

GLOBAL BLOOD SUPPLY

Approximately 3% of severely injured trauma patients will need a massive blood transfusion, and up to 16.5% of patients with postpartum hemorrhage will require a high-volume transfusion and surgical intervention.[79] Although patients in hemorrhagic shock urgently need blood for transfusion, there is a shortfall that makes transfusion scarce or impossible in much of the world. In fact, there is a 114 million unit shortage of blood worldwide annually, and most of the deficit is located in Sub-Saharan Africa, South Asia, and Oceania.[80] With scarcity, blood typically goes to treating more chronic conditions, including oncologic needs and pediatric anemias; lesser amounts are available for emergency obstetric hemorrhage and trauma patients.[81]

The reasons for scarcity are multifactorial. A consistent supply of blood requires complex logistics spanning a continuum from community engagement and donor recruitment to blood collection, blood testing, blood processing, administration, and hemovigilance. With underfunded health systems comes underfunded blood systems and significant challenges with maintenance of each part of this continuum.[82] Further, some challenges specific to low-resource environments would present barriers even with the best resources—high levels of malnutrition drive high levels of chronic anemia, and endemic levels of hepatitis B, C, and human immunodeficiency virus render a significant portion of the population unsuitable for blood donation.

A significant portion of the blood supply in Sub-Saharan Africa and South Asia remains with whole blood as the primary product for transfusion; this presents logistical challenges in cases of providing appropriate resuscitation, as the provision of a 1:1:1 ratio of packed red blood cells to plasma to platelet transfusion requires an organized, well-functioning blood bank with adequate stores of each component and the workforce to thaw, prepare, and deliver adequate quantities of each component for transfusion, on-demand.[17]

Although further investment in health and blood systems is urgently necessary—allowing for optimizations along the entire continuum of transfusion—policy-level changes may also be required that decentralize blood systems and allow for greater stewardship at the community level. Attention must be paid to "disruptive" solutions that can provide more immediate relief in cases of extreme scarcity. Promising strategies include the concept of community walking blood banks, where blood is collected on-demand, tested with rapid diagnostic testing kits, and transfused to those in need; this would be a civilian adaptation of an innovation refined over the past 2 decades by American and Scandinavian militaries.[15,83] Drone-based blood delivery, where blood collection centers are paired with unmanned aerial vehicles for delivery to distant hospitals without blood stores are another recent strategy showing promise in low-resource, blood-deficient areas.[84] Finally, intraoperative autotransfusion—where a patient's blood is collected, filtered, and transfused back to the same patient—is not a new concept in the high-income or low-income setting but is now receiving renewed attention from the low-cost innovation sector.[85] The Hemafuse device by Sisu Global Health is a system designed for the low-resource environment and has shown promise in treating obstetric hemorrhage from ectopic pregnancy and splenic rupture.[86]

SUMMARY

Critical care has and continues to play a key role in the immediate identification of both insidious and overt blood loss, most commonly in the settings of trauma, obstetric hemorrhage, and upper gastrointestinal bleeding. The burden and epidemiology of hemorrhage vary by context, and management depends on the availability of blood products, trained personnel, and the broader health care infrastructure. Hemorrhage remains the cause of almost half of the deaths by trauma, and there is a massive shortage of blood products in many parts of the world, especially in lower-income countries. It is imperative that action is taken soon to decrease the burden of bleeding worldwide and that new alternatives for blood transfusion become readily available to the centers in need.

CLINICS CARE POINTS

- The signs and symptoms of hemorrhagic shock are often subtle, and early diagnosis is critical to prevent the rapid consequences of unrecognized or unchecked bleeding.

- In the setting of trauma, in addition to the key management principles of stopping the bleeding and replacing lost blood volume, identifying hemodynamically significant internal bleeding in all potential spaces will be crucial to guiding further management.

- Postpartum hemorrhage is the leading cause of maternal death worldwide, and its treatment should aim to restore circulatory volume, maintain tissue oxygenation, reverse or prevent coagulopathy, and eliminate the cause of obstetric bleeding.

- Although endoscopy within 24 hours is the standard of care for diagnosis and treatment of upper gastrointestinal bleeding, where endoscopy is not readily available, stratified treatment algorithms established by local governing bodies will guide management to reduce mortality.

- Blood scarcity influences blood administration variably depending on context, but can lead to a redirection of limited available blood products to patients with less urgent conditions, resulting in a large unmet need for blood products for patients experiencing traumatic or obstetric hemorrhage.

DISCLOSURE

The authors have nothing to disclose.

REFERENCES

1. GBD 2015 Maternal Mortality Collaborators. Global, regional, and national levels of maternal mortality, 1990-2015: a systematic analysis for the Global Burden of Disease Study 2015. Lancet 2016;388(10053):1775–812.
2. Curry N, Hopewell S, Dorée C, et al. The acute management of trauma hemorrhage: a systematic review of randomized controlled trials. Crit Care 2011; 15(2):R92.
3. Organization WH. Others the 2016 global status report on blood safety and availability. Available at: https://apps.who.int/iris/bitstream/handle/10665/254987/9789241565431-eng.pdf.
4. Haemorrhage. Available at: https://www.oxfordlearnersdictionaries.com/definition/english/haemorrhage_1. Accessed March 18, 2022.
5.. American College of Surgeons. Committee on trauma. advanced trauma life support: student course manual. 10th Edition. Chicago IL: American College of Surgeons; 2018.
6. Frankel DAZ, Acosta JA, Anjaria DJ, et al. Physiologic response to hemorrhagic shock depends on rate and means of hemorrhage. J Surg Res 2007;143(2):276–80.

7. McGuire D, Gotlib A, King J. Capillary Refill Time. [Updated 2022 Apr 21]. In: StatPearls [Internet]. Treasure Island (FL): StatPearls Publishing; 2022 Jan-. Available from: https://www.ncbi.nlm.nih.gov/books/NBK557753/.

8. Deakin CD, Low JL. Accuracy of the advanced trauma life support guidelines for predicting systolic blood pressure using carotid, femoral, and radial pulses: observational study. BMJ 2000;321(7262):673–4.

9. MacLeod JBA, Winkler AM, McCoy CC, et al. Early trauma induced coagulopathy (ETIC): prevalence across the injury spectrum. Injury 2014;45(5):910–5.

10. Cannon JW. Hemorrhagic shock. N Engl J Med 2018;378(19):1852–3.

11. Wray JP, Bridwell RE, Schauer SG, et al. The diamond of death: hypocalcemia in trauma and resuscitation. Am J Emerg Med 2021;41:104–9. https://doi.org/10.1016/j.ajem.2020.12.065.

12. John M, Ford J, Harper M. Peri-operative warming devices: performance and clinical application. Anaesthesia 2014;69(6):623–38.

13. Hardcastle TC, Stander M, Kalafatis N, et al. External patient temperature control in emergency centres, trauma centres, intensive care units and operating theatres: a multi-society literature review. S Afr Med J 2013;103(9):609–11.

14. Cantle PM, Cotton BA. Balanced resuscitation in trauma management. Surg Clin North Am 2017;97(5):999–1014.

15. Holcomb JB, del Junco DJ, Fox EE, et al. The prospective, observational, multi-center, major trauma transfusion (PROMMTT) study: comparative effectiveness of a time-varying treatment with competing risks. JAMA Surg 2013;148(2):127–36.

16. Holcomb JB, Tilley BC, Baraniuk S, et al. Transfusion of plasma, platelets, and red blood cells in a 1:1:1 vs a 1:1:2 ratio and mortality in patients with severe trauma. JAMA 2015;313(5):471. https://doi.org/10.1001/jama.2015.12.

17. Cap AP, Beckett A, Benov A, et al. Whole blood transfusion. Mil Med 2018; 183(suppl_2):44–51. https://doi.org/10.1093/milmed/usy120.

18. GBD 2016 Causes of Death Collaborators. Global, regional, and national age-sex specific mortality for 264 causes of death, 1980-2016: a systematic analysis for the Global Burden of Disease Study 2016. Lancet 2017;390(10100):1151–210.

19. for Disease Control C, Prevention, Others. Centers for Disease Control and Prevention Web-based injury statistics query and reporting system (WISQARS). National Center for Injury Prevention and Control Retrieved from https://www cdc gov/injury/wisqars/index html. Published online 2017.

20. Organization WH. Others. Injuries and violence: the facts 2014. Available at: https://apps.who.int/iris/bitstream/handle/10665/149798/9789241508018_eng.pdf.

21. Clinical Services, Systems. Guidelines for essential trauma care. 2012. Available at: https://www.who.int/publications/i/item/guidelines-for-essential-trauma-care. Accessed February 23, 2022.

22. Butchart A, Mikton C, Dahlberg LL, et al. Global status report on violence prevention 2014. Inj Prev 2015;21(3):213.

23. Davis JS, Satahoo SS, Butler FK, et al. An analysis of prehospital deaths: who can we save? J Trauma Acute Care Surg 2014;77(2):213–8.

24. Kauvar DS, Lefering R, Wade CE. Impact of hemorrhage on trauma outcome: an overview of epidemiology, clinical presentations, and therapeutic considerations. J Trauma 2006;60(6 Suppl):S3–11.

25. Cannon CM, Braxton CC, Kling-Smith M, et al. Utility of the shock index in predicting mortality in traumatically injured patients. J Trauma 2009;67(6):1426–30.

26. Nunez TC, Voskresensky IV, Dossett LA, et al. Early prediction of massive transfusion in trauma: simple as ABC (assessment of blood consumption)? J Trauma 2009;66(2):346–52.

27. Stengel D, Leisterer J, Ferrada P, et al. Point-of-care ultrasonography for diagnosing thoracoabdominal injuries in patients with blunt trauma. Cochrane Database Syst Rev 2018;12:CD012669.
28. Barbosa RR, Rowell SE, Fox EE, et al. Increasing time to operation is associated with decreased survival in patients with a positive FAST examination requiring emergent laparotomy. J Trauma Acute Care Surg 2013;75(1 Suppl 1):S48–52.
29. Say L, Chou D, Gemmill A, et al. Global causes of maternal death: a WHO systematic analysis. Lancet Glob Health 2014;2(6):e323–33.
30. Maswime S, Buchmann E. A systematic review of maternal near miss and mortality due to postpartum hemorrhage. Int J Gynaecol Obstet 2017;137(1):1–7.
31. Goffman D, Nathan L, Chazotte C. Obstetric hemorrhage: a global review. Semin Perinatol 2016;40(2):96–8.
32. Maternal mortality. Available at: https://www.who.int/news-room/fact-sheets/detail/maternal-mortality. Accessed March 13, 2022.
33. Committee on practice bulletins-obstetrics. Practice bulletin No. 183: postpartum hemorrhage. Obstet Gynecol 2017;130(4):e168–86.
34. Creanga AA, Syverson C, Seed K, et al. Pregnancy-related mortality in the United States, 2011-2013. Obstet Gynecol 2017;130(2):366–73.
35.. Trends in maternal mortality 2000 to 2017: estimates by WHO, UNICEF, UNFPA, world bank group and the united nations population division. Geneva: World Health Organization; 2019.
36. Sheldon WR, Blum J, Vogel JP, et al. Postpartum haemorrhage management, risks, and maternal outcomes: findings from the world health organization multicountry survey on maternal and newborn health. BJOG 2014;121(Suppl 1):5–13.
37. Varouxaki N, Gnanasambanthan S, Datta S, et al. Antepartum haemorrhage. Obstetrics. Gynaecol Reprod Med 2018;28(8):237–42.
38. Amokrane N, Allen ERF, Waterfield A, et al. Antepartum haemorrhage. Obstetrics. Gynaecol Reprod Med 2016;26(2):33–7.
39. Hamadameen AI. The maternal and perinatal outcome in antepartum hemorrhage: a cross-sectional study. Zanco J Med Sci 2018;22(2):155–63.
40. Henriquez DDCA, Henriquez DDC, Bloemenkamp KWM, et al. Management of postpartum hemorrhage: how to improve maternal outcomes? J Thromb Haemost 2018;16(8):1523–34.
41. Vause S, Clark B, Thorne S, Knight M, Nour M, Tuffnell D. Saving Lives, Improving Mothers' Care: Surveillance of Maternal Deaths in the UK 2012-14 and Lessons Learned to Inform Maternity Care From the UK and Ireland Confidential Enquiries Into Maternal Deaths and Morbidity 2009-14. Published online 2016.
42. Hendriks E, MacNaughton H, MacKenzie MC. First trimester bleeding: evaluation and management. Am Fam Physician 2019;99(3):166–74.
43. Dogra V, Paspulati RM, Bhatt S. First trimester bleeding evaluation. Ultrasound Q 2005;21(2):69–85, quiz 149-150, 153-154.
44. Breeze C. Early pregnancy bleeding. Aust Fam Physician 2016;45(5):283–6.
45. Boisramé T, Sananès N, Fritz G, et al. Placental abruption: risk factors, management and maternal–fetal prognosis. Cohort study over 10 years. Eur J Obstet Gynecol Reprod Biol 2014;179:100–4.
46. Li Y, Tian Y, Liu N, et al. Analysis of 62 placental abruption cases: risk factors and clinical outcomes. Taiwan J Obstet Gynecol 2019;58(2):223–6.
47. Gerdessen L, Meybohm P, Choorapoikayil S, et al. Comparison of common perioperative blood loss estimation techniques: a systematic review and meta-analysis. J Clin Monit Comput 2021;35(2):245–58.

48. Hoppenot C, Tankou J, Stair S, et al. Sonographic evaluation for intra-abdominal hemorrhage after cesarean delivery. J Clin Ultrasound 2016;44(4):240–4.

49.. World Health Organization. WHO recommendations for the prevention and treatment of postpartum haemorrhage. Geneva: World Health Organization; 2012.

50. American College of Obstetricians and Gynecologists' Committee on Practice Bulletins—Gynecology. ACOG practice bulletin No. 200: early pregnancy loss. Obstet Gynecol 2018;132(5):e197–207.

51. Bienstock JL, Eke AC, Hueppchen NA. Postpartum hemorrhage. N Engl J Med 2021;384(17):1635–45.

52. Dahlke JD, Mendez-Figueroa H, Maggio L, et al. Prevention and management of postpartum hemorrhage: a comparison of 4 national guidelines. Am J Obstet Gynecol 2015;213(1):76.e1–10.

53. Condous GS, Arulkumaran S. Medical and conservative surgical management of postpartum hemorrhage. J Obstet Gynaecol Can 2003;25(11):931–6.

54. Baskett TF. Acute uterine inversion: a review of 40 cases. J Obstet Gynaecol Can 2002;24(12):953–6.

55. Obore N, Liuxiao Z, Haomin Y, et al. Intraoperative cell salvage for women at high risk of postpartum hemorrhage during cesarean section: a systematic review and meta-analysis. Reprod Sci 2022;13. https://doi.org/10.1007/s43032-021-00824-8.

56. Burtelow M, Riley E, Druzin M, et al. How we treat: management of life-threatening primary postpartum hemorrhage with a standardized massive transfusion protocol. Transfusion 2007;47(9):1564–72.

57. Grimes CE, Bowman KG, Dodgion CM, et al. Systematic review of barriers to surgical care in low-income and middle-income countries. World J Surg 2011;35(5): 941–50.

58. Burke TF, Suarez S, Sessler DI, et al. Safety and feasibility of a ketamine package to support emergency and essential surgery in Kenya when No anesthetist is available: an analysis of 1216 consecutive operative procedures. World J Surg 2017;41(12):2990–7.

59. Jenny HE, Saluja S, Sood R, et al. Access to safe blood in low-income and middle-income countries: lessons from India. BMJ Glob Health 2017;2(2): e000167.

60. Dawson AJ, Buchan J, Duffield C, et al. Task shifting and sharing in maternal and reproductive health in low-income countries: a narrative synthesis of current evidence. Health Policy Plan 2014;29(3):396–408.

61. Burke TF, Ahn R, Nelson BD, et al. A postpartum haemorrhage package with condom uterine balloon tamponade: a prospective multi-centre case series in Kenya, Sierra Leone, Senegal, and Nepal. BJOG: An Int J Obstet Gynaecol 2016;123(9):1532–40.

62. Palmqvist M, Von Schreeb J, Älgå A. Autotransfusion in low-resource settings: a scoping review. BMJ Open 2022;12(5):e056018.

63. Longstreth GF. Epidemiology of hospitalization for acute upper gastrointestinal hemorrhage: a population-based study. Am J Gastroenterol 1995;90(2):206–10.

64. Laine L, Peterson WL. Bleeding peptic ulcer. N Engl J Med 1994;331(11):717–27.

65. Gralnek IM, Jensen DM, Kovacs TO, et al. The economic impact of esophageal variceal hemorrhage: cost-effectiveness implications of endoscopic therapy. Hepatology 1999;29(1):44–50.

66. Rotondano G. Epidemiology and diagnosis of acute nonvariceal upper gastrointestinal bleeding. Gastroenterol Clin North Am 2014;43(4):643–63.

67. Rajan SS, Sawe HR, Iyullu AJ, et al. Profile and outcome of patients with upper gastrointestinal bleeding presenting to urban emergency departments of tertiary hospitals in Tanzania. BMC Gastroenterol 2019;19(1):212.

68. Alema ON, Martin DO, Okello TR. Endoscopic findings in upper gastrointestinal bleeding patients at Lacor hospital, northern Uganda. Afr Health Sci 2012; 12(4):518–21.

69. Garcia-Tsao G, Sanyal AJ, Grace ND, et al. Practice guidelines committee of the American association for the study of liver diseases, the practice parameters committee of the American College of gastroenterology. Prevention and management of gastroesophageal varices and variceal hemorrhage in cirrhosis. Hepatology 2007;46(3):922–38. https://doi.org/10.1002/hep.21907.

70. Elsebaey MA, Elashry H, Elbedewy TA, et al. Predictors of in-hospital mortality in a cohort of elderly Egyptian patients with acute upper gastrointestinal bleeding. Medicine 2018;97(16):e0403.

71. Palmer ED. The vigorous diagnostic approach to upper-gastrointestinal tract hemorrhage. A 23-year prospective study of 1,4000 patients. JAMA 1969; 207(8):1477–80.

72. Piscioneri F, Kluger Y, Ansaloni L, editors. Emergency surgery for low resource regions. Cham (Switzerland): Springer; 2021.

73. Ohmiya N. Management of obscure gastrointestinal bleeding: comparison of guidelines between Japan and other countries. Dig Endosc 2020;32(2):204–18.

74. Mulima G, Qureshi JS, Shores C, et al, Andrén-Sandberg Å. Upper gastrointestinal bleeding at a public referal hospital in Malawi. Surg Sci 2014;05(11):501–7.

75. Tarasconi A, Coccolini F, Biffl WL, et al. Perforated and bleeding peptic ulcer: WSES guidelines. World J Emerg Surg 2020;15:3.

76. Garcia-Tsao G. Current management of the complications of cirrhosis and portal hypertension: variceal hemorrhage, ascites, and spontaneous bacterial peritonitis. Dig Dis 2016;34(4):382–6.

77. Villanueva C, Colomo A, Bosch A, et al. Transfusion strategies for acute upper gastrointestinal bleeding. N Engl J Med 2013;368(1):11–21.

78. Mansoor-Ul-Haq M, Latif A, Asad M, et al. Treatment of bleeding gastric varices by endoscopic cyanoacrylate injection: a developing-country perspective. Cureus 2020;12(2):e7062.

79. Hobday K, Hulme J, Prata N, et al. Scaling up misoprostol to prevent postpartum hemorrhage at home births in Mozambique: a case study applying the Expand-Net/WHO framework. Glob Health Sci Pract 2019;7(1):66–86.

80. Roberts N, James S, Delaney M, et al. The global need and availability of blood products: a modelling study. Lancet Haematol 2019;6(12):e606–15.

81. Butler EK, Hume H, Birungi I, et al. Blood utilization at a national referral hospital in sub-Saharan Africa. Transfusion 2015;55(5):1058–66.

82. Barro L, Drew VJ, Poda GG, et al. Blood transfusion in sub-Saharan Africa: understanding the missing gap and responding to present and future challenges. Vox Sang 2018;113(8):726–36.

83. Kaada SH, Apelseth TO, Hagen KG, et al. How do I get an emergency civilian walking blood bank running? Transfusion 2019;59(S2):1446–52.

84. Nisingizwe MP, Ndishimye P, Swaibu K, et al. Effect of unmanned aerial vehicle (drone) delivery on blood product delivery time and wastage in Rwanda: a retrospective, cross-sectional study and time series analysis. Lancet Glob Health 2022;10(4):e564–9.

85. Sjöholm A, Älgå A, von Schreeb J. A last resort when there is no blood: experiences and perceptions of intraoperative autotransfusion among medical doctors deployed to resource-limited settings. World J Surg 2020;44(12):4052–9.

86. Munoz-Valencia A, Goodwin T, Wesonga B, et al. Implementation of a training program for the intraoperative use of Hemafuse in ruptured ectopic pregnancy in Ghana and Kenya: an innovative whole blood autotransfusion device. In: CUGH 2022 virtual conference. CUGH; 2022. Available at: https://cugh.confex. com/cugh/2022/meetingapp.cgi/Paper/2290.

87. Hasan R, Baird DD, Herring AH, et al. Association between first-trimester vaginal bleeding and miscarriage. Obstet Gynecol 2009;114(4):860–7.

88. Borovac-Pinheiro A, Pacagnella RC, Cecatti JG, et al. Postpartum hemorrhage: new insights for definition and diagnosis. Am J Obstet Gynecol 2018;219(2):162–8.

89. Callaghan WM, Kuklina EV, Berg CJ. Trends in postpartum hemorrhage: United States, 1994–2006. Am J Obstet Gynecol 2010;202(4):353.e1–6.

90. Mehrabadi A, Liu S, Bartholomew S, et al. Temporal trends in postpartum hemorrhage and severe postpartum hemorrhage in Canada from 2003 to 2010. J Obstet Gynaecol Can 2014;36(1):21–33.

91. Singh SP, Panigrahi MK. Spectrum of upper gastrointestinal hemorrhage in coastal Odisha. Trop Gastroenterol 2013;34(1):14–7.

92. Zaltman C, Souza HSP de, Castro MEC, et al. Upper gastrointestinal bleeding in a Brazilian hospital: a retrospective study of endoscopic records. Arq Gastroenterol 2002;39(2):74–80.

93. Savides TJ, Jensen DM, Cohen J, et al. Severe upper gastrointestinal tumor bleeding: endoscopic findings, treatment, and outcome. Endoscopy 1996; 28(2):244–8.

Oxygen as an Essential Medicine

Matthew F. Mart, MD, MSc[a,b,c], Cornelius Sendagire, MBChB, MMed[d], Eugene Wesley Ely, MD, MPH[a,b,c], Elisabeth D. Riviello, MD, MPH[e,1,*], Theogene Twagirumugabe, MD, PhD[f,1]

KEYWORDS

• Oxygen • Critical illness • Global health • COVID-19

KEY POINTS

• Supplemental oxygen is an essential medication for critically ill patients with acute hypoxic respiratory failure and is necessary to maintain normal cellular metabolism.

• The optimal oxygen dose and delivery system remain unknown, and the risks and benefits may differ among disease processes seen in the intensive care unit, with clinical studies demonstrating mixed findings.

• Low- and middle-income countries experience significant disparities in both the global burden of acute hypoxic respiratory failure and oxygen supply. Clinical studies to understand optimal oxygen delivery in these areas are ongoing and are vital to optimal care for patients in resource-limited settings.

• The COVID-19 pandemic has greatly exacerbated health care disparities prevalent in low- and middle-income countries and has accelerated the global response to address shortfalls in oxygen supply.

The authors do not plan to order reprints. Role of the Funder/Sponsor: This material is based upon work supported by the U.S. Department of Veterans Affairs (VA) Office of Academic Affiliations, VA National Quality Scholars Program, and with resources and use of facilities at VA Tennessee Valley Healthcare System in Nashville, Tennessee.

[a] Division of Allergy, Pulmonary, and Critical Care Medicine, Department of Medicine, Vanderbilt University Medical Center, 1161 21st Avenue South, Nashville, TN 37232, USA; [b] Critical Illness, Brain Dysfunction, and Survivorship (CIBS) Center, Vanderbilt University Medical Center, 2525 West End Avenue, Suite 450, 4th Floor, Nashville, TN 37203, USA; [c] Geriatric Research, Education, and Clinical Center (GRECC), Tennessee Valley Healthcare System, 1310 24th Avenue South, Nashville, TN 37212, USA; [d] Anesthesia and Critical Care, Makerere University College of Health Sciences, P.O. Box 7072, Kampala, Uganda; [e] Division of Pulmonary, Critical Care, and Sleep Medicine, Beth Israel Deaconess Medical Center, Harvard Medical School, 330 Brookline Avenue, Boston, MA 02215, USA; [f] Department of Anesthesiology, Kigali University Teaching Hospital, University of Rwanda, College of Medicine and Health Sciences, School of Medicine and Pharmacy, P.O. Box 3286 Kigali, Rwanda
[1] Denotes co-last authorship.
* Corresponding author. 330 Brookline Avenue, Boston, MA 02215.
E-mail address: eriviell@bidmc.harvard.edu

INTRODUCTION

The administration of supplemental oxygen as a medical treatment is among the most common therapies provided to acutely ill patients. This is particularly true in critical care medicine, where up to half of the patients in intensive care units (ICUs) require supplemental oxygen.[1] Oxygen is currently on the World Health Organization's (WHO's) List of Essential Medicines for acutely ill individuals and for people with chronic diseases resulting in hypoxemia.[2] Medical oxygen's status as an essential medicine has become even more prominent given the global COVID-19 pandemic, with the virus' most common and marked clinical manifestation being hypoxemia.

Adequate oxygen availability at the cellular level is vital for normal metabolism in humans, traversing a path from "mouth to mitochondria."[3] Diseases that affect oxygen transfer anywhere along this path, from the pulmonary alveoli to end-organ mitochondria, can cause negative downstream effects and lead to a common array of symptoms. Supplemental oxygen at a concentration greater than atmospheric partial pressure is commonly administered to overcome pathophysiologic barriers in oxygen uptake and delivery. However, oxygen can also be toxic despite its essential nature in maintaining normal aerobic respiration. Excess oxygen can damage proteins, nucleic acids, and other pieces of cellular machinery through increased oxidative stress.[4] Concerns regarding oxygen toxicity in critical care medicine have been noted as far back as the 1960s with descriptions of "respirator lung syndrome" seen in mechanically ventilated patients exposed to high oxygen concentrations.[5] Despite the long-standing evidence of a therapeutic window for supplemental oxygen therapy, the optimal dose and delivery method of oxygen remain a significant scientific gap with varying recommendations from international critical care societies.[6–8]

A significant number of critically ill patients are exposed to high levels of oxygen support in excess of their needs in many ICUs.[9] Yet, undertreatment of hypoxemia also remains a major problem, especially in resource-limited settings. Under-recognition and undertreatment, frequently because of a lack of oxygen supply and monitoring equipment, are associated with a substantial increase in mortality even among patients not admitted to an ICU.[10] Among low- and middle-income countries (LMIC), almost one-quarter of hospitals do not have supplemental oxygen available.[11] The COVID-19 pandemic has exacerbated and highlighted these health care inequities, as multiple LMICs have experienced oxygen shortages during surges of viral transmission, leading to increased preventable mortality and impacting patients with and without COVID-19.[12] These events acted as catalysts for various international efforts to increase oxygen supply.[13] Additionally, unanswered questions remain as to the best approaches to delivering oxygen in LMIC and reduced-resource settings.[14]

In this review, we explore the history of oxygen therapy in medicine and briefly review the important physiology. We subsequently outline the clinical relevance of determining the optimal delivery method and "dose" of supplemental oxygen among critically ill patients. Finally, we explore the impact of oxygen therapy in a global context, discussing the questions and considerations of oxygen therapy in LMICs and highlighting the patient-level and systemic challenges of oxygen supply and a global respiratory pandemic.

HISTORY OF OXYGEN THERAPY IN CRITICAL CARE MEDICINE

The history of oxygen reaches back centuries, with theories regarding molecular oxygen and gas exchange being promulgated as early as the thirteenth century.[3] Yet, the eighteenth century saw an acceleration of scientific knowledge regarding oxygen that laid the framework for its future use as a medical therapy.[3] By the late nineteenth century and early twentieth century, pioneering work by two prominent physicians, Sir William Osler and Jonathan Campbell Meakins, elucidated the role of oxygen therapy in treating hypoxemia caused by pneumonia.[15] Through this work, they established supplemental oxygen therapy as the standard of care for pneumonia and, ultimately, other diseases of hypoxemia in the 1920s.[15]

ICUs were initially developed in Europe in response to the epidemic of respiratory failure secondary to the polio epidemic with the development of negative-pressure ventilators, including the commonly known "iron lung."[16] In the 1960s and 1970s, with the advent of critical care medicine as a specialty and the development of positive-pressure mechanical ventilators, the ability to use supplemental oxygen concentrations above atmospheric levels grew substantially. Positive-pressure ventilators combine the ability to provide ventilation invasively through an endotracheal tube or a tracheostomy tube with the ability to entrain supranormal concentrations of oxygen. Early on, patients routinely received high tidal volumes and high oxygen concentrations in an effort to aggressively normalize patients' physiology.[16] Over the next several decades, however, it was increasingly recognized that high volumes, in conjunction with high oxygen concentrations, were harmful to many patients.[5,17] Efforts to normalize physiology were exchanged for "lung protective ventilation" with lower tidal volumes and increased positive end-expiratory pressures, or PEEP, to avoid many of the untoward effects of high oxygen concentrations.[17,18]

At the same time that invasive mechanical ventilation and oxygen delivery were developing, noninvasive forms of respiratory support were growing in use as well. The use of positive-pressure ventilation through a mask apparatus was known as far back as the 1940s and 1950s; however, it was predominantly limited to patients requiring long-term ventilatory support and oxygen therapy.[19] These devices combine the ability to entrain higher concentrations of oxygen with ventilatory support without the need for an endotracheal tube or tracheostomy, and their use has grown exponentially in the ICU. In the late 1980s and early 1990s, however, multiple studies demonstrated the benefit of noninvasive mechanical ventilation in patients with chronic obstructive pulmonary disease (COPD) and congestive heart failure.[20,21] In the last decade, another noninvasive oxygen delivery method called high-flow nasal cannula (HFNC) has changed practice in treating acute hypoxemic respiratory failure (AHRF) by providing high oxygen flow rates through a nasal cannula apparatus. These noninvasive methods of providing high-level oxygen support have transformed critical care medicine, providing vital tools in the treatment of hypoxemic respiratory failure. Despite revolutionizing critical care medicine and oxygen therapy more broadly, the physiologic and clinical importance of these oxygen delivery systems, and how they may differ in settings with varying resources, is an ongoing area of active research.

PHYSIOLOGIC AND CLINICAL RELEVANCE OF OXYGEN THERAPY
Physiology of Oxygen Therapy

Diatomic oxygen (O_2) is one of the foundational elements on our planet, forming the backbone of bioenergetic function in aerobic organisms. On Earth, the overall oxygen concentration in the atmosphere is approximately 21%, with an inspired partial pressure of roughly 150 mmHg at sea level.[22] At the level of the pulmonary alveoli, the partial pressure of oxygen is approximately 100 mm Hg after accounting for the partial pressure of carbon dioxide and the respiratory exchange ratio. Most of the oxygen that is inspired and traverses the pulmonary capillaries binds to hemoglobin, and a small amount is dissolved in the plasma. The overall concentration of oxygen in the blood can be quantified as follows: Cao_2 (mL O_2/100 mL blood) = (1.36 × Hgb ×

$Sao_2/100) \times 0.003 \times Pao_2$, where Cao_2 is the concentration of oxygen in arterial blood, 1.36 is the carrying capacity of hemoglobin (1.36 mL of O_2 for 1 g of hemoglobin), Hgb is hemoglobin level, Sao_2 is the arterial oxygen–hemoglobin saturation percentage, and Pao_2 is the dissolved partial pressure of oxygen in arterial blood.[22] From the aforementioned equation, it can be discerned that oxygen bound to hemoglobin provides the majority of oxygen available to be delivered to tissues, whereas dissolved oxygen (Pao_2) provides a smaller contribution. The percentage of arterial oxygen bound to hemoglobin at rest in healthy individuals near sea level who are breathing an ambient oxygen concentration of 21% is approximately 98%. By increasing the fraction of inspired oxygen (Fio_2) in patients with impaired oxygen exchange, a greater proportion of available hemoglobin is bound to oxygen. It can then be delivered to tissue, assuming cardiac output and oxygen extraction at the tissue level are normal, with modest increases in the dissolved oxygen concentration. Additionally, increasing the mean pressure in pulmonary alveoli above that of sea-level atmospheric pressure while also increasing the Fio_2 (ie, "hyperbaric" oxygen) provides an even greater increase in available oxygen to tissues, predominantly by increasing the partial pressure of dissolved oxygen.[3] Each of these approaches (increasing Fio_2 and increasing pressure at the pulmonary alveoli) has important clinical uses in increasing the delivery of oxygen.

Clinical Relevance

Oxygen therapy, both in the ICU and outside of the ICU, is a fundamental necessity for the care of acutely ill patients, and there are several different systems available to deliver oxygen. The choice of an oxygen delivery system is multifaceted (**Fig. 1**), impacted by the degree of illness, the necessary "dose" of oxygen, underlying conditions, and patient safety. Each of these factors needs to be carefully considered in the use of oxygen therapy, particularly when resources or settings may also dictate additional limitations on delivery methods.

Low-flow oxygen therapy is perhaps the most frequent delivery method used in hospitals. Low-flow oxygen, at rates from 1 L to 6 L per minute in adults, is commonly

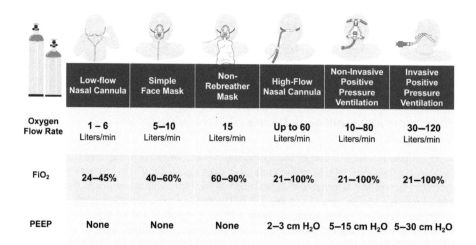

	Low-flow Nasal Cannula	Simple Face Mask	Non-Rebreather Mask	High-Flow Nasal Cannula	Non-Invasive Positive Pressure Ventilation	Invasive Positive Pressure Ventilation
Oxygen Flow Rate	1 – 6 Liters/min	5–10 Liters/min	15 Liters/min	Up to 60 Liters/min	10–80 Liters/min	30–120 Liters/min
FiO_2	24–45%	40–60%	60–90%	21–100%	21–100%	21–100%
PEEP	None	None	None	2–3 cm H_2O	5–15 cm H_2O	5–30 cm H_2O

Fig. 1. Major oxygen delivery systems. FiO_2, fraction of inspired oxygen (percentage); PEEP, positive end-expiratory pressure. (Images courtesy of the OpenCriticalCare.org Project.)

supplied through nasal prongs or by facemask. Because of the lower flow rates, open system design, and patient-level factors, such as respiratory rate, room air (with an oxygen concentration of 21%) mixes with the supplied oxygen, reducing the overall Fi_{o2} delivered to the alveoli to a range of 25% to 40%.[23] Higher Fi_{o2} can be delivered through the use of partial and nonrebreathing masks, which utilize oxygen reservoirs and/or valve systems to limit the entrainment of room air.[24] Over the last 2 decades, the use of HFNC systems that provide heated and humidified flows up to 60 L per minute and supply oxygen concentrations greater than 90% has grown exponentially.[25] Because of the increased flow rates intrinsic to these delivery systems, there is a reduced entrainment of room air, a washout of carbon dioxide with high oxygen concentrations, and small increases in mean airway pressure, providing an effective method of increasing arterial oxygen concentration.[26,27] Providing supplemental oxygen through the use of HFNC devices has been shown to reduce the risk of intubation and death in patients with AHRF,[28] as well as reduce the risk of reintubation in patients who were liberated from invasive mechanical ventilation when compared with conventional oxygen therapy.[29] Lastly, the other predominant form of oxygen delivery system is noninvasive and invasive mechanical ventilation provided through positive pressure ventilation devices. Oxygen can be supplied through these devices across a range of concentrations up to 100%. These devices also provide various methods to increase mean alveolar pressure through the use of positive PEEP or longer durations at peak inspiratory pressures while also providing ventilatory support to facilitate carbon dioxide removal.[16] Although, perhaps, the most efficient method for providing accurate and titratable oxygen concentrations, the use of positive-pressure ventilation systems is resource-intensive and expensive; this can substantially limit their use in certain settings. Noninvasive systems without masks, including tent or hood enclosure systems, exist. Yet, their use is largely limited to a few regions globally, and their effectiveness is actively being studied.[30]

CHOOSING THE RIGHT "DOSE" OF OXYGEN

Regardless of the delivery system, substantial knowledge gaps persist regarding the "dose" of oxygen needed for a variety of conditions treated in critical care medicine. A prime example is the use of supplemental oxygen in patients experiencing acute cardiac ischemia. The previous rationale for using supplemental oxygen, even in patients without hypoxemia, during a myocardial infarction was that it could potentially limit the overall area of infarcted myocardium.[31] However, a large randomized controlled trial (RCT) of continuous supplemental oxygen therapy versus no oxygen in patients with acute myocardial infarction without hypoxemia showed no difference in mortality or rehospitalization.[32] Of note, a systematic review of several RCTs of oxygen therapy found that in patients with cardiac ischemia and no hypoxemia, oxygen therapy was associated with significantly increased mortality.[33] Similarly, in a large clinical trial in patients with acute cerebrovascular accidents, continuous and nocturnal oxygen therapy did not improve outcomes when compared with no oxygen therapy.[34] Changes in the most recent guidelines now reflect the results of these trials in recommending against supplemental oxygen in patients with cardiac or cerebrovascular ischemia who are not hypoxemic.[35]

Several recent RCTs have also shed light on the role of oxygen therapy in general ICU patients. In the OXYGEN-ICU trial, 434 patients at a single hospital in Italy were randomized to conservative oxygen therapy with a target oxygen saturation of 94% to 98% (Pa_{o2} of 70–100 mm Hg) or "standard" oxygen therapy with a target oxygen saturation of 97% to 100% (Pa_{o2} up to 150 mm Hg) with a primary outcome of ICU mortality. The mortality rate was significantly lower in the conservative oxygen arm (11.6% vs. 20.2%). Notably, the study enrolled patients on mechanical ventilation as well as those who were not. The study was also significantly limited by the fact that it was stopped early and did not reach the predetermined sample size. In the more recent, and larger, ICU-ROX trial, mechanically ventilated general ICU patients randomized to a conservative oxygen target of 91% to 96% versus a "usual care" (higher) target had no difference in ventilator-free days nor any difference in 90-day or 180-day mortality.[36] Subgroup analyses in this trial suggested that patients with hypoxic ischemic encephalopathy had better outcomes with conservative oxygen therapy, however. Additionally, patients in the usual care (higher oxygen target) group reported increased difficulties in mobility and self-care. In contrast, in a study of liberal versus conservative oxygen targets in mechanically ventilated patients with acute respiratory distress syndrome (ARDS), there was no difference between the liberal or conservative oxygen therapy arms in terms of survival at 28 days. However, the study was stopped for safety concerns due to five mesenteric ischemia events in the conservative oxygen target group, though this finding of intestinal ischemia was not seen in a subsequent larger follow-up study.[37,38] These studies highlight the ongoing need for further clarity regarding optimal oxygen dosage in critically ill patients. Observational data indicates that well over half of patients treated in ICUs are exposed to excess oxygen concentrations,[39] yet they may also experience clinically significant hypoxemia.[40] These findings have immediate implications for critical illness outcomes, such as patients with COPD,[41] but they also highlight important considerations for oxygen supply, appropriate utilization, and the best approaches to oxygen therapy in resource-limited settings. Given that many hospitals in LMICs lack adequate oxygen supplies and that inadvertent hypoxemia impacts mortality in resource-limited settings,[10,11] appropriate dosing and delivery of oxygen in critically ill patients that maximizes benefit, minimizes harm, and increases availability is of vital importance for global health.

GLOBAL AND PUBLIC HEALTH IMPACT
Epidemiology of Acute Hypoxemic Respiratory Failure and Resource Constraints in Low- and Middle-Income Countries

LMICs account for the majority of the world's population, and the majority of the global burden of disease, including respiratory infections, which are among the most common causes of mortality.[42] Additionally, LMICs experience a proportionally higher rate of critical illness when compared with high-income countries (HICs), and they also experience greater mortality rates in disease processes that would potentially benefit from critical care.[43] AHRF is one of the most common diagnoses in LMICs. Hypoxemia leads to excess mortality in infectious diseases prevalent in some LMICs such as malaria and tuberculosis, as well as noncommunicable diseases, including heart failure and chronic lung disease.[44–46] In one study of 7300 adults presenting to an emergency department in a Ugandan hospital, 4.5% of patients presented with AHRF, most commonly due to pneumonia.[47] Despite being relatively young (median age of 38), the in-hospital mortality for this cohort was 77%. The authors note that only 6% of these patients received mechanical ventilation due to resource limitations, including ICU bed availability. In a similar cross-sectional point prevalence study of adult inpatients admitted to two hospitals in Malawi, 4% of patients had hypoxemia, yet 89% of them were not receiving oxygen therapy.[48] ARDS, an inflammatory form of AHRF, is also highly prevalent in LMICs. In a study of inpatient admissions to one hospital in Rwanda over a 6 week period, 4% of adults met criteria for ARDS using the Kigali modification of the Berlin criteria.[46] Only 31% of patients were admitted to an ICU, however, and in-hospital mortality was 50% for all patients with ARDS.

Despite the burden of critical illness in LMICs, hospitals in these areas are often undersupplied. Caregiving for critically ill patients is a resource-intensive endeavor, fraught with challenges related to the cost of care, staffing, and equipment needs. Supplemental oxygen and pulse oximeters for monitoring oxygen saturation are foundational resources that often have limited availability in LMICs.[11] In a survey of over 200 health care institutions in 12 African countries, less than half had consistent, uninterrupted sources of oxygen, and less than one-quarter had an oxygen concentrator.[49] Whereas the availability of supplemental oxygen, and particularly pulse oximetry, has been shown to improve mortality,[50,51] logistical challenges related to maintenance, electricity, and supply significantly limit oxygen availability in LMICs.[52] In LMICs where the availability of pulse oximetry is limited, inadvertent and undiagnosed hypoxemia is frequent and impacts clinical outcomes and care.[53] Evans and colleagues, in a cross-sectional study of all adult patients admitted to a large teaching hospital in Malawi, found that 14 out of 144 patients needed oxygen therapy due to desaturations lower than 90% during a 24 hour period, but only 4 were receiving oxygen because of the lack of functional oxygen concentrators.[54] A related study found that over half of patients at one Rwandan hospital with hypoxemia received no or limited supplemental oxygen on one or more days of their inpatient admission.[10] This lack of oxygen supply has a direct impact on mortality. Duke and colleagues found that after the introduction of pulse oximeters, oxygen concentrators, and a protocol for detecting and treating hypoxemia in children admitted to 5 hospitals in Papua New Guinea, mortality due to pneumonia fell by 35%.[50]

In contrast, inappropriate oxygen use may also occur frequently and impact oxygen supply downstream for other patients. For example, a retrospective study of pulse oximeter use in pediatric patients at 18 Kenyan hospitals found that 8.6% of patients had oxygen prescribed, but 87% of patients either did not have pulse oximetry performed or did not have oxygen saturations lower than 90%.[55] In situations where oxygen supply is limited, liberal and nontitrated dosing of supplemental oxygen may lead to or exacerbate supply shortages. In a study of patients in the adult emergency department of a Rwandan teaching hospital, Sutherland and colleagues found that 12% of patients were hypoxemic, but on over 80% of days, patients were either over or under-treated with oxygen to achieve a target oxygen saturation of 90% to 95%.[56] Following a targeted educational intervention on appropriate oxygen targets and monitoring, however, the number of oxygen tanks used daily in the emergency department decreased significantly, with concomitant increases in oxygen tank reserves. These studies demonstrate the importance of optimal dosing of oxygen therapy for clinical outcomes and managing supplies of supplemental oxygen in resource-limited settings.

Oxygen Delivery Systems in Low- and Middle-Income Countries

Studies regarding the optimal dose and delivery of oxygen therapy have predominantly been limited to HICs, with inadequate studies regarding oxygen therapy in the care of critically ill patients in LMICs. The use of nasal bubble continuous positive airway pressure (bCPAP) ventilation versus standard low-flow oxygen therapy was trialed in 644 hypoxemic pediatric patients with pneumonia in one hospital in Malawi.[57] There was no difference in in-hospital mortality between the bCPAP group and the nasal low-flow oxygen groups, though the study was stopped early before enrolling its targeted sample size due to futility. Of note, these therapies were provided in a non-ICU setting, and there were more adverse events, including deaths, in the bCPAP group, raising questions regarding the feasibility of providing noninvasive ventilatory support outside of the ICU. A similar multicenter randomized clinical trial named the Children's Oxygen Administration Strategies, or COAST, trial investigated HFNC versus low-flow nasal cannula versus permissive hypoxemia. Maitland and colleagues enrolled 1852 pediatric patients with pneumonia in 4 Ugandan and 2 Kenyan hospitals, stratifying them according to severity of hypoxemia, with severe hypoxemia considered to be oxygen saturations of less than 80%.[58] Patients with severe hypoxemia were randomly assigned to either HFNC or low-flow oxygen therapy, whereas those with less hypoxemia (>80% to 91%) were randomly assigned to either HFNC or low-flow oxygen therapy or were allowed to have permissive hypoxemia down to 80%. The trial was ultimately stopped early by the Trial Steering Committee because of ethical concerns raised regarding randomization to the permissive hypoxemia arm. Although definitive conclusions regarding the efficacy of these approaches to oxygen dosing cannot be drawn from this trial due to its early termination, there are suggestions of potential benefit that require further study. First, at 48 hours, there was a 4% lower mortality in the HFNC arm when compared with low-flow oxygen in the stratum with severe hypoxemia, though this did not quite reach predetermined significance ($P = .076$). Second, in both strata, HFNCs were associated with significantly lower volumes of oxygen used. The finding of oxygen conservation is important and encouraging, as it may suggest that higher flow oxygen delivery may actually reduce overall oxygen requirements. This is likely because of the fact that many children achieved adequate oxygenation from high flows of room air without requiring any oxygen. Whether oxygen conservation may occur through the small amounts of intrinsic PEEP (and thus higher mean alveolar pressure) or reduction of physiologic dead space remains to be proven given the preliminary nature of these findings.

Whether there are clinical benefits to certain oxygen delivery systems for critically ill adults in lower resource settings is unknown. It is also unclear whether delivery systems, such as HFNC oxygen therapy, which have substantially higher flows, can reduce oxygen supply utilization in adults similar to children in the COAST trial given that flow rates in adults can be relatively higher (up to 60 L/min). A handful of upcoming studies may help answer these questions. The Adult Respiratory Failure Intervention Study – Africa (ARISE-Africa), a stepped wedge cluster randomized trial (Clinicaltrials.gov ID: NCT04693403), will study 470 critically ill adults in Uganda with AHRF randomized to HFNC oxygen, continuous positive airway pressure plus oxygen, or standard low-flow oxygen therapy and compare 28-day mortality. Another upcoming trial called the Building Respiratory support in East Africa Through High flow versus low flow oxygen Evaluation (BREATHE), funded by the Wellcome Trust, will evaluate the use of HFNC oxygen therapy versus low-flow oxygen therapy in five hospitals from three East African countries—Rwanda, Kenya, and Malawi. This study will utilize a type 1 effectiveness-implementation hybrid trial design with the primary aim of determining the effectiveness of HFNC oxygen therapy versus low-flow oxygen therapy and a secondary aim of determining the feasibility and utility of protocolized oxygen use with monitoring and titration. Although protocolized low-flow oxygen therapy has been shown to reduce mortality in pediatric patients with pneumonia,[50] it has not been studied in adults and not in comparison with high-flow nasal oxygen therapy, which may have unique benefits due to high flow rates but also impact oxygen utilization and supply. The Circumvent Project in Nigeria is examining helmet noninvasive ventilation using an implementation science framework.[59] These studies, and others, are crucial to improving our understanding of how to best deliver supplemental oxygen in an efficient manner while accounting for the unique context of health care institutions in LMICs.

OXYGEN THERAPY DURING THE COVID-19 PANDEMIC

The arrival of a novel respiratory coronavirus, called severe acute respiratory syndrome-coronavirus 2 (SARS-CoV-2), in 2019 has fundamentally changed critical care medicine as a specialty throughout the world and highlighted existing inequities in ICU resources between countries. In its severe form, coronavirus disease 2019, or COVID-19 as it is commonly named, manifests as severe respiratory distress and AHRF in a substantial percentage of patients infected with SARS-CoV-2 and has strained ICU resources globally. Given the already limited resources present in many LMICs, the pandemic has particularly impacted critical care in LMICs. Medical oxygen was initially the only known therapy for the disease, and remains one of the most important therapies in the treatment of COVID-19 worldwide; limited supply has threatened the lives of thousands of patients in LMICs, both with COVID-19 and those with other diseases that require supplemental oxygen. The WHO continues to highlight oxygen supply in LMIC as a global health emergency.[12,60] A recently developed tool for estimating country and global oxygen needs demonstrates that over 3.6 million oxygen cylinders per day are needed in LMICs for COVID-19 patients alone.[61]

Although inequities in oxygen supply existed long before the arrival of COVID-19, the pandemic has accelerated the global response to oxygen supply. Early on, much of the global focus was on the provision of mechanical ventilators and diagnostic therapies. The WHO's Access to COVID-19 Tools Accelerator (ACT-A) initiative, launched in April of 2020, was designed to coordinate a global effort in the development of tools to fight COVID-19 and ensure access to such resources in LMICs.[62] Although not originally part of the initial pillars of the ACT-A initiative, following several high-profile reports of desperate oxygen shortages and associated mortality in several LMICs, the ACT-A Oxygen Emergency Taskforce was launched in February of 2021. This task force represents an effort by over 20 global health agencies to tackle and prevent medical oxygen shortages that were exacerbated by the pandemic. The task force was able to generate more than $700 million US dollars of funding in an attempt to mitigate the damage of oxygen shortages. This funding, provided by various entities, including The Global Fund, United Nations Children's Fund, Wellcome Trust, and Unitaid, was used for the purchases of oxygen supplies and associated equipment, such as pulse oximeters and monitors as well as providing funding directly to governments in LMIC for the purchase of supplies and in their use and maintenance. In late 2021, the updated ACT-A strategic plan called for an additional 1.4 billion dollars of funding to be obtained to continue efforts in supplying oxygen and supplies to LMICs in 2022.[13] Additionally, the United States Agency for International Development has provided support for the development and delivery of oxygen plants in some countries, in addition to other necessary oxygen supplies.[63] Given the ongoing difficulties in consistent oxygen supply as well as logistical insults to health care infrastructure in LMICs during the COVID-19 pandemic, increased and ongoing support in providing oxygen delivery systems and associated equipment will be vital to saving lives in the pandemic. Additionally, there is a substantial need to train end users (eg, clinicians) on the titration of oxygen based on best practice and for logistical and engineering expertise in the maintenance of oxygen supply, monitoring systems, and pulse oximetry to guarantee the sustainability of oxygen systems in LMICs.

SUMMARY

Medical oxygen therapy is a fundamental cornerstone of critical care medicine. Molecular oxygen is a necessary substrate in normal aerobic metabolism in humans, and it has a vital role in maintaining organ function in both health and disease. As medicine has continued to develop, numerous methods to supply oxygen have been devised, ranging from low flows of concentrated oxygen through nasal cannulas to invasive mechanical ventilation with supplementation of 100% oxygen. Yet, many questions remain regarding the right "dose" and delivery method of oxygen in a number of diseases that lead to critical illness, especially in LMICs. Additionally, the logistics of providing supplemental oxygen in different delivery systems vary and have substantial impacts on LMICs, who bear the greatest burden of disease-related hypoxemia and mortality. LMICs often have inconsistent oxygen supplies, leading to preventable excess mortality. Future studies will help answer questions regarding optimal oxygen delivery approaches and their impact on supply. The COVID-19 pandemic has unearthed and accelerated the inequities in oxygen supply and delivery, increasing international attention to the need but also necessitating further investment and research into the supply and best use of this essential medication.

CLINICS CARE POINTS

- Supplemental oxygen therapy is a vital component in the management of critically ill patients. However, the optimal dose and delivery method of oxygen across the range of critical illness remains unclear.

- Low- and middle-income countries (LMICs) suffer from significant inequities related to oxygen availability and supply, a fact only exacerbated by the COVID-19 pandemic, further confounding decisions regarding optimal approaches to oxygen therapy in these under-resourced settings.

- Further studies addressing the optimal dose and delivery method of supplemental oxygen in LMICs, along with analyses of cost and supply barriers, will guide future public health interventions to reduce impact of acute hypoxemic respiratory failure and oxygen shortages.

DISCLOSURE

Department of Veterans Affairs Tennessee Valley Health Care System Geriatric Research, Education and Clinical Center (GRECC) and VA-MERIT, the National Institutes of Health under awards (R01AG027472, R01AG035117, R01HL111111, R01GM120484, and R01AG058639).

REFERENCES

1. Vincent JL, Akça S, De Mendonça A, et al. The epidemiology of acute respiratory failure in critically ill patients(*). Chest 2002;121(5):1602–9.
2. World Health Organization. The selection and use of essential medicines: report of the WHO Expert Committee, 2017 (including the 20th WHO model list of essential medicines and the 6th WHO Model list of essential medicines for children). Geneva, Switzerland: World Health Organization; 2017.
3. Brugniaux JV, Coombs GB, Barak OF, et al. Highs and lows of hyperoxia: physiological, performance, and clinical aspects. Am J Physiol Regul Integr Comp Physiol 2018;315(1):R1–27.
4. Davies KJA. Oxidative stress: the paradox of aerobic life. In: Rice-Evans C, Halliwell B, Lunt GG, et al, editors. Biochemical Society Symposia, vol. 61. London, United Kingdom: Portland Press; 1995. p. 1–31.
5. Nash G, Blennerhassett JB, Pontoppidan H. Pulmonary lesions associated with oxygen therapy and artifical ventilation. N Engl J Med 1967;276(7):368–74.

6. O'Driscoll BR, Howard LS, Earis J, et al. British Thoracic Society mergency oxygen guideline group, BTS emergency oxygen guideline development group. BTS guideline for oxygen use in adults in healthcare and emergency settings. Thorax 2017;72(Suppl 1):ii1–90.

7. Beasley R, Chien J, Douglas J, et al. T horacic S ociety of A ustralia and N ew Z ealand oxygen guidelines for acute oxygen use in adults: 'Swimming between the flags. ' Respirology. 2015;20(8):1182–91.

8. Fan E, Del Sorbo L, Goligher EC, et al. An official American thoracic society/European society of intensive care medicine/society of critical care medicine clinical practice guideline: mechanical ventilation in adult patients with acute respiratory distress syndrome. Am J Respir Crit Care Med 2017;195(9):1253–63.

9. Suzuki S, Eastwood GM, Peck L, et al. Current oxygen management in mechanically ventilated patients: a prospective observational cohort study. J Crit Care 2013;28(5):647–54.

10. Sutherland T, Musafiri S, Twagirumugabe T, et al. Oxygen as an essential medicine: under- and over-treatment of hypoxemia in low- and high-income nations. Crit Care Med 2016;44(10):e1015–6.

11. Meara JG, Leather AJM, Hagander L, et al. Global Surgery 2030: evidence and solutions for achieving health, welfare, and economic development. Lancet 2015; 386(9993):569–624.

12. Usher AD. Medical oxygen crisis: a belated COVID-19 response. Lancet 2021; 397(10277):868–9.

13. Every Breath Counts Coalition. One year after the launch of the access to COVID-19 tools accelerator (ACT-A) oxygen emergency taskforce, what has been achieved?. Available at: https://stoppneumonia.org/wp-content/uploads/2022/02/ACTAOxygenTaskforceAnniversaryStatement23February2022.pdf. Accessed March 2, 2022.

14. Calligaro GL, Lalla U, Audley G, et al. The utility of high-flow nasal oxygen for severe COVID-19 pneumonia in a resource-constrained setting: a multi-centre prospective observational study. EClinicalMedicine 2020;28:100570.

15. Warren CPW. The introduction of oxygen for pneumonia as seen through the writings of two McGill University professors, William Osler and Jonathan Meakins. Can Respir J 2005;12(2):81–5.

16. MacIntyre N, Rackley C, Khusid F. Fifty years of mechanical ventilation-1970s to 2020. Crit Care Med 2021;49(4):558–74.

17. Acute Respiratory Distress Syndrome Network, Brower RG, Matthay MA, et al. Ventilation with lower tidal volumes as compared with traditional tidal volumes for acute lung injury and the acute respiratory distress syndrome. N Engl J Med 2000;342(18):1301–8.

18. Brower RG, Lanken PN, MacIntyre N, et al. Higher versus lower positive end-expiratory pressures in patients with the acute respiratory distress syndrome. N Engl J Med 2004;351(4):327–36.

19. Pierson DJ. History and epidemiology of noninvasive ventilation in the acute-care setting. Respir Care 2009;54(1):40–52.

20. Meduri GU, Conoscenti CC, Menashe P, et al. Noninvasive face mask ventilation in patients with acute respiratory failure. Chest 1989;95(4):865–70.

21. Brochard L, Isabey D, Piquet J, et al. Reversal of acute exacerbations of chronic obstructive lung disease by inspiratory assistance with a face mask. N Engl J Med 1990;323(22):1523–30.

22. West JB, Luks AM. West's respiratory physiology. Philadelpha, Pennsylvania: Lippincott Williams & Wilkins; 2020.

23. Bazuaye EA, Stone TN, Corris PA, et al. Variability of inspired oxygen concentration with nasal cannulas. Thorax 1992;47(8):609–11.

24. Bateman NT, Leach RM. ABC of oxygen. Acute oxygen therapy. BMJ 1998; 317(7161):798–801.

25. Helviz Y, Einav S. A systematic review of the high-flow nasal cannula for adult patients. Crit Care 2018;22(1):71.

26. Rochwerg B, Granton D, Wang DX, et al. High flow nasal cannula compared with conventional oxygen therapy for acute hypoxemic respiratory failure: a systematic review and meta-analysis. Intensive Care Med 2019;45(5):563–72.

27. Levy SD, Alladina JW, Hibbert KA, et al. High-flow oxygen therapy and other inhaled therapies in intensive care units. Lancet 2016;387(10030):1867–78.

28. Frat JP, Thille AW, Mercat A, et al. High-flow oxygen through nasal cannula in acute hypoxemic respiratory failure. N Engl J Med 2015;372(23):2185–96.

29. Hernández G, Vaquero C, Colinas L, et al. Effect of postextubation high-flow nasal cannula vs noninvasive ventilation on reintubation and postextubation respiratory failure in high-risk patients: a randomized clinical trial. JAMA 2016; 316(15):1565–74.

30. Ferreyro BL, Angriman F, Munshi L, et al. Association of noninvasive oxygenation strategies with all-cause mortality in adults with acute hypoxemic respiratory failure: a systematic review and meta-analysis. JAMA 2020;324(1):57–67.

31. Maroko PR, Radvany P, Braunwald E, et al. Reduction of infarct size by oxygen inhalation following acute coronary occlusion. Circulation 1975;52(3):360–8.

32. Hofmann R, James SK, Jernberg T, et al. Oxygen therapy in suspected acute myocardial infarction. N Engl J Med 2017;377(13):1240–9.

33. Chu DK, Kim LHY, Young PJ, et al. Mortality and morbidity in acutely ill adults treated with liberal versus conservative oxygen therapy (IOTA): a systematic review and meta-analysis. Lancet 2018;391(10131):1693–705.

34. Roffe C, Nevatte T, Sim J, et al. Effect of routine low-dose oxygen supplementation on death and disability in adults with acute stroke: the stroke oxygen study randomized clinical trial. JAMA 2017;318(12):1125–35.

35. Siemieniuk RAC, Chu DK, Kim LHY, et al. Oxygen therapy for acutely ill medical patients: a clinical practice guideline. BMJ 2018;363:k4169.

36. ICU-ROX Investigators and the Australian and New Zealand Intensive Care Society Clinical Trials Group, Mackle D, Bellomo R, et al. Conservative oxygen therapy during mechanical ventilation in the ICU. N Engl J Med 2020;382(11):989–98.

37. Barrot L, Asfar P, Mauny F, et al. Liberal or conservative oxygen therapy for acute respiratory distress syndrome. N Engl J Med 2020;382(11):999–1008.

38. Schjørring OL, Klitgaard TL, Perner A, et al. Lower or higher oxygenation targets for acute hypoxemic respiratory failure. N Engl J Med 2021;384(14):1301–11.

39. Helmerhorst HJ, Schultz MJ, van der Voort PH, et al. Self-reported attitudes versus actual practice of oxygen therapy by ICU physicians and nurses. Ann Intensive Care 2014;4:23.

40. Trial Group SRLF. Hypoxemia in the ICU: prevalence, treatment, and outcome. Ann Intensive Care 2018;8(1):82.

41. Echevarria C, Steer J, Wason J, et al. Oxygen therapy and inpatient mortality in COPD exacerbation. Emerg Med J 2021;38(3):170–7.

42. Rudd KE, Johnson SC, Agesa KM, et al. Global, regional, and national sepsis incidence and mortality, 1990-2017: analysis for the Global Burden of Disease Study. Lancet 2020;395(10219):200–11.

43. Murthy S, Adhikari NK. Global health care of the critically ill in low-resource settings. Ann Am Thorac Soc 2013;10(5):509–13.

44. Bellani G, Laffey JG, Pham T, et al. Epidemiology, patterns of care, and mortality for patients with acute respiratory distress syndrome in intensive care units in 50 Countries. JAMA 2016;315(8):788–800.

45. Stein F, Perry M, Banda G, et al. Oxygen provision to fight COVID-19 in sub-Saharan Africa. BMJ Glob Health 2020;5(6). https://doi.org/10.1136/bmjgh-2020-002786.

46. Riviello ED, Kiviri W, Twagirumugabe T, et al. Hospital incidence and outcomes of the acute respiratory distress syndrome using the kigali modification of the berlin definition. Am J Respir Crit Care Med 2016;193(1):52–9.

47. Kwizera A, Nakibuuka J, Nakiyingi L, et al. Acute hypoxaemic respiratory failure in a low-income country: a prospective observational study of hospital prevalence and mortality. BMJ Open Respir Res 2020;7(1). https://doi.org/10.1136/bmjresp-2020-000719.

48. Kayambankadzanja RK, Schell CO, Mbingwani I, et al. Unmet need of essential treatments for critical illness in Malawi. PLoS One 2021;16(9):e0256361.

49. Belle J, Cohen H, Shindo N, et al. Influenza preparedness in low-resource settings: a look at oxygen delivery in 12 African countries. J Infect Dev Ctries 2010;4(7):419–24.

50. Duke T, Wandi F, Jonathan M, et al. Improved oxygen systems for childhood pneumonia: a multihospital effectiveness study in Papua New Guinea. The Lancet 2008;372(9646):1328–33.

51. Graham HR, Bakare AA, Ayede AI, et al. Oxygen systems to improve clinical care and outcomes for children and neonates: a stepped-wedge cluster-randomised trial in Nigeria. Plos Med 2019;16(11):e1002951.

52. Duke T, Graham SM, Cherian MN, et al. Oxygen is an essential medicine: a call for international action. Int J Tuberc Lung Dis 2010;14(11):1362–8.

53. Foran M, Ahn R, Novik J, et al. Prevalence of undiagnosed hypoxemia in adults and children in an under-resourced district hospital in Zambia. Int J Emerg Med 2010;3(4):351–6.

54. Evans HGT, Mahmood N, Fullerton DG, et al. Oxygen saturations of medical inpatients in a Malawian hospital: cross-sectional study of oxygen supply and demand. Pneumonia (Nathan) 2012;1:3–6.

55. Tuti T, Aluvaala J, Akech S, et al. Pulse oximetry adoption and oxygen orders at paediatric admission over 7 years in Kenya: a multihospital retrospective cohort study. BMJ Open 2021;11(9):e050995.

56. Sutherland T, Moriau V, Niyonzima JM, et al. The "Just right" amount of oxygen. Improving oxygen Use in a Rwandan emergency department. Ann Am Thorac Soc 2019;16(9):1138–42.

57. McCollum ED, Mvalo T, Eckerle M, et al. Bubble continuous positive airway pressure for children with high-risk conditions and severe pneumonia in Malawi: an open label, randomised, controlled trial. Lancet Respir Med 2019;7(11):964–74.

58. Maitland K, Kiguli S, Olupot-Olupot P, et al. Randomised controlled trial of oxygen therapy and high-flow nasal therapy in African children with pneumonia. Intensive Care Med 2021;47(5):566–76.

59. Ahonkhai AA, Musa AZ, Fenton AA, et al. The CircumVent Project: a CPAP/O2 helmet solution for non-invasive ventilation using an implementation research framework. Implement Sci Commun 2021;2(1):93.

60. Skrip L, Derra K, Kaboré M, et al. Clinical management and mortality among COVID-19 cases in sub-Saharan Africa: a retrospective study from Burkina Faso and simulated case analysis. Int J Infect Dis 2020;101:194–200.

61. PATH. COVID-19 oxygen needs tracker. Available at: https://www.path.org/
   programs/market-dynamics/covid-19-oxygen-needs-tracker/. Accessed March
   8, 2022.
62. World Health Organization. The access to COVID-19 tools (ACT) accelerator.
   Available at: https://www.who.int/initiatives/act-accelerator. Accessed March 4,
   2022.
63. United States Agency for International Development (USAID). Usaid ASSIS-
   TANCE to Tajikistan for the COVID-19 CRISIS. Available at: https://www.usaid.
   gov/sites/default/files/documents/2021_10_USAID_Assistance_to_Tajikistan_for_
   the_COVID-19_Crisis_Fact_Sheet.pdf. Accessed March 6, 2022.

Telemedicine to Expand Access to Critical Care Around the World

Krishnan Ganapathy, M Ch (Neurosurgery), FICS, FACS, FAMS, PhD[a],*,
Sai Praveen Haranath, MBBS, MPH, FCCP[b],
Amado Alejandro Baez, MD, MPH, PhD, FCCM[c,d],
Benjamin K. Scott, MD[e]

KEYWORDS

- Tele-intensive care • Tele-critical care • Tele-ICU • COVID and tele-critical care
- Disasters and tele-critical care • India and cross-border tele-critical care
- Telemedicine and critical care • Telemedicine and intensive care

KEY POINTS

- Tele-critical care makes available remote, rapid, cost-effective technology-enabled intensive care in deprived areas. International, cross-border tele-critical care bridging time zones with the assured standard of care is now commonplace.
- COVID-19 pandemic, natural disasters, and wars have resulted in widespread adoption of tele-critical care.
- Tele-critical care requires transparent communication with hardware, software, and connectivity as three important components.
- Barriers in implementing tele-critical care solutions include regulatory policies, compensation structures, network infrastructure costs, and cybersecurity vulnerabilities.
- More research on Tele-Critical implementation and outcomes is required to develop best-practice guidelines, certification, standardization of processes, and clinical training paradigms.

INTRODUCTION

Tele-intensive care units (T-ICU) aim at making available critical care capabilities remotely, using technology. Worldwide, there is an acute shortage of intensivists.

[a] Apollo Telemedicine Networking Foundation, 23 Greames Road, Chennai 600006, India;
[b] Apollo eACCESS TeleICU, Apollo Health City, Jubilee Hills, Hyderabad, TG 500 033, India;
[c] Medical College of Georgia, 1120 15th Street, Augusta, GA 30912, USA; [d] Universidad Nacional Pedro Henriquez Ureña (UNPHU), Avenue John F. Kennedy 1/2, Santo Domingo, Dominican Republic; [e] University of Colorado School of Medicine, Mail Stop B113 Leprino Building, 12401 East 17th Place, Aurora, CO 80045, USA
* Corresponding author.
E-mail address: drganapathy@apollohospitals.com

Crit Care Clin 38 (2022) 809–826
https://doi.org/10.1016/j.ccc.2022.06.007
0749-0704/22/© 2022 Elsevier Inc. All rights reserved.
criticalcare.theclinics.com

Concurrently there has been an unprecedented, exponential growth of audio-visual communication and monitoring systems. Distance has become meaningless. The COVID pandemic has demonstrated that bridging the urban–rural health divide in critical care is eminently doable. With 15% of ICU beds in the United States participating in telemedicine programs, tele-critical care (TCC) seems to have come of age.[1–3] Global TeleICU market will reach USD 7.39 billion by 2027.[4] An intensivist in a Telemedicine-enabled "command center" can remotely monitor patients in smaller suburban or rural areas.[5] Tele-intensivists providing care from points of convenience (eg, home, office mobile devices), rather than from a centralized hub, have the highest impact.[6] T-ICU's have reduced expenditure, ICU/ventilator days, and mortality, improving care, quality, and safety.[7] Reports from India demonstrate that T-ICU is no longer confined to developed countries.[8–10]

HISTORY

As early as 1977, Grundy reported using Telemedicine in critical care.[11] In 1982 Grundy reported on 1548 Telemedicine "visits" made to 395 patients physically located in various states.[12] In 2000, investigators at Johns Hopkins, during a 16-week trial of 24-h remote ICU care showed a reduction in ICU and hospital mortality by 60 and 30%.[13] Stimulus for growth of T-ICU in United States was the Leapfrog Group recommendations in 2000. From 2003 to 2010, hospitals using ICU telemedicine increased from 16 to 213 (0.4% to 4.6% of total) and "Tele ICU beds" from 598 to 5799 (7.9% of total beds). In 2004, 20% of 5 million Americans admitted annually to ICUs died.[14] During the pandemic, Karnataka a state in India established a dedicated command center for critical care support, linking ICUs of COVID-19 hospitals on to a single platform.[15] The first international T-ICU service for hospitals in the United States, from Chennai, India was established in 2010.32,000 h of remote monitoring and consultative services covering 50 hospitals have been carried out.[7]

TELE-CRITICAL CARE SET UP

The key to effective TCC is transparent communication as in aviation practices. This requires state-of-the-art hardware, effective software, and ancillary devices, ensuring seamless transfer of patient data from bedside to provider. Various models have evolved, with advances in telecommunications technology. Legacy systems using dial-up modems have given way to wireless, high-speed two-way audio and video interfaces. The components of a basic T-ICU are given in **Table 1**.

Hardware is a major component, hosting equipment to communicate, enter, retrieve information, and perform audiovisual interaction. Software operates medical, logistic, and communication components. The third constituent is a connectivity network for broadband through an intranet/VPN or the internet. There is a need for data storage in physical or cloud format, power systems with backup power, and disaster mode requirements for downtime procedures and business continuity. Most TCC systems are now real time, enabling subspecialty teleconsultations. Remotely located data are reviewed by the teleconsultant at a convenient time.

T-ICU systems need patient data interfaces, including manually bedside-measured vital signs, and automated transfer of physiologic parameters to Electronic Medical Records. This information is securely visible to the remote command center provider. Electrocardiograms and other physiological waveforms are visible using a direct interface to the central monitor. Web-based systems also allow access to individual monitors eg the General Electric MUSE software. Bandwidth, earlier a challenge is now available inexpensively. 4 Mbps can handle most system requirements. Ensuring

Table 1
Components for a basic or advanced tele-critical care system

Component	Hardware	Software	Connectivity
Essential	• Computer systems (Desktop/laptop/tablet/ mobile device) • AV devices including traditional phones/ internet telephones/ headphones/fixed cameras or cart based cameras	• Proprietary/legacy hospital electronic medical record • Alert systems • Data storage on site/ cloud based • Firewall/cybersecurity	• Redundant systems • At least 4 Mbps bandwidth • Virtual Private Network
Optional	• On site servers • Remote monitoring devices linked to command center directly	Newer modular options for analytics	• Always-on video systems
Future Trends	• Minimal footprint computer systems • Contactless monitoring devices	• Open source software • Advanced artificial intelligence/machine learning • Metaverse	• 5G • IOT-based systems • Virtual presence

network speeds implies planning for increased capacity. A redundant access system used for connectivity increases system reliability.

Newer TCC systems simplify processes by using *off-the-shelf* components like webcams, tablet-based AV connectivity, and video-based monitor review. These systems, though lacking the safety and security of traditional hard-wired enclosed networks, were more deployable during the pandemic. The National Emergency TeleCritical Care Network (NETCCN) system in the United States was developed for rapid deployment during times of disaster and has been used for patient care.[16] Examples of a typical T-ICU setup are shown in **Figs. 1–4**.

Use of Emerging Technologies in Tele-Critical Care

As chips are getting smaller, faster, and more efficient there is great excitement and optimism. Fiberoptic cables and 5G technology have increased the possibility of providing advanced critical care in real time. Interfaces like FaceTime display reasonable fidelity of ultrasound images, with rapidly-trained bedside providers performing an acceptable study.[17] The ubiquitous nature of artificial intelligence (AI) applications has impacted health care. Algorithms identify and label endotracheal tubes on chest x-ray images and predict COVID 19 mortality.[18] Multiple early warning scores of patient deterioration generate automated alerts and trigger a rapid response.

Computer vision and contactless monitoring simplifies patient physical interaction. Using photo-plethysmography, oxygen saturation can be measured. Small wearables to collect cardiac rhythms and other vitals have been developed. Processing terabytes of data generated from the ICU is an active research area. AI has been used to troubleshoot ventilator waveform graphics.

The future of critical care is without boundaries—real and figurative. Patients can become critically ill in any location. TCC can be instantaneously deployed due to its virtual nature. There are anecdotal illustrations of remote domiciliary critical care

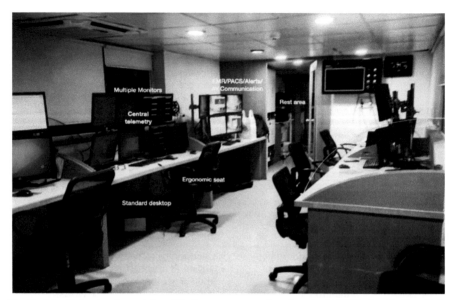

Fig. 1. A typical setup for a tele-critical care command center at eACCESS, Apollo Hospitals, Hyderabad, India. (*Courtesy* of Sai Haranath, MBBS, MPH, FCCP, Telangana, India.)

with remote home monitoring from a command center. The overarching principle of avoiding harm and maximizing benefit has driven innovation to expand the breadth and scope of remote critical care. The process is in its infancy from a global perspective but will remove inequity existing in critical care expertise availability.

Training and Retraining of Consultants, Residents, and Nurses for Running a Tele Intensive Care Unit

Despite agreement that TCC is most effective when clinicians have specific training and competencies, in use of virtual technologies, there is little published research on this topic.[19,20] Descriptions of clinical training in TCC originate primarily from nursing literature. In a 2011 survey of T-ICU programs, Goran[21] found that 85% of those surveyed were using a formal process for orientation, training, and ongoing assessment of core competencies in TCC nursing. This was despite the paucity of professional practice guidelines available at the time. Communication skills,

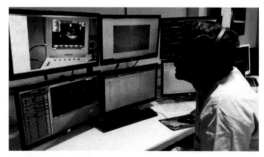

Fig. 2. Viewing remote ultrasound. (*From* Haranath SP, Ganapathy K, Kesavarapu SR, Kuragayala SD. eNeuroIntensive Care in India: The Need of the Hour. Neurol India. 2021;69(2):245–251. doi:10.4103/0028-3886.314591; with permission.)

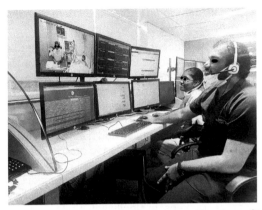

Fig. 3. Interacting with remote ICU from command center. (*Courtesy of* Sai Haranath, MBBS, MPH, FCCP, Telangana, India.)

collaborative decision-making, and effective use of telemedicine tools and technologies were considered. The American Association of Critical Care Nurses created the CCRN-E, a specialty nursing certification for nurses providing TCC.[22] Certification requires a clinical practice component and a certifying examination. As of January 2022, nearly 500 registered nurses have been certified through this pathway in the United States.[23]

For physicians, training is likely to be *ad hoc* and on-the-job. In 2021 the Association of American Medical Colleges released a report describing "Telehealth Competencies Across the Learning Continuum".[24] In both the United States and United Kingdom, several groups have reported successful implementation of structured telemedicine skills curricula.[25,26]

For those in practice, the American Telemedicine Association offers certificate training in Telehealth (https://www.americantelemed.org/resource).[27] The National Consortium of Telehealth Resource Centers (https://telehealthresourcecenter.org)[28] and professional societies such as The Society of Critical Care Medicine (SCCM; https://www.sccm.org/Clinical-Resources/Disaster/COVID19/Telemedicine-and-COVID-19)[29] offer informal guidance and educational resources but more formal practice guidelines and assessment strategies are needed.

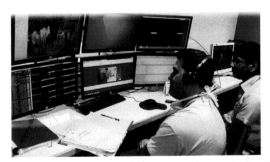

Fig. 4. Interacting with remote ICU. (*From* Haranath SP, Ganapathy K, Kesavarapu SR, Kuragayala SD. eNeuroIntensive Care in India: The Need of the Hour. Neurol India. 2021;69(2):245–251. doi:10.4103/0028-3886.314591; with permission.)

Policy and Regulatory Challenges in Interstate and International Deployment of Tele-Crictical Care Services

COVID-19 has necessitated the acceptance and utilization of telemedicine.[30] However, existing policy, regulatory, and financial barriers have proven challenging due to the paucity of well-established definitions, practice guidelines, and standards of care. In the United States, medical licensing and legal liability are regulated by state governments. Medical privileging and credentialing are administered at the local level. The US Centers for Medicare and Medicaid Services, which sets standards recognized by private insurance companies and health systems, requires that medical professionals be licensed and credentialed to practice at a physician's physical location. Limited opportunities exist for credentialling-by-proxy arrangements between health systems. Interstate medical licensing compacts have been adopted by only half of all states. Legal precedents to guide TCC services are limited. Obtaining malpractice coverage remains a significant obstacle to providing interstate TCC.[31]

Despite significant cost reductions in technology and tools required, provision of TCC services, parallelly using large centralized hub-and-spoke care-delivery models, remains expensive.[32,33] In the United States, no specific billing codes are available to offset TCC services. Fees for critical care services still require physical presence. TCC programs have demonstrated labor-savings compared with in-person coverage. Improvements in quality, safety, and efficiency of care have been documented.[34] Many services charge what amounts to a subscription fee for coverage, but alternative compensation strategies would improve uptake.

During the pandemic, emergency waivers were granted, allowing billing of critical care codes using telemedicine. Many states and localities simplified and expedited licensing and credentialing processes. Many TCC programs initially elected to defer billing for their expanded services, in part due to pervasive uncertainty about the duration of the emergency conditions.[35–37]

International delivery of TCC is complicated. Although the World Health Organization and the United Nations' International Telecommunications Union have made efforts to improve interoperability and access to mobile health, little formal guidance or international law is available regarding TCC.[38] Licensing, credentialing, and compensation are generally dependent on ad-hoc arrangements. Most deployments have involved either circadian-concordant ICU coverage by US-trained physicians living abroad, or limited volunteer services provided during disasters.[9,39] Pandemic-induced temporary volunteer deployments could weaken foundations for future necessary regulations.

International Cross Border Tele-Critical Care: a Perspective from India

Cross-border remote critical care was an uncommon use of technology in critical care, until 2010. The United States has a large requirement for critical care, as many institutions followed the Leapfrog group recommendations for staffing.[40] Commencing in Baltimore,[41] the concept expanded, necessitating the need for after-hours coverage and expanded resources.[42] Simultaneously another social factor was in a play where critical care providers trained, licensed, board-certified, and credentialed in various US states, were moving back to their home countries-primarily Israel and India. Entrepreneurs in both countries quickly designed safe, secure, and profitable businesses that provided remote critical care to the United States, in the same manner as a TCC provider in the United States would function. Different time zones created a workforce primarily working during *their* daytime. *On-call* provider shortages have been a long-standing problem. This virtual model overcomes supply problems as well as issues of night, weekend, and holiday coverage. 5000 ICU patients are probably being monitored nightly from overseas. These systems should be studied to understand logistics, challenges, and opportunities.

CASE STUDIES—ILLUSTRATIONS

It has been the experience of the authors from India that many ICU emergencies and management dealt with remotely are not reported. These include post-cardiac arrest resuscitation, management of sepsis, septic shock, hemorrhagic shock, respiratory failure, cardiac emergencies, postoperative care as well as clinical trials.

ILLUSTRATIONS

A 79-year-old woman was admitted with pancreatitis in a small suburban hospital with limited services in India. She was revived following a cardiac arrest and was subsequently evaluated remotely. A diagnosis of hemorrhagic conversion of pancreatitis was made. Immediate lab work confirmed severe anemia and blood product resuscitation advised. Transfer to an advanced center was initiated. Communication with bedside teams at both locations, close follow-up of pending tests and regular updates ensured advanced level care, even before being shifted. At the same time, a call was received from another ICU discussing arterial blood gas values in a patient with acute respiratory failure, secondary to pneumonia. Adjustment of the noninvasive ventilator was viewed on camera and immediate feedback was obtained on the changes made. In a typical 12-h shift, a teleconsultant may have 30 interactions. This varies widely depending on day, time, unit capacity, hospital features, and staff engagement with the Tele-ICU.

DOMINICAN REPUBLIC COVID-19 TELE-INTENSIVE CARE UNIT—ILLUSTRATIONS

On March 31, 2020, the Dominican presidency (Decree 140–20) created the Presidential COVID-19 Committee and tasked it with creating public–private partnerships (PPP) as well as developing public policy, strategies, and operations to combat COVID-19 at a national level. The committee, on April 5, 2020, presented a comprehensive technology utilization, hospital capacity augmentation, and test–trace–treat strategy with a focus on strengthening local government capacities via PPP including ICU capacity augmentation *via* use of telematic technologies.[43]

The Tele-ICU Project was developed as a capacity-building and force-multiplying effort to support hospitals with basic ICUs but lacked human resources. An initial data-driven needs assessment noted that access gaps existed in health services outside of Santo Domingo (the capital) and Santiago (second largest city). Rural municipalities referred patients to these two cities, creating an unwanted additional surge that overwhelmed care services. Referrals could have been handled in a regional hospital, with a simplified training solution and TCC provided by urban intensivists. The Dominican Republic Tele-ICU Project sought to improve the quality, diagnosis, and treatment of COVID-19, by connecting subject matter experts in provincial hospitals to medical centers having advanced ICUs. The Dominican health system improved the reference pathway and flow of COVID-19 patients to health care centers of higher levels. Through this first-of-a-kind initiative, doctors were able to share *via* teleconference, best practices proving their effectiveness. A total of 2500 nurses and general/primary care physicians were trained in principles of critical care, via a 10-h, 3-day program using the Society for Critical Care Medicine COVID-19 resources.

In September 2020 the first Dominican TeleICU project was launched using a crowdfunding model. This comprised 14 donors, belonging to the Council of Directors of the Dominican Republic American Chamber of Commerce who contributed to the development of the Project. This was the first example of effective health-related crowdfunding. Private sector support guaranteed the care continuum for patients requiring medical specialists expanding their coverage virtually, facilitating the second opinion for difficult cases. This pilot project is led by the Ministry of Public Health, National Health Service (SNS), and the Emergency and Sanitary Management Committee for the fight against COVID-19. This T-ICU project demonstrated the effectiveness of PPP with alliances between local government and private entities. Working from a local perspective, entrepreneurs worked to control the pandemic and keep their employees healthy.

Illustrations from Haiti: On August 14, 2021, a 7.2 magnitude earthquake rattled the nation, killing 2200 and leaving thousands of Haitians injured, in need of assistance. In addition to casualties, 66 health facilities were damaged or destroyed, placing an impossible burden on an already fragile health care system.[44] Haiti is the poorest country in the Western Hemisphere. Even before the earthquake, there were drastic health inequities, limited access to care, and a shortage of physicians and nurses. Further impediments included the assassination of Haiti's President Jovenel Moïse before the earthquake, civil unrest, government instability, and the pandemic. Parts of Haiti are still recovering from the 2010 earthquake (250,000 deaths).[45]

With the Society for Critical Care Medicine, an ICU capacity-building program was developed for Haiti. The goals of the project were to (a) optimize human resources in acute and critical care, responding to patients affected by the earthquake directly or indirectly (b) improve referral system to higher-level care centers to decongest the existing health system. This pilot, included implementation of a virtual Fundamental Critical Care Support course (16 h) directed to general nursing staff and nonintensivist physicians, thus providing working ICU knowledge. This program empowered the University Hospital in Mirebalais to care for critically ill patients remotely, limiting patients sent to bigger referral hospitals in Port-au-Prince. Using an inexpensive web-based Health Insurance Portability and Accountability Act (HIPAA) compliant platform, Haiti-National ICU physicians living outside of Haiti provided T-ICU support to their compatriots remotely.

Earthquakes are catalysts for technological solutions.[46] Before the earthquake, Haiti needed this project. During the pandemic, critically ill patients needed a higher level of care. This project is catalyzing change based on immediate needs. Developing nations like Haiti, with inadequate critical care services, can use this model.

CASE STUDY: UNITED STATES AND INTERNATIONAL TELE-CRITICAL CARE

In the early months of the pandemic, in response to unprecedented strain on critical care resources, the Army's Center for Telemedicine and Advanced Technology Research partnered with the Society of Critical Care Medicine (SCCM), the office of the Assistant Secretary for Preparedness and Response (ASPR) and the Medical Technology Enterprise Consortium (MTEC) to develop an all-hazards NETCCN. Through a competitive funding process, multi-organizational teams were asked to design and build a lightweight, rapidly deployable platform for the delivery of TCC services to any bedside, temporary hospital, or home, using any web-enabled device at the point of care. The minimum viable product would meet cybersecurity and patient privacy standards, and provide synchronous and asynchronous communication tools, a basic electronic medical record system, and a patient cohorting and triage system for the creation of scalable virtual wards. Three teams were then selected for clinical pilot deployments and an additional team to provide logistics and dashboarding support. Over the next year, in response to successive regional COVID surges, NETCCN provided care to hundreds of patients in 61 sites across 18 US states and one US territory, including many critical access hospitals without local critical care capability. Results are being analyzed. Future directions for the program include participation in a national disaster medicine data commons, incorporation of autonomous and remotely controlled medical devices through the Technology in Disaster Environments program, and potential integration with other emergency systems such as the Regional Disaster Health Response System and the National Disaster Medical System.[47]

INDIA AND INTERNATIONAL TELE-CRITICAL CARE

India and Israel were the initial hubs for international TCC. With more intensivists moving out of the United States, this has expanded to other countries. India has a unique time-zone advantage. The high-intensity work of TCC requires strict standards of quality, safety, and system security. In an analogous fashion, a few providers in India began TCC. Initially, these included monitoring of distant hospitals in their own health system. Subsequently, pilot programs and, later, commercial contracts with smaller hospitals in near and distant locations, were initiated. Difficulty in convincing hospitals to adopt a TCC program and making it a viable business proposition remain the biggest barriers to widespread adoption.

The pandemic has allowed many models of TCC to be used. Expansion of existing systems to cover broader geography, as well as a greater range of serious clinical conditions, was noted. As hospitals increased bed capacity, TCC programs adapted, by simplifying documentation requirements, to focus on patient care. As patients increased, complexity of care also rose. Managing critically ill COVID patients with ARDS is time-consuming requiring a considerable degree of coordination with bedside teams. The benefit of remote connectivity was seen in virtual *rounding*, a form of "near" tele-CC though beneficiaries were physically distanced.

India now has multiple organizations providing TCC in various formats. Some are focused on, higher volume public sector hospitals; some are focused on internal patients and others are reaching out to remote locations, with overlapping strategies. Given the as yet niche market, processes and protocols are evolving. Effective use of TCC during the pandemic in India showed its doability.[48] eNeurointensive care has also been documented.[6] Traction and calls to action are building, given the clear utility of TCC in resource-constrained settings.[8] In the TELESCOPE trial in Brazil, TCC-based rounding and outcomes are being studied in a cluster-randomized manner.[49] Increased confidence in handling COVID patients using a hybrid model in a US–Mexico set of border hospitals has been documented.[9]

Tele-Critical Care in Disasters

The first large-scale attempt to provide international telemedicine support to disaster victims was in 1989, in the aftermath of the devastating Spitak earthquake in Russian Armenia. A pioneering National Aeronautics and Space Administration-supported "Spacebridge to Armenia" provided telemedicine consultation using a combination of facsimile, two-way audio, and one-way video.[50] In the subsequent decades, a number of programs have provided support for victims of earthquakes, hurricanes, and other disasters using large, centralized command centers, and lightweight distributed mobile health technologies.[51,52]

Continuous growth in computing power, network coverage, and communications bandwidth has normalized transmission of near real-time monitor and electronic health record data and two-way high-fidelity audiovisual communications platforms. These TCC technologies promise rapid, cost-effective, and scalable support, particularly in unexpected resource-strained disaster areas.[53–56] Systems utilizing existing commercially available communications software and web-based or downloadable applications, working on personal devices of any clinician, caregiver, or patient are necessary.[57] These ad-hoc approaches proliferated in response to the pandemic[58–61] and subsequently in response to Russia's 2022 invasion of Ukraine.[62]

As communications tools, TCC programs are well-positioned to provide logistical support before disasters occur. A logical framework for the coordination of disaster simulation exercises, development of formal disaster contingency plans, and establishment of higher-level networking functions between local entities are provided. TCC networks facilitate large-scale training simulations and monitor resource allocation and strategic medical stockpiles. Real-time surveys are done regarding clinical and material resource strains. This information could be combined with other data streams to help predict clinical surges, and rapidly mobilize or shift resources to the point of need, ensuring early dissemination of clinical information. Lessons learned are likely to benefit future patients and care teams.[63]

In addition, TCC support, while focused primarily on managing critically ill or injured patients, helps mitigate numerous knock-on effects that accumulate in the aftermath of a disaster. Tele-triage supports help identify patients, who could be managed at home. This reduces unnecessary transfers, saving hospital beds. During the pandemic, numerous TCC programs participated in home monitoring of infected and chronically ill patients, minimizing patient transfer.[64–67]

Excepting pandemics, most large-scale disasters are likely to disrupt the communications infrastructure basis of TCC platforms. Allocating bandwidth for emergency response systems and design of drop-in mobile ad-hoc networks and satellite-based internet systems reduce the impact of legacy communications disruptions.[68–71] A second looming threat involves the weaponization of information technologies and increased risks to patient privacy and cybersecurity. This accompanies moves toward distributed systems–especially in the context of war or disaster. Block-chain or other encryption technologies may provide adequate information security.[72,73]

How COVID-19 Changed the Role of Telemedicine in Critical Care

T-ICU is a telemedicine application that has gained strength recently. The objective is to integrate critical care units with intensivists providing highly specialized remote services to centers without trained personnel.[74–77] The main driver for T-ICU is evidence supporting the positive impact of the "intensivist" model. T-ICU is a cost-effective tool that successfully addresses access and level of care opportunities, through efficient resource allocation.[78,79] Telemedicine enables the exchange of knowledge between teams, as well as the training and education of multidisciplinary teams. With advances in medical care, the number of critical patients has been increasing significantly. This affects day-bed occupancy in critical care units.[47,80–82] Despite the use of digital technology, telemedicine deployment had been low before the pandemic. Benefits for institutions implementing a care system based on T-ICU is shown in **Box 1**.

The pandemic has had a devastating impact on global health. Traditionally, public health emergencies expose health system challenges and opportunities. Telehealth has been proposed and utilized as a solution in various health specialties. It is particularly suited for scenarios in which access to care is challenging, such as in rural areas with limited resources. Telehealth can help manage the surge in various conditions

---

Box 1
Benefits of tele-intensive care unit

- Increased survival indicators
- Decrease in referrals
- Efficient bed rotation/utilization, ensuring greater coverage
- Caring for a greater number of patients
- Significant cost reduction

---

and help improve the quality diagnosis and treatment of COVID-19. T-ICU can ensure retention with remote support and help triage appropriate patients to higher levels of care.

Hospitals had to address various multiple components of critical care capacity. Significant disparities already existed in the distribution of access to critical care expertise across the world. In developing countries, patients far exceeded available ICU beds.[83–87] This surge required hospitals to expand capacity and implement tiered staffing models. Physicians without formal critical care training were often caring for severely ill patients, including those mechanically ventilated. For COVID-19, telemedicine has been utilized for same-site care to conserve health care resources such as personal protective equipment. Same-site telemedicine ensured safe and high-quality patient care while maintaining social distancing to minimize virus spread. For remote site care, T-ICU has been utilized to augment the workforce, reducing unnecessary referrals and optimizing level of care in underserved areas as shown in **Table 2**.[88–92]

With telemedicine, physicians and nurses can maintain continuity of patient care, simultaneously triaging patients preparing for an anticipated case backlog, after crisis abatement. From a pandemic perspective, T-ICU programs have been implemented to appropriately allocate resources and prevent virus exposure while maintaining safe and effective patient care. In disasters and large emergency scenarios, from a utilitarian perspective for COVID-19 and non-COVID 19 cases, T-ICU can be used for ethical/triage decisions. When there is a high probability of morbidity, a T-ICU consult can be used for resource allocation and palliative care decision-making. Resource utilization could be optimized favoring patients with a higher probability of survival.[93]

Table 2
Tele-ICU Applications during the pandemic

Same Site Applications	Remote Site Applications	Remote Site Applications
1. Personal Protective Equipment Conservation	1. Human Capacity Force Multiplier	2. Intensive Care Specialist Availability
2. Physical Distancing tool	3. Other Specialist Consultant availability	4. Rural/Resource Limited Hospital Support
3. Family Access/ Consultation	5. Tele-Education/Quality Assurance (QA)/Quality Improvement (QI)	6. Health System Triage/ Transfer tool
4. Specialist Consultant Protection	7. ICU Resource Conservation	8. Triage at initial remote site
	9. Dissemination of information to health care teams, and to the general population	10. From triage to Providing patient care

The pandemic has provided immense opportunities for telehealth and telemedicine solutions. Telemedicine services have become a critical asset, with important implications across the whole health care delivery continuum. Telemedicine offers several advantages, especially in nonurgent/routine care and situations where services do not require direct provider-patient interaction. This reduces resource use, improves access to care, and minimizes risk of person-to-person transmission of the infectious agent. In addition, telemedicine solution providers can remotely identify patients requiring further care, using tailored approaches. Telemedicine is a powerful monitoring and coordinating tool ensuring appropriate use of provider facilities. It covers a greater number of patients in remote areas who have no access to specialists or ICU beds. Telemedicine is a safe and efficient care modality with levels of acceptance and improvement of quality of care, now proven worldwide.

SUMMARY

COVID-19 has turned the world upside down. The exponential deployment of communication technology in making available critical care is a global phenomenon. Wireless miniaturization of equipment and real-time remote monitoring has significantly reduced the time for clinical decisions. Training, retraining, and relearning for nurses, residents, and consultants working in T-ICUs have started. Interstate and international deployment of TCC services has led to policy, regulatory, and reimbursement challenges. Interestingly, TCC is an organizational innovation rather than a clinical or technological advance.[94] Resource-intensive and expensive critical care accounts for 15% of hospital costs in the United States (1% of US gross domestic product).[95] Hopefully with TCC, this will significantly come down. The optimal "dose" of remote providers appears to be one nurse per 30 to 35 ICU beds and one intensivist for 100 to 130 patients.[96]

THE FUTURE

With Telehealth eventually becoming the new normal, smart hospitals of the future will be restricted to carrying out complex procedures and handling serious trauma. Specialized ICU's may constitute 40 to 50% of standalone beds in single-specialty hospitals. Alternatively, with location becoming irrelevant, any bed may be converted into a virtual critical care bed. Multispecialty teleconsultants will be virtually available 24/7. A "lab/doctor" in your pocket will be a reality. Noninvasive sensors and breath analysis will simplify wireless telemonitoring. Miniaturized extracorporeal membrane oxygenation and extracorporeal CO_2 removal devices will reduce the need for mechanical ventilation.[97] Personalized, patient-centric, technology-enabled, remote intensive care will be commonplace. The T-ICU market in 2028 is expected to reach USD 5 billion with a compound annual growth rate of 17.64% over the previous years.[98] With a manned mission to Mars possibly occurring by the end of the decade, extending TCC to space may not be science fiction.[99,100]

CLINICS CARE POINTS

- Lung dynamics such as plateau pressure and evaluation of autoPEEP using ventilator graphics is preferably evaluated with a respiratory therapist As in face-to-face care, the bedside team verbally repeating the order given by the remote teleconsultant will ensure accuracy.

- Time zone differences is helpful in utilizing remote critical care services. Formally ending a shift and starting shift handover is helpful.

- Immediate communication between the bedside team and the remote monitoring team is critical, whenever there is a change in clinical condition or parameters monitored.
- Sepsis reassessment and evaluation of perfusion parameters like lactic acid can be done through remote care assistance.
- Evidence based best practices including DVT (deep venous thrombosis) prophylaxis, stress ulcer prophylaxis, early appropriate antibiotic use when indicated and head of bed elevation. These can be remotely instituted and monitored.

ACKNOWLEDGMENTS

Ms. Lakshmi rendered secretarial assistance

DISCLOSURE

The authors confirm that no competing financial interests exist and there are nil source(s) of support in the form of grants, equipment, etc.

REFERENCES

1. Caples SM. Intensive care unit telemedicine care models. Crit Care Clin 2019; 35:479–82.
2. Becker C, Frishman WH, Scurlock C. Telemedicine and Tele-ICU: the evolution and differentiation of a new medical field. Am J Med 2016;129:e333–4.
3. Davis TM, Barden C, Dean S, et al. American telemedicine association guidelines for TeleICU operations. Telemed J E Health 2016;22:971–80.
4. The Rise of tele-ICU. In: RemoteICU. 2020. Available at: https://www.remoteicu.com/blog/tele-hospitalist/the-rise-of-teleicu/. Accessed April 06, 2022.
5. Guinemer C, Boeker M, Weiss B, et al. Telemedicine in intensive care units: protocol for a scoping review. JMIR Res Protoc 2020;9:e19695.
6. McLeroy RD, Ingersoll J, Nielsen P, et al. Implementation of tele-critical care at general leonard wood army community hospital. Mil Med 2020;185:e191–6.
7. Haranath SP, Ganapathy K, Kesavarapu SR, et al. eNeuroIntensive care in India: the need of the hour. Neurol India 2021;69:245–51.
8. Ramakrishnan N, Vijayaraghavan BK, Venkataraman R. Breaking barriers to reach farther: a call for urgent action on Tele-ICU services. Indian J Crit Care Med 2020;24:393–7.
9. Ramnath VR, Hill L, Schultz J, et al. An In-person and telemedicine "hybrid" system to improve cross-border critical care in COVID-19. Ann Glob Health 2021; 87:1.
10. Sidney Hilker S, Mathias S, Anand S, et al. Operational model to increase intensive care unit telemedicine capacity rapidly during a pandemic: experience in India. Br J Anaesth 2022;128(6):e343–5. https://doi.org/10.1016/j.bja.2022.02.036. Online ahead of print.
11. Grundy BL, Crawford P, Jones PK, et al. Telemedicine in critical care: an experiment in health care delivery. JACEP 1977;6:439–44.
12. Grundy BL, Jones PK, Lovitt A. Telemedicine in critical care: problems in design, implementation, and assessment. Crit Care Med 1982;10:471–5.
13. Rosenfeld BA, Dorman T, Breslow MJ, et al. Intensive care unit telemedicine: alternate paradigm for providing continuous intensivist care. Crit Care Med 2000;28:3925–31.

14. Angus DC, Barnato AE, Linde-Zwirble WT, et al. Robert wood Johnson foundation ICU end-of- Life peer group. Use of intensive care at the end of life in the United States: an epidemiologic study. Crit Care Med 2004;32:638–43.

15. Iyengar K, Garg R, Jain VK, et al. Electronic intensive care unit. Lung India 2021; 38:S97–100.

16. National emergency tele-critical care network - about. In: National emergency tele-critical care network (NETCCN). 2021. Available at: https://www.tatrc.org/netccn/#:~:text=NETCCN%20is%20an%20evolving%20network,to%20use%20and%20readily%20available. Accessed April 06, 2022.

17. Robertson TE, Levine AR, Verceles AC, et al. Remote tele-mentored ultrasound for non-physician learners using FaceTime: a feasibility study in a low-income country. J Crit Care 2017;40:145–8.

18. Kar S, Chawla R, Haranath SP, et al. Multivariable mortality risk prediction using machine learning for COVID-19 patients at admission (AICOVID). Sci Rep 2021; 11:12801.

19. Becker CD, Fusaro MV, Scurlock C. Telemedicine in the ICU: clinical outcomes, economic aspects, and trainee education. Curr Opin Anaesthesiol 2019;32:129–35.

20. Kahn JM, Rak KJ, Kuza CC, et al. Am J Respir Crit Care Med 2019;199:970–9.

21. Goran SF. A new view: tele-intensive care unit competencies. Crit Care Nurse 2011;31:17–29.

22. Davis TM, Barden C, Olff C, et al. Professional accountability in the tele-ICU: the CCRN-E. Crit Care Nurs Q 2012;35:353–6.

23. CCRN-E certificates by state. In: American association of critical-care nurses. 2022. Available at: https://www.aacn.org/certification/get-certified/ccrne-certificants-by-state. Accessed April 06, 2022.

24. Telehealth competencies across the learning continuum series. In: Association of american medical colleges - new and emerging areas in medicine, Washington, DC. 2021. Available at: https://www.aamc.org/what-we-do/mission-areas/medical-education/cbme/competency. Accessed April 06, 2022.

25. Mulcare M, Naik N, Greenwald P, et al. Advanced communication and examination skills in telemedicine: a structured simulation-based course for medical students. MedEdPORTAL 2020;16:11047.

26. Gunner CK, Eisner E, Watson AJ, et al. Teaching webside manner: development and initial evaluation of a video consultation skills training module for undergraduate medical students. Med Educ Online 2021;26:1954492. https://doi.org/10.1080/10872981.2021.1954492.

27. Discover resources - accelerate program implementation & performance. In: American telemedicine association. 2022. Available at: https://www.americantelemed.org/resource. Accessed April 06, 2022.

28. The national Consortium of telehealth resource centers provides trusted consultation, resources & news at No cost to help you plan your experience. In: National consortium of telehealth resource centers. 2022. Available at: https://telehealthresourcecenter.org. Accessed April 06, 2022.

29. Tele-critical care and COVID-19. In: Society of critical care medicine. 2022. Available at: https://www.sccm.org/Clinical-Resources/Disaster/COVID19/Telemedicine-and-COVID-19. Accessed April 06, 2022.

30. Friedman AB, Gervasi S, Song H, et al. Telemedicine catches on: changes in the utilization of telemedicine services during the COVID-19 pandemic. Am J Manag Care 2022;28:e1–6.

31. Subramanian S, Pamplin JC, Hravnak M, et al. Tele-critical care: an update from the society of critical care medicine Tele-ICU committee. Crit Care Med 2020;48: 553–61.
32. Kumar G, Falk DM, Bonello RS, et al. The costs of critical care telemedicine programs: a systematic review and analysis. Chest 2013;143:19–29.
33. Sim I. Mobile devices and health. N Engl J Med 2019;381:956–68.
34. Becker CD, Fusaro MV, Scurlock C. Deciphering factors that influence the value of tele-ICU programs. Intensive Care Med 2019;45:1046–51.
35. Krouss M, Allison MG, Rios S, et al. Rapid implementation of telecritical care support during a pandemic: lessons learned during the coronavirus disease 2020 surge in New York city. Crit Care Explor 2020;2:e0271.
36. Singh J, Green MB, Lindblom S, et al. Telecritical care clinical and operational strategies in response to COVID-19. Telemed J E Health 2021;27:261–8.
37. Chandra S, Hertz C, Khurana H, et al. Collaboration between Tele-ICU programs has the potential to rapidly increase the availability of critical care physicians- our experience was during coronavirus disease 2019 nomenclature. Crit Care Explor 2021;3:e0363.
38. Bhaskar S, Bradley S, Chattu VK, et al. Telemedicine across the globe-position paper from the COVID-19 pandemic health system resilience PROGRAM (REPROGRAM) International Consortium (Part 1). Front Public Health 2020;8: 556720.
39. Moughrabieh A, Weinert C. Rapid deployment of international tele-intensive care unit services in war-torn Syria. Ann Am Thorac Soc 2016;13:165–72.
40. Milstein A, Galvin RS, Delbanco SF, et al. Improving the safety of health care: the leapfrog initiative. Eff Clin Pract 2000;3:313–6.
41. Philips eCareManager. In: Philips professional health care. 2021. Available at: https://www.usa.philips.com/healthcare/product/HC865325CM/ecaremanager-enterprise-telehealth-software. Accessed April 06, 2022.
42. Reynolds HN. The tele-ICU: formative or out-of-date or both? Practice models and future directions. In: Koenig M, editor. Telemedicine in the ICU. Cham: Springer; 2019. p. 3–19.
43. Santo Domingo. Danilo appoints amado alejandro báez as adviser to the executive branch on public health. In: Listin diario. In: .. 2020. Available at: https://listindiario.com/la-republica/2020/03/31/611222/danilo-designa-a-amado-alejandro-baez-como-asesor-del-poder-ejecutivo-en-salud-publica. Accessed April 06, 2022.
44. 2021 Haiti Earthquake situation report #1 - september 1, 2021 – fast facts. In: OCHA Services - reliefweb. 2021. Available at: https://reliefweb.int/report/haiti/2021-haiti-earthquake-situation-report-1-september-1-2021. Accessed April 06, 2022.
45. Juin S, Schaad N, Lafontant D, et al. Strengthening national disease surveillance and response-Haiti, 2010-2015. Am J Trop Med Hyg 2017;97:12–20.
46. Callaway DW, Peabody CR, Hoffman A, et al. Disaster mobile health technology: lessons from Haiti. Prehospital Disaster Med 2012;27:148–52.
47. Pamplin JC, Scott BK, Quinn MT, et al. Technology and disasters: the evolution of the national emergency tele-critical care network. Crit Care Med 2021;49: 1007–14.
48. Haranath SP, Udayasankaran JG. Tele-intensive care unit networks: a viable means for augmenting critical care capacity in India for the COVID pandemic and beyond. Apollo Med 2020;17:209–16.

49. Noritomi DT, Ranzani OT, Ferraz LJR, et al. Telescope trial investigators. Tele-Critical care versus usual care on ICU performance (telescope): protocol for a cluster-randomised clinical trial on adult general ICUs in Brazil. BMJ Open 2021;11:e042302.

50. Houtchens BA, Clemmer TP, Holloway HC, et al. Telemedicine and international disaster response: medical consultation to Armenia and Russia via a Telemedicine Spacebridge. Prehospital Disaster Med 1993;8:57–66.

51. Benner T, Schachinger U, Nerlich M. Telemedicine in trauma and disasters–from war to earthquake: are we ready? Stud Health Technol Inform 2004;104:106–15.

52. Latifi R, Tilley EH. Telemedicine for disaster management: can it transform chaos into an organized, structured care from the distance? Am J Disaster Med 2014; 9:25–37.

53. Scott BK, Miller GT, Fonda SJ, et al. Advanced digital health technologies for COVID-19 and future emergencies. Telemed J E Health 2020;26:1226–33.

54. Ieronimakis KM, Colombo CJ, Valovich J, et al. The trifecta of tele-critical care: intrahospital, operational, and mass casualty applications. Mil Med 2021;186: 253–60.

55. Winterbottom FA. The role of tele-critical care in rescue and resuscitation. Crit Care Nurs Clin North Am 2021;33:357–68.

56. Rolston DM, Meltzer JS. Telemedicine in the intensive care unit: its role in emergencies and disaster management. Crit Care Clin 2015;31:239–55.

57. Lilly CM, Greenberg B. The evolution of Tele-ICU to tele-critical care. Crit Care Med 2020;48:610–1.

58. Webb H, Parson M, Hodgson LE, et al. Virtual visiting and other technological adaptations for critical care. Future Healthc J 2020;7:e93–5.

59. Wittbold KA, Baugh JJ, Yun BJ, et al. iPad deployment for virtual evaluation in the emergency department during the COVID-19 pandemic. Am J Emerg Med 2020;38:2733–4.

60. Barayev E, Shental O, Yaari D, et al. WhatsApp Tele-Medicine – usage patterns and physicians views on the platform. Isr J Health Policy Res 2021;10:34.

61. Khan S, Mallipattu SK. Monitoring hospitalized dialysis patients with COVID-19: repurposing baby monitors for patient and staff safety. Kidney Med 2021;3: 136–8.

62. O'Neill T. US doctors provide free telehealth for Ukrainian soldiers, civilians, refugees. In: New York Post. Available at: https://nypost.com/2022/03/11/us-doctors-provide-free-telehealth-for-ukrainian-soldiers-civilians-refugees/. Accessed April 06, 2022.

63. Litvak M, Miller K, Boyle T, et al. Telemedicine use in disasters: a scoping review. Disaster Med Public Health Preparedness 2021;1–10. https://doi.org/10.1017/dmp.2020.473. Online ahead of print.

64. Adly AS, Adly MS, Adly AS. Telemanagement of home-isolated COVID-19 patients using oxygen therapy with noninvasive positive pressure ventilation and physical therapy techniques: randomized clinical trial. J Med Internet Res 2021;23:e23446.

65. Lukas H, Xu C, Yu Y, et al. Emerging telemedicine tools for remote COVID-19 diagnosis, monitoring, and management. ACS Nano 2020;14:16180–93.

66. Martínez-Riera JR, Gras-Nieto E. Home Care and COVID-19. Before, in and after the state of alarm. Enferm Clin (Engl Ed) 2021;31:S24–8. Spanish.

67. Alsharif AH. Cross sectional E-health evaluation study for telemedicine and M-health approaches in monitoring COVID-19 patients with chronic obstructive pulmonary disease (COPD). Int J Environ Res Public Health 2021;18:8513.

68. Wong A, Chow YT. Solar-supplied satellite internet access point for the internet of things in remote areas. Sensors (Basel) 2020;20:1409. https://doi.org/10.3390/s20051409.

69. Careless J. How FirstNet Will broaden communications. The wireless broadband network will connect police, fire and EMS through mobile devices. EMS World 2015;44:36–7.

70. Guillen-Perez A, Cano MD. Flying Ad Hoc networks: a new domain for network communications. Sensors (Basel) 2018;18:3571. https://doi.org/10.3390/s18103571.

71. Lwin MT, Yim J, Ko YB. Blockchain-based lightweight trust management in mobile Ad-Hoc Networks. Sensors (Basel) 2020;20:698.

72. Al-Hawawreh M, Moustafa N, Slay J. A threat intelligence framework for protecting smart satellite-based healthcare networks. Neural Comput and Applic 2021. https://doi.org/10.1007/s00521-021-06441-5.

73. Santos JA, Inácio PRM, Silva BMC. Towards the use of blockchain in mobile health services and applications. J Med Syst 2021;45:17.

74. Schaffler-Schaden D, Mergenthal K, Avian A, et al. COVI-Prim longitudinal survey: experiences of primary care physicians during the early phase of the COVID-19 pandemic. Front Med (Lausanne) 2022;9:761283.

75. Varlas VN, Borş RG, Pop AL, et al. Oncofertility and COVID-19: at the crossroads between two time-sensitive fields. J Clin Med 2022;11:1221.

76. Charlot A, Baudin F, Tessier M, et al. Mobile telemedicine screening for diabetic retinopathy using nonmydriatic fundus photographs in burgundy: 11 years of results. J Clin Med 2022;11:1318.

77. Cvietusa PJ, Goodrich GK, Steiner JF, et al. Transition to Virtual Asthma Care During the COVID-19 Pandemic: An Observational Study. J Allergy Clin Immunol Pract 2022;10(6):1569–76.

78. Bolster MB, Chandra S, Demaerschalk BM, et al. Virtual care and medical educator group. crossing the virtual chasm: practical considerations for rethinking curriculum, competency, and culture in the virtual care era. Acad Med 2022. https://doi.org/10.1097/ACM.0000000000004660. Online ahead of print.

79. Dooley MJ, Simpson KN, Simpson AN, et al. A modification of time-driven activity-based costing for comparing cost of telehealth and in-person visits. Telemed J E Health 2022. https://doi.org/10.1089/tmj.2021.0338.

80. Nguyen MT, Garcia F, Juarez J, et al. Satisfaction can co-exist with hesitation: qualitative analysis of acceptability of telemedicine among multi-lingual patients in a safety-net health care system during the COVID-19 pandemic. BMC Health Serv Res 2022;22:195. https://doi.org/10.1186/s12913-022-07547-9.

81. Lurie N, Carr BG. The role of telehealth in the medical response to disasters. JAMA Intern Med 2018;178:745–6.

82. Yoo BK, Kim M, Sasaki T, et al. Selected use of telemedicine in intensive care units based on severity of illness improves cost-effectiveness. Telemed J E Health 2018;24:21–36.

83. Pierce M, Gudowski SW, Roberts KJ, et al. The rapid implementation of ad hoc tele-critical care respiratory therapy (eRT) service in the wake of the COVID-19 surge. J Clin Med 2022;11:718.

84. Macedo BR, Garcia MVF, Garcia ML, et al. Implementation of tele-ICU during the COVID-19 pandemic. J Bras Pneumol 2021;47:e20200545. https://doi.org/10.36416/1806-3756/e20200545.

85. Srinivasan SR. Editorial: tele-ICU in the age of COVID-19: built for this challenge. J Nutr Health Aging 2020;24:536–7.

86. Williams D Jr, Lawrence J, Hong YR, et al. Tele-ICUs for COVID-19: a look at national prevalence and characteristics of hospitals providing teleintensive care. J Rural Health 2021;37:133–41.

87. Song X, Liu X, Wang C. The role of telemedicine during the COVID-19 epidemic in China-experience from Shandong province. Crit Care 2020;24:178. https://doi.org/10.1186/s13054-020-02884-9.

88. Conroy I, Murray A, Kirrane F, et al. Key requirements of a video-call system in a critical care department as discovered during the rapid development of a solution to address COVID-19 visitor restrictions. JAMIA Open 2021;4:ooab091. https://doi.org/10.1093/jamiaopen/ooab091.

89. Noritomi DT, Ranzani OT, Ferraz LJR, et al. TELE-critical Care versus usual Care on ICU Performance (TELESCOPE): protocol for a cluster-randomised clinical trial on adult general ICUs in Brazil. BMJ Open 2021;11:e042302.

90. Jalilian Khave L, Vahidi M, Shirini D, et al. Clinical and epidemiological characteristics of post discharge patients with COVID-19 in tehran, Iran: protocol for a prospective cohort study (Tele-COVID-19 Study). JMIR Res Protoc 2021;10: e23316.

91. Sakusic A, Markotic D, Dong Y, et al. Rapid, multimodal, critical care knowledge-sharing platform for COVID-19 pandemics. Bosn J Basic Med Sci 2021;21:93–7.

92. Pierce M, Gudowski SW, Roberts KJ, et al. Establishing a telemedicine respiratory therapy service (eRT) in the COVID-19 pandemic. J Cardiothorac Vasc Anesth 2021;35:1268–9.

93. Ram-Tiktin E. Ethical considerations of triage following natural disasters: the IDF experience in Haiti as a case study. Bioethics 2017;31:467–75.

94. Vranas KC, Slatore CG, Kerlin MP. Telemedicine coverage of intensive care units: a narrative review. Ann Am Thorac Soc 2018;15:1256–64.

95. Halpern NA, Pastores SM. Critical care medicine in the United States 2000-2005: an analysis of bed numbers, occupancy rates, payer mix, and costs. Crit Care Med 2010;38:65–71.

96. Berenson RA, Grossman JM, November EA. Does telemonitoring of patients - the eICU -improve intensive care? Health Aff (Millwood) 2009;28:w937–47.

97. Vincent JL, Creteur J. Critical care medicine in 2050: less invasive, more connected, and personalized. J Thorac Dis 2019;11:335–8.

98. Global tele-intensive care unit (ICU) market – industry trends and forecast to 2028. In: Data bridge market research. 2021. Available at: https://www.databridgemarketresearch.com/reports/global-tele-intensive-care-unit-icu-market. Accessed April 06, 2022.

99. Critical care medicine in space. In: ICU management in practice. 2019. Available at: https://healthmanagement.org/c/icu/news/isicem19-critical-care-medicine-in-space. Accessed April 06, 2022.

100. Formanek AR III. Anesthesiology and critical care medicine in space: a clear and present need. In: ASA monitor. In: .. 2018. Available at: https://pubs.asahq.org/monitor/article-abstract/82/7/52/6371/Anesthesiology-and-Critical-Care-Medicine-in-Space?redirectedFrom=fulltext. Accessed April 06, 2022.

Focused Cardiac Ultrasound Training for Non-cardiologists

An Overview and Recommendations for a Lower Middle-Income Country

Wangari Waweru-Siika, MBChB, MMed, FRCA[a,b,]*,
Annette Plüddemann, PhD[c], Carl Heneghan, MA, MRCGP, DPhil[c]

KEYWORDS

• Focused cardiac ultrasound • Low- and middle-income countries • Point of care

KEY POINTS

• The shortage of experts in low- and middle-income countries (LMICs) leads to diagnostic delays in patients in urgent need of echocardiography.
• Training non-cardiologists to perform focused cardiac ultrasound (FoCUS) is a possible solution to this problem.
• Evidence to support training delivery and competence assessment following brief trainings in FoCUS is required before these trainings are scaled up.

INTRODUCTION

Mortalities in intensive care units (ICUs) in low- and-middle-income countries (LMICs) are among the highest in the world, with more than 50% of critically ill patients in some not surviving their ICU stay.[1,2] Although the causes of these poor outcomes are multifactorial, diagnostic equipment shortages and lack of skilled personnel are thought to be significant contributory factors.[3,4] Poor quality of care in patients with underlying cardiovascular disease is the leading cause of mortality in these settings, accounting for 84% of amenable deaths.[5]

[a] Department of Anaesthesia, Aga Khan University, 3rd Parklands Avenue, PO Box 30270, Nairobi-00100, Kenya; [b] Department for Continuing Education, University of Oxford, 1 Wellington Square, Oxford OX1 2JA, United Kingdom; [c] Nuffield Department of Primary Care Health Sciences, University of Oxford, Oxford OX2 6GG, United Kingdom
* Corresponding author. Department of Continuing Education, University of Oxford, 1 Wellington Square, Oxford OX1 2JA, United Kingdom.
E-mail address: wangari.waweru-siika@kellogg.ox.ac.uk

Crit Care Clin 38 (2022) 827–837
https://doi.org/10.1016/j.ccc.2022.06.015
0749-0704/22/© 2022 Elsevier Inc. All rights reserved.

Prolonged hypotension is a recognized cause of increased morbidity and mortality among the critically ill, and timely intervention to restore organ perfusion is key to improving outcomes.[6–10] Previous work has demonstrated an unacceptably high mortality in hypotensive patients admitted to critical care, with a retrospective cohort study of 450 ICU patients at a public, tertiary hospital in western Kenya revealing an adjusted odds ratio for mortality of 7.98 ($P<.001$) in patients in need of vasopressor support.[4] Although management is mainly supportive, uncovering the underlying cause is crucial, as delays in diagnosis may lead to loss of life.[9,11–13] Echocardiography is a useful, noninvasive diagnostic tool for undifferentiated hypotension at the point of care, reducing diagnostic uncertainty and guiding interventions.[9,12,14] Bedside echocardiography influences intensive care management decisions in up to 49% of patients.[15] LMICs are however constrained in their ability to meet the needs of acutely ill patients in urgent need of echocardiographic evaluation.[16]

In 2018, Kenya launched its Universal Health Coverage program[17] based on Sustainable Development Goal Number 3 of the World Health Organization (WHO),[17–19] the basic tenets of which are equity in access and quality of health services for all by the year 2030.[19] Kenya has only 60 cardiologists and 30 sonographers for a population of more than 50 million.[19–21] In addition, competency in echocardiography takes years to acquire.[20,22] With an insufficient number of echocardiography experts to meet the needs of the critically ill, diagnostic delays in time-critical emergencies will be difficult to overcome in the near future.[21,23] Focused Cardiac Ultrasound (FoCUS), an abbreviated, cardiac ultrasound examination performed at the point of care for a narrow range of possible diagnoses, is easier to perform, with a lower training burden.[24] FoCUS could hold the key to mitigating diagnostic delays caused by the shortage of echocardiography experts in LMICs. What is less clear is what FoCUS curriculum is recommended for low-resource settings, training delivery, and objective competency assessment for non-cardiologists caring for the critically ill.

THE DEVELOPMENT AND APPLICATION OF POINT-OF-CARE APPLICATIONS

Point-of-care applications were primarily developed to shorten test result turnaround time, reduce time to diagnosis, and increase efficiency of care.[25–27] Point-of-care imaging became possible when bulky machines became smaller, lighter, and therefore more portable.[27] This was particularly beneficial in emergency departments (EDs) and critical care areas where patients are often unstable, yet quick decision making is crucial. Perilous journeys to the computed tomographic (CT) scanner that led to these being dubbed the "doughnuts of death" were averted without compromising diagnostic accuracy.[28,29] The popularity of point-of-care ultrasound (PoCUS) has grown exponentially in recent years, a process accelerated for the most part by the advent of miniaturization.[27] Compared with other imaging modalities, such as CT scans and MRIs, ultrasound is less costly, safer, and nonionizing, enabling repeat assessments in a broad variety of patients.[30]

THE SCOPE OF FOCUSED CARDIAC ULTRASOUND

FoCUS is not intended to replace comprehensive echocardiography by an expert.[24,31] It instead refers to an abbreviated, qualitative assessment of the heart using ultrasound, often by the treating clinician, to answer a specific clinical question. The American College of Echocardiography therefore strongly advises that a FoCUS examination always be followed by a comprehensive echocardiogram by an expert.[32] Various other professional societies have been instrumental in the provision of practice standards and guidelines to guide the growth and development of FoCUS over the years. Recognizing the key role played by ultrasound in medical practice, training in this modality has now been incorporated into several specialty training curricula, such as emergency medicine, critical care, and anesthesia.[33,34] This has mostly occurred for fellowship and residency training programs, although some accrediting bodies have lobbied to have this training included at the undergraduate level.

FoCUS has a wide range of applications and can safely be applied to a broad range of patients in a variety of emergency and nonemergency settings.[31] In the pre-hospital emergency setting, FoCUS has been used to quickly evaluate acutely ill patients wherever they may be found, including at the scenes of a disaster.[35] In the ED, emergency medicine physicians have been at the forefront of using FoCUS for the initial assessment of unstable patients on arrival for years, including those in cardiac arrest.[36–38] In pediatrics, FoCUS applications range from their use in utero, to their use in neonates, in the pediatric emergency medicine department, and in intensive care.[39–41] In primary care and general internal medicine, FoCUS has been used by internists to assess patients in surgeries and on hospital rounds.[42] In cardiology, FoCUS by cardiologists has been used for the evaluation of patients with heart failure, primarily to assess their volume status and establish diuretic dose requirements. Some have gone on to train heart failure nurses specifically for this purpose.[43,44] In perioperative areas, FoCUS has been used by surgeons and anesthetists to guide the optimization of cardiac function preoperatively and guide interventions intraoperatively and postoperatively.[15,45–47] In intensive care, FoCUS is widely used to define the presence and the extent of cardiac dysfunction among the critically ill.[48] The ongoing COVID pandemic has in addition highlighted the utility of FoCUS in a variety of acute care settings.

The place of FoCUS as a basic screening tool in emergency settings is reflected in the hierarchical proposal by the World Interactive Network Focused on Critical Ultrasound (WINFOCUS) for echocardiography competence in critical care (**Fig. 1**).

With respect to distinct conditions or entities, the use of FoCUS for the assessment of volume status in patients with septic shock was first endorsed in the 2016 Surviving Sepsis Campaign guidelines.[49] Fluid resuscitation was previously guided by static measures, such as central venous pressure,[10] but these have been shown to be inaccurate measures of cardiac preload.

SCANNING PROTOCOLS

Scanning protocols are necessary to ensure that a standardized approach is followed, using a validated combination of views. A FoCUS protocol provides a predefined approach to scanning, with specific views and, in some cases, a prescribed order in which these views are to be obtained. The 4 basic cardiac views in FoCUS are the parasternal long-axis view, parasternal short axis, apical 4-chamber, and subcostal views (inferior vena cava and/or 4-chamber). There are numerous protocols but none that can be described as "universal."[24] Clinicians have over the years therefore designed a variety of FoCUS protocols in an attempt to meet specific clinical needs.

Scanning protocols may be multiorgan or single organ, depending on the number of organ systems scanned.[50,51] A single-organ protocol involves just 1 organ system, such as the heart or lungs, whereas a multiorgan protocol includes 2 or more organ systems. Multiorgan protocols are often used to address the needs of complex patients, such as those with trauma or hypotensive patients, specifically those with undifferentiated hypotension. Recent evidence suggests that multiorgan scanning protocols, such as the RUSH (Rapid Ultrasound in Shock and Hypotension) protocol, may have greater diagnostic utility than single-organ protocols in shock etiology.[51]

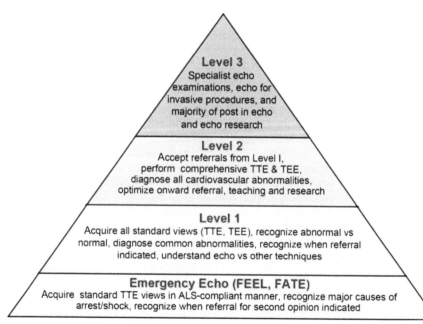

Fig. 1. Hierarchical proposal by the WINFOCUS for echocardiography competence in critical care. ALS, advanced life support; FATE, focus assessed transthoracic echocardiography; FEEL, focused echocardiography in emergency life support; TEE, transesophageal echocardiography (*From* Price S, Via G, Sloth E, et al. Echocardiography practice, training and accreditation in the intensive care: document for the World Interactive Network Focused on Critical Ultrasound (WINFOCUS). Cardiovasc Ultrasound. 2008;6:49. Published 2008 Oct 6. https://doi.org/10.1186/1476-7120-6-49.)

Scanning protocols differ in the combination of organs scanned and cardiac views obtained. In the emergency or trauma setting, for instance, a classic scanning protocol is the FAST scan (or extended FAST, e-FAST).[52] The utility of a FAST scan was first described in the 1990s when it was demonstrated that surgeons could perform this ultrasound protocol to detect occult hemorrhage in trauma patients with a reasonable degree of accuracy, compared with direct peritoneal lavage and CT scanning.[29] This trauma protocol was widely accepted thereafter and is in use in many EDs around the world. The RUSH protocol was developed in 2006 by Weingart and colleagues.[53] Summarized as "pump, tank, and pipe," the protocol is typically performed for the diagnosis of shock etiology, systematically examining the heart, lungs, abdomen, pelvis, and even deep veins. The basic FATE (Focus Assessed Transthoracic Echocardiography) protocol includes cardiac views (parasternal, apical 4-chamber, and subcostal) and pleural scans in a prescribed order.[54] The FEEL (Focused Echocardiography in Emergency Life Support),[55] FUSE (Focused Ultrasound in Echocardiography), and FEER (Focused Echocardiographic Evaluation in Resuscitation)[56] protocols are primarily designed for use in cardiac arrest scenarios. BLEEP (Basic Echocardiography in Emergency Pediatrics) is specifically designed for use in pediatrics. Lung-based scanning protocols in current use include FALLS (Fluid Administration Limited by Lung Sonography)[57] and BLUE (Basic Lung Ultrasound Evaluation).[58]

FOCUSED CARDIAC ULTRASOUND TRAINING CURRICULA

Given the variety of protocols and the lack of a "universal protocol," there is no one way of delivering FoCUS training, with curricula differing depending on the specific protocol in question. The basic structure for the vast majority of these, however, is similar, comprising a didactic component, delivered face to face or electronically, and a hands-on component, in the form of workshops or proctored training.

In 2018, the European Association for Cardiovascular Imaging (EACVI) issued a position paper regarding the need to harmonize FoCUS training among the various specialties.[24] The summary was produced in consultation with the European Society of Anaesthesiologists, the European Association of Cardiothoracic Anaesthesiology, the Acute Cardiovascular Care Association of the European Society of Cardiology, and the WINFOCUS and referenced documents previously issued by the American Society of Echocardiography and the American College of Emergency Physicians. The intention of the EACVI was to provide a document to guide the ongoing training in FoCUS by various specialties, thus ensuring that certain core elements were met regardless of curriculum followed. Accepting the myriad of protocols that currently exist, emphasis was placed on the need to outline a core curriculum that would ensure that core tenants were met by all proposed syllabuses.

COMPETENCY ASSESSMENT METHODS WITHIN DIFFERENT CLINICAL SPECIALTIES

Competency in FoCUS is not uniformly assessed, an issue further compounded by the fact that the definition of FoCUS competence is itself undefined.[59] Some have chosen to use formative assessments, such as supervised scans and logbooks, whereas others have adopted summative assessments, such as Observed Structured Clinical Examinations and triggered assessments. Furthermore, competency assessment varies by specialty, with notable differences in the approach by emergency medicine, critical care, and anesthesia. Finally, FoCUS skills are not uniformly acquired, and although some novices quickly learn to demonstrate good image quality after a brief training, they may struggle with image interpretation.[59] The definition of competence in FoCUS therefore depend on the extent to which emphasis is laid on technical versus cognitive skills, and how these are evaluated.

Some accrediting bodies prescribe a number of scans that a novice must perform and correctly interpret to be deemed competent in FoCUS. The range for these may be as low as 30 and as high as 60, depending on the accrediting body.[59] On the other hand, no less than 150 to 200 scans are required for competency in level 1 echocardiography.[60] Other groups have been less prescriptive of number of scans, defining instead a timeframe within a given clinical setting as a surrogate for sufficient exposure and practice. There is growing interest now in the role of simulation-based competency assessment as an objective, reproducible tool for this purpose.[59] There has been concern, however, that practitioners do not continue to practice FoCUS as required following brief trainings.[61]

One of the major reasons PoCUS in general and FoCUS in particular has been met with fear and trepidation by some clinicians is the fear of diagnostic errors; the fear of causing harm to patients who are scanned by those who are not competent to do so. Various researchers have demonstrated that diagnostic accuracy in the hands of novices of different cadres can vary, leading to diagnostic errors.

FOCUSED CARDIAC ULTRASOUND IN THE CRITICALLY ILL

Although FoCUS enables rapid diagnosis at the point of care,[37,62,63] there is no evidence of a mortality benefit from the use of POCUS in general and FoCUS in particular. Most studies demonstrate a tendency toward improved diagnostic accuracy, reduction of diagnostic uncertainty, and reduced time to decision/efficiency of diagnosis. Studies based in Ghana, Iran, India, and Egypt that have looked at the use of PoCUS in the ED or critical care have demonstrated a reduction in diagnostic uncertainty resulting from its use. In LMICs where critical care mortality is particularly high, it is not inconceivable that any attempts to improve diagnostic efficiency have the potential to improve critical care outcomes.

The 2018 SHOC-ED trial, a randomized multisite clinical trial of 273 patients with undifferentiated shock in EDs across 6 centers in Canada and South Africa found a multiorgan PoCUS that included FoCUS to have no impact on mortality.[64] This study, however, was performed in well-resourced institutions in Canada and South Africa, where the standard of care is superior to that in Kenya. In addition, many physicians in the South African site faced challenges generating PoCUS images, leading to inconclusive views, potentially leading to the lack of a mortality benefit in this trial. Finally, the trial faced significant recruitment challenges because of perceived ethical concerns among ED clinicians for many of whom PoCUS in shock is current standard of care and was terminated early.[64] The findings of this study are therefore not generalizable, and the adoption of FoCUS in low-resource settings, such as are found in Kenya where echocardiography experts are in short supply, may have a measurable impact on outcomes.

RESEARCH IMPLICATIONS AND SUGGESTIONS FOR THE FUTURE

The diagnostic utility of FoCUS performed by non-cardiologists has been advocated, highlighting the impact of task-shifting traditional cardiologist roles.[44,65] Modifying the scope of practice of nurses is a possible solution to the shortage of cardiologists and other echocardiography experts in LMICs. The shortage of nurses in Kenya, for instance, is not as dire as that of its physicians, with 8.3 active nurses per 10,000 population against the recommended 25 per 10,000, compared with 5 doctors per 10,000 population against the recommended 36 per 10,000 by WHO standards. Task-shifting traditional physician roles to nurses has successfully been implemented in 27 countries in North America, Europe, Australia, and New Zealand.[66,67]

The 2018 EU-MUNROS study assessing the perception of health care workers across 9 European countries to task-shifting noted that partial task-shifting from physicians to nurses had occurred in acute myocardial infarction care in The Netherlands, England, and Scotland, allowing advanced nurse practitioners (ANPs) or practice nurses to conduct assessments and select appropriate protocols to apply.[66] In the United Kingdom, the presence of ANPs in an acute hospital setting was noted to lead to a reduction in the workload of junior doctors, and to have a positive impact on patient outcomes.[68] A 2018 study from the Aga Khan University Nairobi tested the ability of collaborative task-sharing to provide access to PoCUS among pregnant women and found 96.6% accuracy of midwife scans following a 5-week training in obstetric ultrasound.[69]

Introducing a nurse-led FoCUS service in LMICs has the potential to reduce diagnostic delays, increase efficiency of care, and improve outcomes among the critically ill. The diagnostic test accuracy of FoCUS in patients with nontraumatic hypotension by operators with limited experience is, however, uncertain.[70] Before this complex intervention is scaled up in LMICs, its diagnostic test accuracy following brief trainings should be carefully examined, particularly among the critically ill.

SUMMARY

FoCUS by non-cardiologists in LMICs is a potential solution to the shortage of echocardiography experts in these settings. Understanding who to train, how, and for how long should be based on robust evidence before such trainings are rolled out on a larger scale.

CLINICS CARE POINTS

- Focused cardiac ultrasound by non-cardiologists is a useful screening tool in a variety of clinical settings.
- FoCUS however does not replace the need for comprehensive echocardiography by an expert.
- Training non-cardiologists in LMICs to perform FoCUS could mitigate the shortage of echocardiography experts in these settings.
- FoCUS training in LMICs should ensure diagnostic accuracy of this investigation in the hands of non-cardiologists.An evidence-based approach to FoCUS training and competency assessment for non-cardiologists in LMICs is key to ensuring patient safety.

REFERENCES

1. Lalani H, Waweru-Siika W, Mwogi T, et al. Evaluation of intensive care unit outcomes and mortality at a referral hospital in Western Kenya. Am J Respir Crit Care Med 2017;195.
2. Smith Z, Ayele Y, McDonald P. Outcomes in critical care delivery at Jimma University Specialised hospital, Ethiopia. Anaesth Intensive Care 2013;41(3):363.
3. Hospital KN. The proposed KNH private hospital PPP project. Project Information Memorandum; 2019.
4. Lalani HS, Waweru-Siika W, Mwogi T, et al. Intensive care outcomes and mortality prediction at a national referral hospital in western Kenya. Ann Am Thorac Soc 2018;15(11):1336–43.
5. Kruk ME, Gage AD, Joseph NT, et al. Mortality due to low-quality health systems in the universal health coverage era: a systematic analysis of amenable deaths in 137 countries. The Lancet 2018;392(10160):2203–12.
6. Reaume M, Di Felice C, Melgar T. Point of care echocardiography: An essential extension of the physical exam in shock. American Journal of Respiratory and Critical Care Medicine Conference: American Thoracic Society International Conference, ATS. 2018;197(Meeting Abstracts).
7. Cecconi M, De Backer D, Antonelli M, et al. Consensus on circulatory shock and hemodynamic monitoring. Task force of the European Society of Intensive Care Medicine. Intensive Care Med 2014;40(12):1795–815.
8. Jones AE, Yiannibas V, Johnson C, et al. Emergency department hypotension predicts Sudden Unexpected in-hospital mortality: a prospective cohort study. Chest 2006;130(4):941–6.
9. Shokoohi H, Boniface KS, Pourmand A, et al. Bedside ultrasound reduces diagnostic uncertainty and guides resuscitation in patients with undifferentiated hypotension. Crit Care Med 2015;43(12):2562–9.
10. Rivers E, Nguyen B, Havstad S, et al. Early goal-directed therapy in the treatment of severe sepsis and septic shock. New Engl J Med 2001;345(19):1368–77.
11. Islam M, Levitus M, Eisen L, et al. Lung ultrasound for the diagnosis and management of acute respiratory failure. Lung 2020;198(1):1–11.
12. Laursen CB, Sloth E, Lambrechtsen J, et al. Focused sonography of the heart, lungs, and deep veins identifies missed life-threatening conditions in admitted patients with acute respiratory symptoms. Chest 2013;144(6):1868–75.
13. Wallbridge P, Steinfort D, Tay TR, et al. Diagnostic chest ultrasound for acute respiratory failure. Respir Med 2018;141:26–36.

14. Heiberg J, El-Ansary D, Canty DJ, et al. Focused echocardiography: a systematic review of diagnostic and clinical decision-making in anaesthesia and critical care. Anaesthesia 2016;71(9):1091–100.

15. Heiberg J, El-Ansary D, Canty DJ, et al. Focused echocardiography: a systematic review of diagnostic and clinical decision-making in anaesthesia and critical care. Anaesthesia 2016;71(9):1091–100.

16. Becker TK, Tafoya CA, Osei-Ampofo M, et al. Cardiopulmonary ultrasound for critically ill adults improves diagnostic accuracy in a resource-limited setting: the AFRICA trial. Trop Med Int Health 2017;22(12):1599–608.

17. Government TK. Vision 2030 2020.

18. Organisation WH. Kenya Rolls Out Universal Health Coverage. 2018.

19. Organisation WH. Sustainable Development Goals. 2018.

20. England NHE. Training and development (cardiology).

21. B J. GE, Kenya Cardiac Society collaborate to train cardiac health professionals. 2018.

22. Institute JHMHaV. Cardiac Sonography Training Programme.

23. Health KMo. Kenya Health Workforce Report: The Status of Healthcare Professionals in Kenya, 2015. 2015.

24. Neskovic AN, Skinner H, Price S, et al. Focus cardiac ultrasound core curriculum and core syllabus of the European Association of Cardiovascular Imaging. Eur Heart J Cardiovasc Imaging 2018;19(5):475–81.

25. Chaisirin W, Wongkrajang P, Thoesam T, et al. Role of point-of-care testing in reducing time to treatment decision-making in urgency patients: a randomized controlled trial. West J Emerg Med 2020;21(2):404–10.

26. Kozel TR, Burnham-Marusich AR. Point-of-care testing for infectious diseases: past, present, and future. J Clin Microbiol 2017;55(8):2313–20.

27. Díaz-Gómez JL, Mayo PH, Koenig SJ. Point-of-care ultrasonography. New Engl J Med 2021;385(17):1593–602.

28. L L. Act now to ensure the CT is not the doughnut of death in trauma. April 2012;11.

29. Rozycki GS, Shackford SR. Ultrasound, what every trauma surgeon should know. J Trauma 1996;40(1):1.

30. Clevert D-A, Nyhsen C, Ricci P, et al. Position statement and best practice recommendations on the imaging use of ultrasound from the European Society of Radiology ultrasound subcommittee. Insights into Imaging 2020;11(1):115.

31. Spencer KT, Kimura BJ, Korcarz CE, et al. Focused cardiac ultrasound: recommendations from the American Society of Echocardiography. J Am Soc Echocardiography 2013;26(6):567–81.

32. Doherty JU, Kort S, Mehran R, et al. ACC/AATS/AHA/ASE/ASNC/HRS/SCAI/SCCT/SCMR/STS 2019 appropriate Use criteria for multimodality imaging in the assessment of cardiac structure and function in Nonvalvular heart disease : a report of the American College of cardiology appropriate Use criteria task force, American Association for Thoracic Surgery, American heart Association, American society of echocardiography, American society of Nuclear cardiology, heart Rhythm society, society for cardiovascular Angiography and interventions, society of cardiovascular computed tomography, society for cardiovascular magnetic resonance, and the society of Thoracic surgeons. J Nucl Cardiol 2019;26(4):1392–413.

33. Ma IWY, Arishenkoff S, Wiseman J, et al. Internal medicine point-of-care ultrasound curriculum: consensus recommendations from the Canadian internal medicine ultrasound (CIMUS) Group. J Gen Intern Med 2017;32(9):1052–7.

34. Mizubuti GB, Allard RV, Ho AMH, et al. Knowledge retention after focused cardiac ultrasound training: a prospective cohort pilot study. Braz J Anesthesiology (English Edition) 2019;69(2):177–83.

35. Busch M. Portable ultrasound in pre-hospital emergencies: a feasibility study. Acta Anaesthesiol Scand 2006;50(6):754–8.

36. Del Rios M, Colla J, Kotini-Shah P, et al. Emergency physician use of tissue Doppler bedside echocardiography in detecting diastolic dysfunction: an exploratory study. Crit Ultrasound J 2018;10(1):4.

37. Donham C, Dinh V, Selden N, et al. The contribution of nursing point-of-care ultrasound on septic emergency department patients. J Invest Med 2019;67(1):128.

38. Dwyer KH, Rempell JS, Stone MB. Diagnosing centrally located pulmonary embolisms in the emergency department using point-of-care ultrasound. Am J Emerg Med 2018;36(7):1145–50.

39. O' Brien AJ, Brady RM. Point-of-care ultrasound in paediatric emergency medicine. In. Vol 522016:174-180.

40. Longjohn M, Wan J, Joshi V, et al. Point-of-care echocardiography by pediatric emergency physicians. Pediatr Emerg Care 2011;27(8):693–6.

41. Poon WB, Wong KY. Neonatologist-performed point-of-care functional echocardiography in the neonatal intensive care unit. Singapore Med J 2017;58(5):230–3.

42. Bhagra A, Tierney DM, Sekiguchi H, et al. Point-of-Care ultrasonography for primary care physicians and general internists. Mayo Clin Proc 2016;91(12):1811–27.

43. Gundersen GH, Norekval TM, Haug HH, et al. Adding point of care ultrasound to assess volume status in heart failure patients in a nurse-led outpatient clinic. A randomised study. Heart 2016;102(1):29–34.

44. Hjorth-Hansen A, Graven T, Holmen Gundersen G, et al. Feasibility and reliability of focused echocardiographic imaging by nurses supported by interpretation via telemedicine in an outpatient heart failure clinic. Eur Heart J Cardiovasc Imaging 2017;18(Supplement 3):iii319.

45. Lee LKK, Tsai PNW, Ip KY, et al. Pre-operative cardiac optimisation: a directed review. Anaesthesia 2019;74:67–79.

46. Diaz-Gomez JL, Via G, Ramakrishna H. Focused cardiac and lung ultrasonography: implications and applicability in the perioperative period. Rom J Anaesth Intensive Care 2016;23(1):41–54.

47. Faris JG, Veltman MG, Royse CF. Limited transthoracic echocardiography assessment in anaesthesia and critical care. Best Pract Res Clin Anaesthesiol 2009;23(3):285–98.

48. Dudzinski DM, Picard MH. Handheld echocardiography: its role in intensive care units. Curr Cardiovasc Imaging Rep 2013;6(4):301–4.

49. De Backer D, Dorman T. Surviving sepsis guidelines: a continuous move toward better care of patients with sepsis. JAMA 2017;317(8):807–8.

50. Nazerian P, Vanni S, Volpicelli G, et al. Accuracy of point-of-care multiorgan ultrasonography for the diagnosis of pulmonary embolism. Chest 2014;145(5):950–7.

51. Volpicelli G, Lamorte A, Tullio M, et al. Point-of-care multiorgan ultrasonography for the evaluation of undifferentiated hypotension in the emergency department. Intensive Care Med 2013;39(7):1290–8.

52. Zaharie LC, Pasc M. Focused assessment with sonography for trauma. Clujul Med 2016;89(Supplement 2):S40.

53. Perera P, Mailhot T, Riley D, et al. The RUSH exam: rapid Ultrasound in SHock in the evaluation of the critically Ill. Emerg Med Clin 2010;28(1):29–56.

54. Laursen CB, Jakobsen CJ, Lassen AT, et al. Focus assessed transthoracic echo-cardiography (FATE) in patients acutely admitted with respiratory symptoms. Appl Cardiopulmonary Pathophysiology 2012;16(SUPPL. 1):187.

55. Breitkreutz R, Price S, Steiger HV, et al. Focused echocardiographic evaluation in life support and peri-resuscitation of emergency patients: a prospective trial. Resuscitation 2010;81(11):1527–33.

56. Breitkreutz R, Walcher F, Seeger FH. Focused echocardiographic evaluation in resuscitation management: concept of an advanced life support-conformed algorithm. Crit Care Med 2007;35(5 Suppl):S150–61.

57. Lichtenstein D. Fluid administration limited by lung sonography: the place of lung ultrasound in assessment of acute circulatory failure (the FALLS-protocol). Expert Rev Respir Med 2012;6(2):155–62.

58. Lichtenstein D. Lung ultrasound in the critically ill: the BLUE protocol. Anaesthesiology Intensive Ther 2014;46(SUPPL. 2):147–8.

59. Bowcock EM, Morris IS, McLean AS, et al. Basic critical care echocardiography: how many studies equate to competence? A pilot study using high fidelity echocardiography simulation. J Intensive Care Soc 2017;18(3):198–205.

60. Echocardiography BSo. Level 1 accreditation. 2022. Available at: https://www.bsecho.org/Public/Accreditation/Personal-accreditation/Level-1/Public/Accreditation/Accreditation-subpages/Personal-accreditation-subpages/Level-1-accreditation.aspx?hkey=6099b4b8-5cb9-4425-a201-1874aadcb73f. Accessed April 1, 2022.

61. Hayward M, Chan T, Healey A. Dedicated time for deliberate practice: one emergency medicine program's approach to point-of-care ultrasound (PoCUS) training. CJEM 2015;17(5):558–61.

62. Daley J, Dwyer K, Grunwald Z, et al. Utility of focused cardiac ultrasound for pulmonary embolism in emergency department patients with abnormal vitals. Acad Emerg Med 2019;26(Supplement 1):S51–2.

63. Shokoohi H, Boniface KS, Zaragoza M, et al. Point-of-care ultrasound leads to diagnostic shifts in patients with undifferentiated hypotension. Am J Emerg Med 2017;35(12):1984 e1983–7.

64. Atkinson PR, Milne J, Diegelmann L, et al. Does point-of-care ultrasonography improve clinical outcomes in emergency department patients with undifferentiated hypotension? An International Randomized Controlled Trial From the SHoC-ED Investigators. Ann Emerg Med 2018;72(4):478–89.

65. Steinwandel U, Gibson N, Towell A, et al. Can a renal nurse assess fluid status using ultrasound on the inferior vena cava? A cross-sectional interrater study. Hemodialysis Int 2018;22(2):261–9.

66. Maier CB, Köppen J, Busse R, et al. Task shifting between physicians and nurses in acute care hospitals: cross-sectional study in nine countries. Hum Resour Health 2018;16(1):24.

67. Maier CB, Aiken LH. Task shifting from physicians to nurses in primary care in 39 countries: a cross-country comparative study. Eur J Public Health 2016;26(6):927–34.

68. McDonnell A, Goodwin E, Kennedy F, et al. An evaluation of the implementation of Advanced Nurse Practitioner (ANP) roles in an acute hospital setting. J Adv Nurs 2015;71(4):789–99.

69. Vinayak S, Brownie S. Collaborative task-sharing to enhance the Point-Of-Care Ultrasound (POCUS) access among expectant women in Kenya: the role of midwife sonographers. J Interprof Care 2018;32(5):641–4.
70. Becker DM, Tafoya CA, Becker SL, et al. The use of portable ultrasound devices in low and middle-income countries: a systematic review of the literature. Trop Med Int Health 2016;21(3):294–311.

Facility-Oriented Simulation-Based Emergency Care Training in Kenya
A Practical Approach for Low- and Middle-Income Countries

Nelson Nyamu, MD, MRCEM[a],*, Janet Sugut, MBCHB[a],
Trufosa Mochache, MBCHB[a], Pauline Kimeu, MBCHB[a],
Grace Mukundi, B.S.N.[a], David Ngugi, Diploma Nursing[a],
Sally Njonjo, B.S.N.[a], Adan Mustafa, MBCHB[a], Paul Mbuvi, MBCHB[a],
Emily Nyagaki, M.S. Digital Business[a], Gatebe Kironji, MD, MPH[b],
Grace Wanjiku, MD, MPH[c], Benjamin Wachira, MBCHB, MD[d]

KEYWORDS

- Emergency care • Simulation training • Clinical mentoring • Emergency departments

KEY POINTS

- Simulation-based emergency care training allows health care providers to learn and practice real-world activities in an accurate, realistic, safe, and secure environment.
- The emergency care course is a facility-oriented, simulation-based emergency care training program developed in Kenya to train teams of health care providers currently working in emergency departments across the country on a systematic approach to assessing critically ill or injured patients.
- Local health care providers in Low-and-Middle-Income Countries can model and develop similar facility-oriented simulation-based emergency care training programs to upskill existing health care providers already working in emergency departments without any formal training in emergency medicine.

[a] Emergency Medicine Kenya Foundation, P. O. Box 1023-00200, Nairobi, Kenya; [b] Vituity Emergency Medicine, St. Agnes Hospital, 900 South Caton Avenue, Baltimore, MD 21229, USA; [c] The Warren Alpert Medical School of Brown University, 55 Claverick Street, Suite 100, Providence, RI 02903, USA; [d] Aga Khan University, Nairobi; P. O. Box, 30270 - 00100, Nairobi, Kenya
* Corresponding author.
E-mail address: nelsonfundi@gmail.com

Crit Care Clin 38 (2022) 839–852
https://doi.org/10.1016/j.ccc.2022.06.012
0749-0704/22/© 2022 Elsevier Inc. All rights reserved.
criticalcare.theclinics.com

INTRODUCTION

The development of emergency care systems and emergency medicine (EM) as a specialty is crucial to addressing global morbidity and mortality.[1] However, there is a significant gap between the need and availability of emergency care from specially trained providers, particularly in low- and middle-income countries (LMICs). Developing facility-oriented, simulation-based emergency care training programs grounded in principles of teamwork training for an emergency response is an important strategy for improving the quality of emergency care.[2–4]

Simulation-based training (SBT) has been shown to be superior and more effective than traditional modes of training, such as lecture-based and problem-based training.[5–10] SBT provides a more realistic and authentic learning environment where learners practice their skills, allowing room for mistakes without patient risk.[11] This allows the learners to internalize the educational principles, self-reflect on their practice, and improve their performance and mastery of knowledge and skills by incorporating psychomotor activities with the cognitive aspect of problem-based learning. With its immersive techniques, it can also be used to prepare entry-level providers by equipping them with the skills needed in the real world.[11–13] SBT can be employed to test adherence to algorithms or enhance knowledge in a particular area of interest. It also allows for training of both technical and nontechnical skills, such as leadership, team dynamics, communication, situation awareness, decision-making, and awareness of their limitations. In health care, this leads to fewer medical errors and increased patient safety.[14]

Emergency care is uniquely suited to learning through simulation as it is procedure oriented and comprises the whole range of medical specialties as well as a wide range of patient groups and disease pathology.[3,15] SBT has been extensively used in emergency care training, especially in trauma and cardiac arrest team training[3] Combining an emergency care simulator with problem-based teaching leads to enhanced awareness, skills, teamwork, and improved analytical skills in clinical settings[16] Simulation-based teamwork training for emergency department staff has also been shown to improve clinical team performance when added to an existing didactic curriculum.[4]

In LMICs, SBT is particularly useful as it offers a way to broaden the skills of various subsets of health care workers, including those who may be serving remote communities with little assistance from other specialists.[11] Using the local environment and available equipment to simulate health care workers' day-to-day settings enable them to learn new skills within a familiar setting.[17] Thus, SBT can be conducted within the health care workers' regular facility with simulated or standardized patients, making it a cost-effective and efficient training approach.[18] Simulated patients refer to people who have no illness and have been coached on how to display a certain presentation, whereas standardized patients actually have the disease but have also been trained on how to respond during the simulation. Doing this could also improve teamwork and communication, contributing to improved patient outcomes.[19,20] SBT can also be used to train health care workers on disaster preparedness and mass casualty events, such as road traffic accidents, which are common in LMICs.[19,21] Unfortunately, many health care training institutions in LMICs have yet to fully adopt and integrate the use of SBT.[22] There is a general lack of awareness of SBT as a learning option, including lack of context-specific curriculums and trained instructors.[22] Other hindrances to SBT uptake include limited funding, lack of equipment, and lack of well fitted training spaces/simulation laboratories.[22]

In Kenya, multiple studies have noted the lack of coordinated emergency care and recommended the training of emergency department staff (nurses, clinical officers, and medical officers) through short courses.[13,23] The majority of these health care workers do not have specific training in emergency care because of a shortage of emergency care training programs for nurses and mid-level providers, and a lack of postgraduate EM training programs for doctors.[13,23] Existing emergency care short courses are usually focused on individual providers and are based on either American or European standards.[13,23]

The emergency care course (TECC) is a 5-day facility-oriented, simulation-based emergency care training program that was developed to train teams of health care providers currently working in Kenyan emergency departments on a systematic approach to assessing critically ill or injured patients.[24] We describe the development and implementation of this program and the strengths, weaknesses, opportunities, challenges, and recommendations for other LMICs.

The Emergency Care Course

The emergency care course (TECC) was developed in 2018 by a team of local emergency care experts and practitioners as a course that would reflect the day-to-day needs of emergency departments across Kenya. It was designed to enable emergency care teams (nurses, clinical officers, and doctors) to develop the skills and knowledge needed to deliver safe and evidence-based quality emergency care for critically ill or injured patients in their own facilities.[24]In-facility training ensures knowledge and skills are context-specific and also allow the nurses, clinical officers, and doctors to work through scenarios together.

Participants
From February 2019 to July 2021, the course has been taught at 21 emergency departments across Kenya. A total of 240 health care providers have been trained, as shown in **Table 1**.

TECC is divided into the following components that focus on triage, systemic assessment, and stabilization of the critically ill or injured patients who present to the emergency department:

Precourse reading
Trainees receive electronic copies of the emergency care algorithms developed by the Emergency Medicine Kenya Foundation.[25] These are evidence-based, context-specific emergency care guidelines that have been in use in Kenya since 2013. These algorithms provide standardized care pathways with the additional goals of conserving resources and reducing medical errors. Trainees have about 2 weeks to review materials before the training. During the training, participants use printed copies of the algorithms for reference.

The emergency care course workshop
This is a five-day full-day in-person workshop held at the participant's facility. It incorporates various modes of content delivery, such as simulations, skill stations, video presentations, and focused discussions covering adult, pediatric, and obstetric emergencies as well as trauma.

The participating emergency department selects 12 health care providers for the training, who are led by a team of TECC faculty comprised of two emergency doctors and two emergency nurses. The faculty is emergency department health care providers who have undergone training on the administration of the TECC simulation-based curriculum.

Table 1
Training per facility and distribution of participants by cadre

	Emergency Departments	Clinical Officers	Doctors	Nurses	Grand Total
1	Port Reitz Sub-County Hospital; Mombasa County	4	2	4	10
2	Garissa County Referral Hospital Garissa	3	4	5	12
3	Machakos Level 5 Hospital	3		5	8
4	Makindu Sub-County Hospital	4	2	6	12
5	Makueni County Referral Hospital				12
6	Karatina Sub-County Hospital	8		8	3
7	Mt Kenya Sub-County Hospital				2
8	Mukurwe-ini Hospital				2
9	Nyeri County Referral Hospital				3
10	Moi Teaching and Referral Hospital	3	3	6	12
11	Nakuru Level 5 Hospital	2	2	8	12
12	Kakamega County General Teaching & Referral Hospital	1	2	8	11
13	Vihiga County Referral Hospital	4	2	6	12
14	Jaramogi Oginga Odinga Teaching & Referral Hospital	2	3	7	13
15	Ahero County Hospital				1
16	Kisumu County Referral Hospital				1
17	Kisii Teaching & Referral Hospital	3	3	6	12
18	Kenyatta National Hospital	4	59	33	81
19	Mama Lucy Kibaki Hospital				7
20	Mbagathi County Hospital				6
21	Lodwar County Referral Hospital	5	1	9	15
	Grand Total	46	83	111	240

Simulations. Simulations are locally referenced patient scenarios that trainees manage as a group of six under the facilitation of the faculty. The workshop consists of a total of 24 simulated patient scenarios, as shown in **Table 2**.

These scenarios were developed to reflect the day-to-day reality of emergency care in Kenyan emergency departments with local patients' names, explanations, and resources to enhance fidelity and suspension of reality.

Each case is designed to highlight the different phases of delivering emergency care, which correspond with steps in the emergency care algorithm. Participants are encouraged to actively reference the emergency care algorithms during the simulations to entrench their regular use. The faculty customizes the content and expectations of the scenario to the level of training and expectations of performance for the different participants.

Low fidelity adult, infant, child, and obstetric mannequins (**Fig. 1**) are used in the scenarios to enhance realism, and android tablets with a simulator app are used to simulate a cardiac monitor. In some instances, equipment from the participant's emergency department is incorporated in the training.

Early in the course, the faculty emphasizes the need to suspend reality so that participants treat the simulations as real patient encounters. Participants are asked to

Table 2
Simulated patient scenarios

Theme	Subthemes	Patient Scenarios
Adult resuscitation	Approach to the unconscious patient	(1) Adult cardiac arrest (VF[a]/pVT[b]) and post-cardiac arrest care (2) Adult cardiac arrest (asystole/PEA[c], Hs[d], and Ts[e]), post-cardiac arrest care and electrolyte abnormalities (hyperkalaemia)
	Approach to the patient with difficulty in breathing	(3) Choking (4) Anaphylaxis (5) Acute asthma
	Approach to the patient with chest pain	(6) Acute coronary syndrome (7) Pulmonary embolism
	Approach to the patient with an altered level of consciousness (AEIOU TIPPS)	(8) Approach to a patient with seizures (9) Approach to a stroke patient (10) Sepsis and septic shock (11) DKA[f] (12) Toxicology 　(a) Organophosphate poisoning 　(b) Methanol poisoning 　(c) Bites and stings (snake bites)
Trauma resuscitation	Management of the trauma patient	(13) Airway management in trauma (14) Chest trauma (15) Abdominal trauma and shock in trauma (16) Crush injury (17) Burns & electrical injuries resuscitation
Obstetric resuscitation		(18) Maternal cardiac arrest (19) Maternal trauma (20) Pre-eclampsia/Eclampsia
Pediatric resuscitation		(21) Approach to the sick child (22) Pediatric resuscitation (23) Pediatric trauma resuscitation (24) Neonatal resuscitation

a= ventricular fibrillation; b= pulseless ventricular tachycardia; c= pulseless electrical activity; d= hypoxia, hypovolemia, hyperkalemia and hypokalemia; hypothermia; e= tension pneumothorax, cardiac tamponade, toxins, thrombosis (both cardiac and pulmonary)

perform activities, such as actual taking of vital signs, placing of an electrocardiogram (ECG) electrodes, insertion of intravenous access lines, and dignified handling of the mannequin throughout the course.

For facilitation and scoring purposes, the trainers refer to faculty guides that were developed specifically for the workshops. These guides contain the clinical vignette, case narrative, case learning objectives, critical actions, equipment needed, a step-

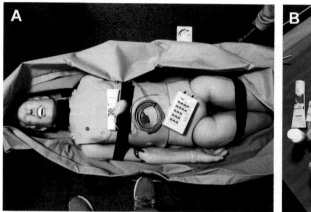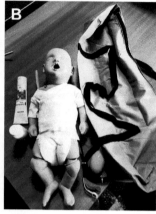

Fig. 1. Low-fidelity simulators. (*A*) adult mannequin and (*B*) pediatric mannequin.

by-step case simulation guide, and guidance for debriefing. The facilitation of the simulation is described in **Fig. 2**.

Skill stations. The skill stations are designed to provide training on key emergency care procedures. The workshop consists of a total of 17 skill stations, as shown in **Table 3**.

Local materials, for example, goat ribs to simulate chest tube insertion, chicken legs for intraosseous access, and locally available plaster or preformed splints are utilized to develop and enhance the skills stations (**Fig. 3**).

All of the medical equipment used by the participants in skill stations is locally acquired and reflects the resources available in the emergency departments in which the trainees work. The faculty utilizes a standardized skills station guide to ensure that the objectives of the stations are achieved by each participant.

Before each practice-based scenario, the faculty select a team leader. The team leader role is rotated amongst the participants who thereafter assigns roles to the other participants of the team. The faculty then convey the title of the simulation, the objectives and review the relevant emergency care algorithm with the team and highlight the fidelity features of the simulation.

Once the scenario starts, the faculty use a facilitative approach during the simulation with the delivery of hints and cues and encouragement of the team leader and the other participants to make reference to the emergency care algorithms to manage the patient appropriately.

At the end of the scenario, the faculty debrief the entire team using standard debriefing guides. The debriefing guides are case-specific and utilise the Gather-Analyse -Summarize (GAS) model i.e. review of the facts of the case (Gather), ask questions to understand the learner thought process (Analyze) and review of the take-home points (Summarize)

Fig. 2. Simulation facilitation.

Table 3
Skill stations

Themes	Skill Stations
Adult resuscitation	(1) Airway management (basic, advanced, and difficult airway) (2) Basic electrocardiogram skills & ST elevation myocardial infarction electrocardiogram skills (3) Adult cardiopulmonary resuscitation and defibrillation

Trauma resuscitation	(4) C-spine stabilization (manual in-line stabilization), helmet removal, Llogrolling & application of head-blocks
	(5) Glasgow Coma scale assessment
	(6) Extended focused assessment using sonography in trauma
	(7) Three-way chest seal and chest tube insertion
	(8) Radiology
	   (a) Head computed tomography scan (traumatic bleeds) practice
	   (b) C-Spine X-ray practice
	   (c) Airway management in trauma
	   (d) Chest X-ray practice
	   (e) Extremities X-ray practice
	   (f) Pelvis X-ray practice
	(9) Pelvic fracture stabilization
	(10) Fracture stabilization (femur, radial–ulnar, tib–fib)
	(11) Mass casualty triage

Obstetric resuscitation	(12) Shoulder dystocia (13) Breech delivery (14) Postpartum hemorrhage (15) Early & late pregnancy scanning
Pediatric resuscitation	(16) Intraosseous access (17) Umbilical vein catheterization

Video presentations and focused discussions. The course incorporates selected video presentations curated to illustrate various elements of emergency care knowledge and practice, for example, condom placement for postpartum hemorrhage. Case discussions based on clinical practice reflection are also included to enhance adult learning and ground the training in local reality.

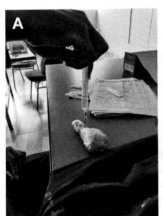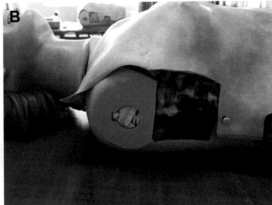

Fig. 3. (*A*) Chicken leg used in the intraosseos access skills station and (*B*) goat ribs in the chest tube insertion station.

Knowledge and skills assessment. The participants take a multiple choice pretest with 30 questions at the beginning of the workshop, which offers a baseline assessment of the participants' knowledge, and a similar post-test at the end of the workshop to evaluate changes in knowledge. The pass mark for the post-test is 70%. Trainees who are not successful are given a second chance to re-evaluate the questions that they missed and provide the correct answers. Failure to achieve the pass mark despite the remediation results in the participant not passing the post-test. The average pretest score so far is 57.3% [interquartile range (IQR) = 20, n = 240], whereas the average post-test score is 76.9% (IQR = 13.3, n = 240) and the difference between the means has been found to be statistically significant using the paired samples t-test (P <0.0001).

The participants are also assessed on the last day as the team leader in one of five standardized simulated patient scenarios that they would have participated in during the workshop. The team leader is assessed based on a set of critical actions that must be performed to pass the simulated patient scenario assessment. Those who are not successful in the assigned scenario are remediated and given a second scenario, failure of which results in the participant not passing the simulated patient scenario assessment. The pass rate for the simulated patient scenario assessment so far is 97.9% (n = 240), with only 5 (2.1%, n = 240) who have not been successful so far.

A 2-year recertifiable certificate is issued to participants who pass both the post-test and the simulated patient scenario assessment. So far, 97.9% (235; n = 240) have been certified in TECC.

Course evaluation. The participants complete an evaluation form to assess each aspect of the course, including the simulation experience, the performance of the facilitators, the learning environment, and the delivery of the content. The assessment is done on a Likert scale with the response anchors ranging from "strongly disagree" to "strongly agree." The feedback is mainly positive, with most items assessed as "agree" or "strongly agree." Themes captured in the qualitative feedback include those on course content (eg, "a lot of knowledge was gained from the training"), case discussions (eg, "'it's good we discuss all the case scenarios"), practical simulations ("Practical cases were realistic and they helped in the learning process," "I like the skills demonstration. Each learner is given a chance to practice."), and future recommendations (eg, "we need more than 5 days of training," "I recommend the training to be done frequently at our institution"). We use this feedback to improve the course.

Post-training mentorship

At the beginning of the course, a WhatsApp group is created with the course participants and the faculty. This allows for online mentorship during and after the course. The participants are encouraged to share interesting cases for discussion and to consult with the faculty at any time through the group. This creates an avenue for continued learning post-course.

DISCUSSION

Development and implementation of local, facility-oriented, simulation-based emergency care training for teams of emergency health care providers with no formal training has the potential to strengthen the emergency health care system in low-resource settings. The success of the participants taking TECC clearly demonstrates that SBT using the local environment and available equipment to simulate the health care workers' day-to-day settings can be used to train teams of health care providers on a systematic approach to assessing critically ill or injured patients in LMIC settings.

LMICs have unique challenges and limitations that SBT should consider during the design stage.[26] Such considerations include the availability of simulation training centers, the pool of trainers, financing, logistical costs of the attendees, and collaboration with the local health authorities.[22,27] Local health care providers, as well as hospital leadership teams and policymakers, must be included in the process of identifying training gaps and contextualizing the training curriculum.[27] This will ensure local buy-in and contribute to the course's sustainability.

Emergency care involves high anxiety and high-risk situations with dire consequences if a failure occurs.[28] This has the potential to create a feeling of being exposed or threatened by the simulation exercise, which may be a barrier to learning.[29] Involvement of local health care providers in the development of the training program can provide local context to ensure practices that uphold psychological safety are appropriately included, for example, setting clear course objectives, the establishment of fiction contrast, giving attention to logistical details, and conveying cultural respect for the learners.[29]

Facility-oriented, simulation-based emergency care training is best taught to practicing health care providers and thus must incorporate various andragogy principles that capture how adults learn.[30] These principles, according to the Knowles andragogy theory, include self-directedness, need to know, use of experience in learning, readiness to learn, orientation to learning, and internal motivation. In SBT, this involves constant learner involvement in the simulation-based scenarios, clinical case discussions, and the incorporation of their experiences. Moreover, the course must largely be problem-centered and focused on issues pertinent to the participant's day-to-day life in the emergency department. The provision of the precourse materials allows for self-directed preparation and prebriefing. Thus, learners are aware of the learning objectives and the ground rules for SBT.[31]

The high cost of simulation equipment and mannequins is a key factor leading to hesitancy in the uptake of SBT in LMICs.[29] The use of low-fidelity simulation equipment and using locally available materials is cost-effective and sustainable.[18] Previous studies have also demonstrated that the use of low-fidelity mannequins is not inferior to that of high-fidelity mannequins.[32] Focus on the psychological fidelity of the simulation rather than on the physical fidelity of the mannequins or other training material has been shown to be effective in achieving skill mastery.[33] Low-fidelity mannequins are effective in enhancing the suspension of reality, particularly when their use is supplemented by other learning methods, such as videos, simulated patients, and locally adapted patient scenarios.[18,27] We have successfully implemented low-cost locally available materials, such as the use of blood transfusion needles and fresh chicken thighs to train intraosseous needle insertion skills and goat ribs for chest tube insertion.

Facility-oriented simulation-based emergency care training is also useful for health care workers to advocate for emergency equipment necessary in their settings, such as ECG machines, vital sign monitors, and defibrillators. In some cases, it also leads to innovation among the trained health care workers to improvise sustainable solutions. For instance, the importance of having a crash cart with clearly labeled equipment and medication was identified during the training, and some facilities improvised by either demarcating already existing cabinets or making some from cardboard.

The major challenge arising from this facility-oriented, simulation-based emergency care training is financing. TECC has been largely financed through short-term grants, and this model is not sustainable. There is a definite need to have buy-in from the hospital administration and policymakers to ensure budget allocation for the continuous training of emergency care workers, especially when there is high staff turnover.[27]

Long-term partnerships with private institutions or external funding organizations are also needed to support the training.[27]

The pool of trainers with the skillset for facility-oriented, simulation-based emergency care training is limited.[22,34] This often results in over-reliance on the few available trainers who are still engaged in clinical practice at their own facilities. Incorporating new trainees in the continuous development of the program and also providing additional training for them to become faculty can assist in addressing this gap. Health care providers with a keen interest in emergency care and a demonstrated desire to teach can undergo certification and re-certification to grow the faculty and ensure consistency with their teaching approach.[27,35]

The variance in the baseline level of emergency care knowledge and training amongst the trainees often results in the slowing down of the course in an attempt to address the various learning gaps. In addition, we have noted that most participants do not go through the precourse reading materials as reflected in their pretest scores and the discussions held. Although this may be viewed as a limitation, it creates an opportunity for increased interaction between the faculty and the participants to enhance learning and ensure the participants grasp the concepts.

Cultural variations must be taken into account during simulations.[27] Scene setting and debriefing exercises must consider the cultural idiosyncrasies of the particular area.[27] Additionally, language and literacy barriers between trainers and trainees, and between the trainees and their future patients, must be taken into consideration. Health care workers in LMICs often have to deal with patients and families with cultural beliefs that impact their acceptance of various aspects of medical care.[27] Debriefing during simulation could also be impacted by cultural beliefs, such as the belief in some communities that the outcome of a patient is always determined by God's will.[27,36] Robust preimplementation surveys on the potential impact of socio-cultural differences on the planned SBT sessions could be conducted to inform strategies on the delivery of the content to ensure the training objectives are achieved.

Post-training mentorship is key and should be followed up by refresher courses. Post-training mentorship would serve to reinforce adherence to evidence-based care and provide an avenue to assess the impact of the training on patient care.[27] In TECC, this has been done through social media groups, for example, WhatsApp. Frequent training and continued education have been shown to improve clinical knowledge and skills as well as boost the morale and confidence of clinicians, which in turn improves patient outcomes.[6]

Future work could explore the use of technology in the form of telesimulation or mHealth in offering both post-training mentorship and refresher courses.[27] Telesimulation is a novel teaching method where the instructor teaches new techniques to a trainee located in a different place using basic videoconferencing software and simulators connected through the Internet.[27] This could be used to target clinicians in far-flung areas who find it difficult to travel to major cities to attend training. Telesimulation enhances affordability, flexibility, and convenience and could be considered for implementation in LMICs.[37]

The majority of health care providers working in the emergency departments in LMICs are junior doctors, clinical officers, and nurses who have no formal training in emergency care.[13,23,38] The introduction of simulation-based emergency care training in medical schools and colleges can act as a bridge toward building the training capacity for SBT in LMICs.[22,39] Further, a shift from traditional methods of learning to more integrated training with an emphasis on simulation-based learning will increase students' enthusiasm, build confidence, and increase clinical competence. This will in turn produce a more knowledgeable and skilled clinician who can train existing health care workers who have not received similar training. This will also have the benefit of reducing the variability in emergency care knowledge between the different cadres working in the emergency departments.

Our article has some limitations. We have focused on how facility-oriented, simulation-based emergency care training is conducted in the TECC course. More data on team performance metrics need to be obtained to assess the impact of the study on team dynamics.[40] Moreover, more research needs to be conducted to assess the impact of the course on patient outcomes as well as on knowledge and skill retention in the long term.[34]

SUMMARY

Development and implementation of a local facility-oriented simulation-based emergency care training program for teams of health care providers with no formal EM training is possible and has the potential to strengthen the emergency health care system in LMICs. Local needs assessment, the use of local emergency care algorithms, consideration of resource limitations, and cultural variation are key to the success of these emergency care training programs. Implementation and continued evaluation of simulation-based emergency care courses is necessary to determine their impact on the emergency health care system in LMICs.

CLINICS CARE POINTS

- In low- and middle-income countries (LMICs), simulation-based emergency care training must be contextualized to local needs and experiences.
- Andragogy principles need to be incorporated into the training of health care providers currently in practice to enhance learning.
- Low-fidelity simulation and incorporation of locally available materials is as effective as high-fidelity equipment when used appropriately.
- Some of the obstacles to the uptake of simulation-based training (SBT) in LMICs include insufficient financing and an inadequate number of trainers.
- Telesimulation has been shown to be as effective as in-person simulation-based training and presents an opportunity to further SBT for emergency medicine in LMICs.

ACKNOWLEDGMENTS

The Emergency Medicine Kenya Foundation which runs the training.

DISCLOSURE

The authors have nothing to disclose.

REFERENCES

1. Reynolds TA, Sawe H, Rubiano AM, et al. Strengthening Health Systems to Provide Emergency Care. In: Jamison DT, Gelband H, Horton S, et al., editors. Disease Control Priorities: Improving Health and Reducing Poverty. 3rd edition. Washington (DC): The International Bank for Reconstruction and Development / The World Bank; 2017 Nov 27. Chapter 13. Available from: https://www.ncbi.nlm.nih.gov/books/NBK525279/ doi: 10.1596/978-1-4648-0527-1_ch13

2. Gaba DM. What does simulation add to teamwork training?. 2006. Available at: https://psnet.ahrq.gov/perspective/what-does-simulation-add-teamwork-training#ref1. Accessed February 24, 2022.

3. Weile J, Nebsbjerg MA, Ovesen SH, et al. Simulation-based team training in time-critical clinical presentations in emergency medicine and critical care: a review of the literature. Adv Simul (Lond) 2021;6(1):3.

4. Shapiro MJ. Simulation based teamwork training for emergency department staff: does it improve clinical team performance when added to an existing didactic teamwork curriculum? Qual Saf Health Care 2004;13(6):417–21.

5. Walker DC, Fritz J, Olvera M, et al. Team training in obstetric and neonatal emergencies using highly realistic simulation in Mexico: impact on process indicators. BMC Pregnancy Childbirth 2014;14:367.

6. Mduma E, Ersdal H, Svensen E, et al. Frequent brief on-site simulation training and reduction in 24-h neonatal mortality–an educational intervention study. Resuscitation 2015;93:1–7.

7. Shrestha R, Shrestha AP, Shrestha SK, et al. Interdisciplinary in situ simulation-based medical education in the emergency department of a teaching hospital in Nepal. Int J Emerg Med 2019;12(1):19.

8. Patterson MD, Geis GL, LeMaster T, et al. Impact of multidisciplinary simulation-based training on patient safety in a paediatric emergency department. BMJ Qual Saf 2013;22(5):383–93.

9. Owen H, Mugford B, Follows V, et al. Comparison of three simulation-based training methods for management of medical emergencies. Resuscitation 2006; 71(2):204–11.

10. Langhan TS, Rigby IJ, Walker IW, et al. Simulation-based training in critical resuscitation procedures improves residents' competence. CJEM 2009;11(6):535–9.

11. Andreatta P. Healthcare simulation in resource-limited regions and global health applications. Simul Healthc 2017;12(3):135–8.

12. Ouma PO, Maina J, Thuranira PN, et al. Access to emergency hospital care provided by the public sector in sub-Saharan Africa in 2015: a geocoded inventory and spatial analysis. Lancet Glob Health 2018;6(3):e342–50.

13. Wachira B, Martin IBK. The state of emergency care in the Republic of Kenya. Afr J Emerg Med 2011;1(4):160–5.

14. Sweeney LA, Warren O, Gardner L, et al. A simulation-based training program improves emergency department staff communication. Am J Med Qual 2014;29(2): 115–23.

15. Davis DW JS. Simulation training and skill assessment in emergency medicine. 2021 [Updated 2021 May 9]. Available at: https://www.ncbi.nlm.nih.gov/books/NBK557695/. Accessed November, 22, 2021.

16. Wang XP, Martin SM, Li YL, et al. [Effect of emergency care simulator combined with problem-based learning in teaching of cardiopulmonary resuscitation]. Zhonghua Yi Xue Za Zhi 2008;88(23):1651–3.

17. Ker JM L, Bradley P. Early introduction to interprofessional learning: a simulated ward environment. Med Educ 2003;37(3):248–55.

18. Gaba DM. The future vision of simulation in health care. Qual Saf Health Care 2004;13(Suppl 1):i2–10.

19. Abass AS, Odufeko TG. Medical simulation a tool yet untapped in most developing nations in Africa. Int J Computer Appl 2014;97(5):1–4.

20. Hunt EA, Shilkofski NA, Stavroudis TA, et al. Simulation: translation to improved team performance. Anesthesiol Clin 2007;25(2):301–19.

21. WHO. Global status report on road safety 2018. Geneva (Switzerland): World Health Organization; 2018.

22. Umoren RA, Ezeaka C, Fajolu I, et al. Simulation-based training in low resource settings: a survey of healthcare providers and learners in Nigeria. Pediatrics 2020;146(1_MeetingAbstract):277.

23. Lee JA, Wanjiku G, Nduku N, et al. The status and future of emergency care in the Republic of Kenya. Afr J Emerg Med 2022;12(1):48–52.

24. Emergency Medicine Kenya Foundation. The emergency care course (TECC). 2022. Available at: https://www.emergencymedicinekenya.org/tecc/. Accessed 17 January, 2022.

25. Emergency Medicine Kenya Foundation. Emergency care algorithms. 2022. Available at: https://www.emergencymedicinekenya.org/algorithms/. Accessed 17 January, 2022.

26. Dieckmann PT K, Qvindesland SA, Thomas L, et al. The use of simulation to prepare and improve responses to infectious disease outbreaks like COVID-19: practical tips and resources from Norway, Denmark, and the UK. Adv Simulation 2020;5(3):1–10.

27. Shilkofski NA, Meaney PA. Simulation in limited-resource settings. In: Grant VC A, editor. Comprehensive healthcare simulation: pediatrics. Cham: Springer; 2016. p. 315–28.

28. Weaver SJ, Salas E, Lyons R, et al. Simulation-based team training at the sharp end: a qualitative study of simulation-based team training design, implementation, and evaluation in healthcare. J Emerg Trauma Shock 2010;3(4):369–77.

29. Rudolph JW, Raemer DB, Simon R. Establishing a safe container for learning in simulation: the role of the presimulation briefing. Simul Healthc 2014;9(6):339–49.

30. Chang S. Applications of andragogy in multi-disciplined teaching and learning. J Adult Education 2010;39(2):25–35.

31. INACSL Standards Committee, McDermott SL, Horsley E, et al. Healthcare simulation standards of best practice TM prebriefing: preparation and briefing. Clin Simulation Nurs 2021;58:9–13.

32. Massoth C, Roder H, Ohlenburg H, et al. High-fidelity is not superior to low-fidelity simulation but leads to overconfidence in medical students. BMC Med Educ 2019;19(1):29.

33. Maran NJ, Glavin RJ. Low- to high-fidelity simulation - a continuum of medical education? Med Educ 2003;37(Suppl 1):22–8.

34. Kivlehan SM, Dixon J, Kalanzi J, et al. Strengthening emergency care knowledge and skills in Uganda and Tanzania with the WHO-ICRC basic emergency care course. Emerg Med J 2021;38(8):636–42.

35. Rybarczyk MM, Ludmer N, Broccoli MC, et al. Emergency medicine training programs in low- and middle-income countries: a systematic review. Ann Glob Health 2020;86(1):60.

36. Rashed GT and Hussien GM. Culture and Health: A study in Medical Anthropology in Kenya. Presented on the 30th Annual International Conference of the Institute of African Research and Studies themed Human Security in Africa in May 2015; Cairo, Egypt.

37. Mikrogianakis A, Kam A, Silver S, et al. Telesimulation: an innovative and effective tool for teaching novel intraosseous insertion techniques in developing countries. Acad Emerg Med 2011;18(4):420–7.

38. Roshana S, Lisa A, Shaza A, et al. Simulation education to advance emergency medicine and pediatric critical care in Nepal. Int J Crit Care Emerg Med 2020; 6(3):1–4.

39. Umoren R, Ezeaka VC, Fajolu IB, et al. Perspectives on simulation-based training from paediatric healthcare providers in Nigeria: a national survey. BMJ Open 2020;10(2):e034029.

40. Shapiro MJ, Gardner R, Godwin SA, et al. Defining team performance for simulation-based training: methodology, metrics, and opportunities for emergency medicine. Acad Emerg Med 2008;15(11):1088–97.

Living on the Edge of Possibility

Ethical Issues in the Care of Critically Ill Patients in Resource-Limited Settings

Immaculate Kariuki-Barasa, MB, ChB, MMed[a],
Mary B. Adam, MD, MA, PhD[a,b],*

KEYWORDS

- Ethical challenges • Critical care medicine • Low-resource settings

KEY POINTS

- Ethical challenges are experienced frequently in critical care service provision and to varying extents depending on levels of growth and complexity.
- Although there are similarities on how these challenges present in both low-resource and high-resource settings, some unique differences emerge that are highlighted in this article.
- Moral distress of healthcare workers (HCW) in low resource contexts (LRC), is an ever present challenge, when pushing the boundaries to offer critically ill patients more complex care in the interest of averting preventable deaths.

BACKGROUND

Ethical challenges have been present in the care of critically ill patients since intensive care medicine was birthed in the height of the 1950s' polio epidemic.[1] The successful transfer of knowledge from anesthesia (where positive pressure ventilation was used) and surgery (where tracheostomies had been done for only about 4 years) to innovate to save the life of a 12-year-old girl with polio in respiratory failure and with bulbar palsy opened the possibility to prevent the death of hundreds of children and adults who were suffocating in their own secretions. Using the combined "new" technology and locally available resources (a tracheostomy performed just below the larynx, a cuffed rubber tube, and a rubber bag), ventilation was delivered manually, and a death was prevented.

[a] AIC Kijabe Hospital, PO Box 20, Kijabe 00220, Kenya; [b] ACQUIRE Africa Mission Healthcare Corporate Offices P.O Box 2320-00621 Nairobi 00621, Kenya.
* Corresponding author. AIC Kijabe Hospital, PO Box 20, Kijabe 00200, Kenya.
E-mail address: Mary.b.adam@gmail.com

Crit Care Clin 38 (2022) 853–863
https://doi.org/10.1016/j.ccc.2022.06.009
0749-0704/22/© 2022 Elsevier Inc. All rights reserved.

criticalcare.theclinics.com

Before this innovation, the Blegham Hospital in Copenhagen was completely unable to support the respiratory needs of patients that the polio epidemic presented.[2] The institutional response to this successful innovation was to keep trying to prevent death. This led to hiring 250 medical students who worked 24/7 to hand ventilate patients. Recognition of the success in terms of lives saved stimulated new thinking about other possibilities to address potentially preventable deaths. The idea of caring for all such patients in a dedicated ward grew so that in 1953, the specialty of intensive care was born.[2]

Historically, the growth in the technical ability to care for critically ill patients in high-income countries (HIC) grew incrementally, step by step, as trials of new technology unfolded. Monitoring, invasive procedures, and disagreement on the correct way to use scarce resources were part of that process.[3] There was a corresponding growth of availability of the "stuff" needed (monitoring, ventilators outside the anesthesia suite) as well as the "staff" (physician, nurses, pharmacists, respiratory therapists, physical therapists) to provide more complex care, as the evidence demonstrated patient's benefiting with successful prolonging of life and recovery of function. However, that growth was uneven. Not all institutions did things the same way.[4] Each stage along the journey brought new ethical concerns and required ethical reflection.[1,5,6]

In each era of development, pushing the technical boundaries of medicine in order to care for critically ill patients presented a wealth of ethical issues. At each step, the questions, "What can we do?" and "What should we do?" produced ethical tension as innovations continued to push the boundaries of technical possibility.[7–10] The questions of "What can we do?" and "What should we do?" are now being asked across the globe. The search for a global consensus on issues such as end of life care, withholding or withdrawing treatment is evidence that the ethical issues present in caring for patients with critical illness is no longer just an HIC problem.[11,12] The ethical challenges in low-resource countries (LRC) mirror those faced in HIC, but with a caveat. In HIC settings, intensive care growth happened incrementally over decades. LRC are able to leapfrog decades of slower technical skill development with faster methods of knowledge transfer, policy pushes, and transparency initiatives. This accelerates access to critical care forward on institutional and national agendas as the burden of chronic disease expands.[10,13–21]

The speed of change means limited time for ethical reflection. There is minimal support from legal systems that are under development in building a framework of case law to respond to these types of questions.[17,22] The challenge is compounded in LRC whereby cultural understanding and meaning of certain procedures may clash with published data reflecting evidenced-based medical probabilities of success.[22,23] For health care workers (HCWs) in LRC, even the best data may not apply well to the patient in front of you. The scope of medical options are an unstudied "in-between" what is available in published data in HIC and national Ministry of Health guidelines.[15,24]

Ethical reflection on caring for critically ill patients (outside the HIV/AIDS sector) is in its infancy within the African context and LRCs in general.[25] Development of capacity to address ethical issues as well as capacity in delivering critical care services is uneven. Addressing moral questions embedded in the care of critically ill patients is now a skill set required in LRCs.[26] Previously, the ethical questions were unnecessary, as there were no other options to address the needs of the patient. Now, however, as capacity to provide care to critically ill patients expands, these ethical questions are becoming more and more a part of everyday practice, further increasing the workload and moral burden on HCWs in LRC. The duty to care and the duty to do no harm, foundational ethical principles, are placed in tension at the edges of possibility.[27,28] This moral tension is palpably present wherever the scientific, technological, and human resource boundaries of care are pushed. Where the questions of what is potentially possible somewhere on the globe, what is possible here and now, and what is possible if we tried one more thing, is an exhausting moral tension HCWs feel acutely in LRCs.

HCWs in LRCs must make decisions in the face of uncertainty, ethical uncertainty, and medical uncertainty. The perspectives on how to best address this uncertainty may vary. Nevertheless, the overarching moral duty to care and the fundamentals of ethical principles are no different anywhere on the globe.

Aim

In this article, we address the ethical issues arising in the care of critically ill patients in LRC using our own experience at AIC Kijabe Hospital, Kenya as a case study. In this case study, we hope to illustrate both similarities and differences in approaches to ethical issues in LRC and allow HCWs across the globe to identify themes common within their own settings. We describe how preserving the value and human dignity of each patient requires ethical reflection based on the context in which care occurs.[29] In addition, we share perspectives on the importance of addressing the moral distress of HCWs in LRC, a challenge ever present, when pushing the boundaries to offer critically ill patients more complex care in the interest of averting preventable deaths.[30]

We organize our case study around a 4D framework, identifying controversial questions that arise in the care of critically ill patients. We address ethical issues in (1) development, (2) delivery, (3) decision making (from policy to cultural perspectives), and (4) moral distress. We phrase questions as HCWs would raise them. In this approach, we describe the pragmatic, the what is, and reflect on how to cope when working on the edge of possibility, the stage of "almost, but not yet."

Development
What do I do now? I don't have an IV pump or a monitor for this preemie. Is doing this halfway better than not trying at all?

The intensive care unit (ICU) at AIC Kijabe Hospital initially arose to support more complex surgical cases where there was need for continuous monitoring postoperatively. Gradually, this extended to additional care for critically ill patients, first to adults, and later to children. In the process, we have learned what is possible with what we have, and we dream of how we push farther and reduce preventable deaths. Crisis and caring drive innovation at the bedside, just as it did in Blegham Hospital in the polio epidemic. The need to improve our services with bigger spaces, more beds, newer machines, and more qualified staff is relentless. We have seen first hand how using local data to develop a context-relevant protocol for treating newborn hypernatremia or adapting low-cost technology like Bubble CPAP dramatically changed our ability to support critically ill patients. The ability to leapfrog technological innovation and adapt it exists. However, this calls for continuous refining and interrogation of health system processes and addressing the ever-emerging ethical issues that arise. As the edge of possibility moves, the answer to the questions of "What can I do?" versus "What should I do?" moves. Do we now resuscitate 600-g infants or keep policy at 700 g?[31]

The uneven growth of ICU services is common in LRC. It may present as a fully equipped ICU or dialysis unit that may be open but not does not have a full-time (or even part-time) critical care specialist or any specialty trained nurses to run it. Other times, trained staff may be available but may not have the infrastructural support to put their knowledge and skills to work. A critical service may expand without the ancillary services, nutrition, physiotherapy, and so forth, to support it. Although most growth will eventually lead to overall quality improvement, it presents new ethical challenges to both staff and institutions. Is it fair of patients and clinicians to ask generalists in a hospital with an ICU to attempt to give critical care in the newly minted ICU or renal unit? Is it ethical to lock the doors of a critical service in the face of dire need, as we wait for the appropriate staff to get trained or hired? The navigation of this in-between state and an attempt to define boundaries for the staff and patients are tedious, difficult, and energy consuming. In addition to clinical decision making, it presents a challenge in moral/ethical decision making. What is an acceptable nurse:patient ratio in ICU if the textbook recommended one cannot be met? How about an ICU design? What are practical physician or nursing staffing patterns for a resource-constrained setting?[32] Do the staffing patterns make a difference in outcomes, and how significant is that difference? These ongoing struggles experienced in HIC during the COVID crises times are more reflective of the ongoing daily struggles in LRCs.

Although improvements have occurred as physicians have wrestled with these questions, they present an extra burden to the already stretched HCWs. Trying to sort out what is aspirational and what is a bare minimum acceptable level of care is an exhausting part of the daily struggle when caring for patients with critical illnesses in LRC.[33]

Delivery of critical care services

Where can I refer this patient? If only they had come earlier.

They need ICU care and cannot afford the expensive private options where there is a bed.

OR

They need post-ICU physical therapy and rehabilitation services, and none even exist in our region/county. What will happen to them now?

OR

What's a general pediatrician like me doing running insulin drips on a 750-g preemie? This is way above my pay grade!

The care process for any health care system, especially care for critically ill patients, is an intersection of many pathways that may include protocols for disease management, admission, and referral criteria as well as ancillary support services.[34,35] Even in settings that have had ICU care for decades, evaluating outcomes and process of care is ongoing because critical care services are expensive and limited in supply. Ethical issues of resource allocation are dominant in the continuous improvement process. Which level of expertise needs to be bedside 24/7 to make key decisions? Where can task shifting be safely implemented? What protocols or bundles of care improve outcomes and patient safety and keep costs manageable? Does doing more make it better?[36]

Although the question in an HIC might be, "Is there evidence for improved outcomes with continuous presence or timely availability of an intensivist in an ICU?" In our setting, there are very few trained intensivists. In Kenya, we have just recently started the training of Fellows in Pediatric Critical Care. The cadre of staff manning the ICU is usually a generalist or a critical care clinical officer. The feeling of being required to make decisions "way above my pay grade" is a common stressor.

In addition, established ICU treatment protocols frequently do not fit our context. Although there are many well-investigated protocols and bundles of care known to improve outcomes or manage costs, they often do not fit the patient you have in front of you or the setting we are working in at Kijabe. This poses the ethical issue of how much is enough? In our experience, having worked in both HIC and LRC, the questions are different, but the ethical themes are the same. When in the HIC, the question is more often when withholding treatment is ethically permissible, not who get ICU care. While in the LRC, the ethical tensions are more often about who gets ICU care. This is because more is available in HIC. However, more does not always mean better. The value and dignity of human beings do not change based on age, location, gender, race, education, or economic status. Good enough for Africa but not good enough for HIC is ethically abhorrent. Context-specific capacity does not change the presence of ethical issues of resource allocation even as the implementation capacity changes. Which adult in respiratory failure with COVID gets extracorporeal membrane oxygenation in the West, where capacity is greater, is an ethical question of resource allocation paralleled in our setting by who gets the ventilator? As COVID began, our institution made a hard decision that we would not intubate COVID patients over 50 years of age, even if they were staff. This was a military triage type of decision because we only had 3 critical care spaces and 2 ventilators that were available in the COVID unit.

There will be many instances when what is known to be best practice will not be feasible in our setting. Faced with this reality, the clinician must address the challenge as a *provision level* allocation problem, not a *policy level* dilemma. For us at Kijabe, this took the form of creating a rehydration protocol for newborns with hypernatremia who in HIC would have gone straight into a renal unit for dialysis. It looked like building training programs to upskill midlevel providers called clinical officers to be able to offer 24/7 coverage in the ICU. There are ethical issues that come in this innovation phase: Are we doing the right thing? Should we close this ICU if we don't have intensivists? Is trying this rehydration protocol since I don't have dialysis better than doing nothing? Historically these questions have been asked as technology and service options to care for critically ill patients expand.[37] These are difficult allocation questions because who gets scarce services may determine who lives and who dies.[38]

Away from the bedside, the ancillary support services and multidisciplinary teams that are necessary to have fully integrated and efficient critical care services and rehabilitative post-ICU care services are often unavailable or rudimentary in many LIC settings.[39] This has repercussions on the outcomes of patients who have lower potential to obtain full functional recovery because of lower quality of care owing to ancillary services. We see this in Kijabe's neonatal ICU (NICU) where the absence of comprehensive post-NICU care dooms surviving neonates and their families to suboptimal long-term outcomes. Our technical capacity to support 600- to 1000-g infants is stunted because of the uneven development of prenatal care (especially for poor women) in addition to the minimal availability of post-NICU rehabilitative care.

Decision making: policy level tradeoffs at macro (national) and micro (institution) level systems

What are these policymakers thinking? Why did they "baptize" this facility as ICU but not bring the trained staff we need? Who here even knows how to use that ventilator or to suction out a tracheostomy?

Why are they expanding the ICU when in our country we can't even get children fully immunized for real preventable lifesaving things like measles and rotavirus?

There is no perfect blueprint that creates an ideal health care system.[40] The structuring of health financing and resource allocation is an ethical question at both institutional and national levels. "Who pays" and "how" is a question across the globe.[41]

In most HIC, health care is financed by governments and or private health care insurance, protecting families from catastrophic financial cost. In our setting, most of the health care costs are transferred to household budgets with catastrophic impact on families.[42,43]

Significant ethical issues related to financing and resource allocation arise in the decision-making pathway when expanding care for critically ill patients. At the macro and the meso level, the process and framework for health care priority setting are mostly ad hoc rather than systematic. Policymakers may have to hold the tension of prioritization of preventable illnesses versus critical care services.[44,45] There is evidence that early presentation of patients or timely referrals would lead to patient improvement with minimal and less costly interventions. Theoretically, a focus on more well-integrated primary health services and referral pathways is likely to reduce downstream influx of critically ill patients. However, institutional, state, and even household budgets do not often reflect this in part because primary care and referral services in our context are weaker. There can be a feeling of a mismatch of national and institutional strategy weighted toward technology for advanced disease care and not preventive care. For health care leaders, the development of good health care processes at both extremes of the disease spectrum when resources are scarce is challenging. Should we aspire to growing both simultaneously or in one direction at a time? What is a good prioritization strategy? When there is a huge variance in the level/quality of care received from one institution to another, how do you make appropriate comparisons or extract data for population-level decision making? What is a good measure of success? Is it in a state-of-the-art, evidence-based health system that cares for few or is it in benefits accrued to many? Our big question at Kijabe has been, "What is expensive but still worth doing?" while also asking, "What is possible with what we have?"

At the national health policy level, whether to train more trauma surgeons, open surgical ICUs, or deploy more road safety enforcers to prevent morbidity and mortality from trauma are dimensions of health system growth that are in tension. In a perfect world, all parts should receive all the resources they need to grow simultaneously. However, we do not live in a perfect world. Ethical challenges fall on both HCWs and policy makers as they grapple with what to prioritize. At Kijabe, these tensions may play out in deciding where to allocate its few physicians. Is it to the diabetic/hypertension clinic to provide optimum outpatient care or to the ICU unit to manage the complications of diabetes/hypertension? How does the leadership navigate a course and direction to address the complexity of the problems?

External donors often drive the agenda without meeting the prioritized institutional or population needs.[45] This has an opportunity cost and often contributes to the uneven growth of care available for the critically ill patient and for the patient with routine illnesses. Donor-driven agendas meet important needs like subsidized specialist surgical services at Kijabe. However, the care needed is not evenly subsidized for all patients even within the same institution. This type of inequality brings added stress on providers who work across the units and must function where donor funding makes critical care services possible as well as needing to care for patients who need but are not benefited by the subsidized critical care (can we, yes; should we, no, because there are no financial means). Forcing physicians to explain we cannot offer this care to a patient because of finances, when across the hall finances are not the determining factor is very stressful, contributing to the moral burden of caring for critically ill patients.

When we interrogate admission protocols and referral systems, common themes emerge. Are our critical care units admitting the right patients? Who shall we try to save in this facility? If not here, where shall we refer them to? Where do we get the appropriate ambulance to transfer them? Can the patient afford this type of care? Is there a pathway for referring patients to facilities with a lower and less expensive level of care once they are stabilized? Is there space in the "referral" center whatever the level? How do we decide? What is the opportunity cost and risk (for patient, family, and HCWs) of taking care of a patient beyond our capabilities? The answers to these questions in LRC contexts are ill defined in part because they are ever changing. For example, within Kijabe at the unit level, we can schedule very complex head and neck surgical cases based on a daily bed availability assessment in the ICU, offering the option of complex care opening without "turning patients away." This places the moral and ethical burden of decision making more on the individual HCWs staffing the ICU/head and neck unit rather than the system.

Distress
Please, I beg you, I will work anywhere, just don't put me back in the ICU. I can't see one more patient die. I can't take it anymore. They already call me the "body packager."

How can I stop? The family says do everything, but nothing we can do will change the clinical outcome. Continuing will liquidate resources that the family needs to feed the other children.

I was so angry when the doctor said stop the resuscitation after 3 rounds of epinephrine! I get it, but the child was the same age as my daughter. How do I play with my 3-year-old and not cry when I get home?

High clinical workload and care for seriously ill patients are known risk factors for diminished well-being of HCWs especially in settings with resource constraints.[46] Diminished personal well-being may present as emotional distress, compassion fatigue, or burnout in addition to other mental health challenges.[47] Because HCWs do not make clinical decisions in a vacuum, the overall resource pressure resulting from institutional and national policy themes may also exacerbate distress. Recognition of this reality and creation of safety nets to protect patients and staff are paramount.[48]

As more families have more access to care (including ICU care), deaths that would have otherwise occurred at home are now occurring in the hospital. In settings where robust and fully developed palliative services are minimal, hospitalists have to grapple with good end-of-life care processes. In our context at Kijabe, we are just beginning to examine questions like, What does a good death in a critical care unit look like? When can the natural process of death be allowed to occur in absence of advance patient directives? How do we create a pathway for more collaborative decision making in our communitarian context,[8] when the patient is incapacitated, especially as cultural norms (firstborn son) do not line up with legal surrogate decision makers (spouse)? We often wonder what is determining family decisions: patients' wishes or resource availability?

The best application of recognized ethical principles like respect and patient autonomy requires a thorough understanding of social cultural issues. For example, kin caregivers are a recognized pillar in the health care provision to children in many African contexts and exert substantive influence during decision making, including in the ICU.[49] Family harmony, with elder input, is often essential to a good decision, even when the parent alone is the legal decision maker for the child. This is highly nuanced. There are also distinct cultural differences and approaches to health in the different microcosms (ie, urban vs rural, low- vs high-income households, and different ethnic communities).[50] The cultural factors that drive ethical tensions may differ from patient to patient, but the moral responsibility to uphold patient's value and dignity still stands.

SUMMARY

The birth of critical care medicine as a specialty and the subsequent progress in HIC in the ability to care for critically ill patients shows recurring patterns. Themes, such as pushing the boundaries of possibility, the drive for innovation, combining new skills and locally available resources, or uneven progress based on region, look to a possibility in the hope of preventing death. These themes are now present in LRCs as the ability to care for critically ill patients is expanding across the globe. In LRC, the additional resource pressure in an effort to improve, innovate, and provide quality care in immature/incomplete/growing health care systems can easily be a source of moral distress to the clinicians. We have just described layers of ethical challenges that HCWs in low- to middle-income countries experience as part of their daily reality: working in a context with few safety nets. Even in this scenario, preserving the value and human dignity of each patient is essential and possible. At AIC Kijabe Hospital, the development of an ethics committee and the training of HCWs on ethical approaches to the issues is one of the ways we hope to reduce the moral distress present for families and clinicians and to support ethical institutional decision making. Although we are yet to develop or use validated institutional strategies (such as routine debriefing) to promote personal or team self-care, we recognize that growth in services for critically ill patients has to move beyond the bedside to include the development, decision making, and delivery of services that demonstrate consistent implementation of moral and ethical principles permeating care for both patient and clinician.

CLINICS CARE POINTS

- The duty to care and the duty to do no harm, foundational ethical principles, are placed in tension at the edges of possibility
- Proactive approaches to addressing moral distress among health care workers in critical care contexts is necessary.

FUNDING

There was no funding for this work.

DISCLOSURE

Neither author has any commercial or financial interest to declare.

REFERENCES

1. Luce JM, White DB. A history of ethics and law in the intensive care unit. Crit Care Clin 2009;25(1):221–37, x.
2. Kelly FE, Fong K, Hirsch N, et al. Intensive care medicine is 60 years old: the history and future of the intensive care unit. Clin Med 2014;14(4):376–9.
3. Weil M, Shubin H. The new practice of critical care medicine. Chest 1971;59(5): 473–4.

4. Weil MH, Tang W. From intensive care to critical care medicine: a historical perspective. Historical Article Support and AuthorAnonymous, Research Support, Non-U.S. Gov't. Am J Respir Crit Care Med 2011;183(11):1451–3. https://doi.org/10.1164/rccm.201008-1341OE.

5. Placencia FX, McCullough LB. The history of ethical decision making in neonatal intensive care. J Intensive Care Med 2011;26(6):368–84.

6. Cohen CB. Ethical problems of intensive care. Anesthesiology 1977;47(2):217–27.

7. Liu J, Chen XX, Wang XL. Ethical issues in neonatal intensive care units. Research Support, Non-U.S. Gov't. Review. J Matern Fetal Neonatal Med 2016;29(14):2322–6. https://doi.org/10.3109/14767058.2015.1085016.

8. Lantos JD. Ethical problems in decision making in the neonatal ICU. N Engl J Med 2018;379(19):1851–60.

9. Neville TH, Wiley JF, Kardouh M, et al. Change in inappropriate critical care over time. Research Support, N.I.H., Extramural. J Crit Care 2020;60:267–72. https://doi.org/10.1016/j.jcrc.2020.08.028.

10. Losonczy LI, Papali A, Kivlehan S, et al. White paper on early critical care services in low resource settings. Ann Glob Health 2021;87(1):105.

11. Sprung CL, Truog RD, Curtis JR, et al. Seeking worldwide professional consensus on the principles of end-of-life care for the critically ill. The consensus for worldwide end-of-life practice for patients in intensive care units (WELPICUS) study. Consensus development conference. Am J Respir Crit Care Med 2014;190(8):855–66. https://doi.org/10.1164/rccm.201403-0593CC.

12. Myburgh JMDP, Abillama FMD, Chiumello DMD, et al. End-of-life care in the intensive care unit: report from the task force of world federation of societies of intensive and critical care medicine. J Crit Care 2016;34:125–30.

13. Murthy S, Leligdowicz A, Adhikari NK. Intensive care unit capacity in low-income countries: a systematic review. PLoS One 2015;10(1):e0116949.

14. Slusher TM, Kiragu AW, Day LT, et al. Pediatric critical care in resource-limited settings-overview and lessons learned. Front 2018;6:49. https://doi.org/10.3389/fped.2018.00049.

15. Riviello ED, Letchford S, Achieng L, et al. Critical care in resource-poor settings: lessons learned and future directions. Crit Care Med 2011;39(4):860–7.

16. Schell CO, Khalid K, Wharton-Smith A, et al. Essential emergency and critical care: a consensus among global clinical experts. BMJ Glob Health 2021;6(9):e006585.

17. Monsudi KF, Oladele TO, Nasir AA, et al. Medical ethics in sub-Sahara Africa: closing the gaps. Afr Health Sci 2015;15(2):673–81.

18. Tumukunde J, Sendagire C, Ttendo SS. Development of intensive care in low-resource regions. Curr Anesthesiology Rep 2019;9(1):15–7.

19. Bjorklund A, Slusher T, Day LT, et al. Pediatric Critical care in resource limited settings—lessening the gap through ongoing collaboration, advancement in research and technological innovations. Front 2022. https://doi.org/10.3389/fped.2021.791255.

20. Pronovost P, Thompson DA, Holzmueller CG, et al. Impact of the Leapfrog Group's intensive care unit physician staffing standard. J Crit Care 2007;22(2):89–96.

21. Milestone D, Ashok M, Dobos D. Leapfrog to value. Global development incubator. 2022. Available at: https://www.leapfrogtovalue.org/flagship-report. Accessed Feburary 7, 2022.

22. Stonington SD. The debt of life–Thai lessons on a process-oriented ethical logic. N Engl J Med 2013;369(17):1583–5.
23. Nyman DJ, Sprung CL. International perspectives on ethics in critical care. Review. Crit Care Clin 13(2), 1997, 409-415.
24. Vineis P. Evidence-based medicine and ethics: a practical approach. J Med Ethics 2004;30(2):126–30.
25. Moodley K, Kabanda SM, Kleinsmidt A, et al. COVID-19 underscores the important role of clinical ethics committees in Africa. BMC Med Ethics 2021;22(1):131.
26. Moodley K, Rennie S, Behets F, et al. Allocation of scarce resources in Africa during COVID-19: utility and justice for the bottom of the pyramid? Developing World Bioeth 2021;21(1):36–43.
27. Pellegrino ED. For the patient's good: the restoration of beneficence in health care, 100. Oxford University Press; 1988. p. 434–6.
28. Schumann JH, Alfandre D. Clinical ethical decision making: the four topic approach. Semin Med Pract 2008;11:7.
29. Kilner JF. Dignity and destiny: humanity in the image of God. New Haven CT: Wm. B. Eerdmans Publishing Company; 2015.
30. Fourie C. Moral distress and moral conflict in clinical ethics. Research Support, Non-U.S. Gov't. Bioethics 2015;29(2):91–7. https://doi.org/10.1111/bioe.12064.
31. Basnet S, Adhikari N, Koirala J. Challenges in setting up pediatric and neonatal intensive care units in a resource-limited country. Pediatrics. Oct 128(4), 2011, E986-E992.
32. Pronovost PJ, Angus DC, Dorman T, et al. Physician staffing patterns and clinical outcomes in critically ill patients: a systematic review. JAMA 2002;288(17): 2151–62.
33. Vincent J-L. Critical care-where have we been and where are we going? Crit Care 2013;17(1):1–6.
34. Diaz JV, Riviello ED, Papali A, Adhikari NKJ, Ferreira JC. Global Critical Care: Moving Forward in Resource-Limited Settings. Ann Glob Health. 2019;22:85(1):3 Available at: https://annalsofglobalhealth.org/articles/10.5334/aogh.2413/. Accessed July 20, 2022
35. Craig J, Kalanxhi E, Hauck S. National estimates of critical care capacity in 54 African countries. medRxiv 2020. https://doi.org/10.1101/2020.05.13.20100727.
36. Weled BJ, Adzhigirey LA, Hodgman TM, et al. Critical care delivery: the importance of process of care and ICU structure to improved outcomes: an update from the american college of critical care medicine task force on models of critical care. Crit Care Med 2015;43(7):1520–5.
37. Kilner JF. A moral allocation of scarce lifesaving medical resources. J Relig Ethics 1981;17(2):245–85.
38. Kilner JF. Who lives? Who dies?: ethical criteria in patient selection. New Haven, CT: Yale University Press; 1990.
39. Louw Q, editor. Collaborative capacity development to complement stroke rehabilitation in Africa [Internet]. Cape Town (ZA): AOSIS; 2020. PMID: 34606188. Accessed July 21, 2022
40. Mills A. Health care systems in low-and middle-income countries. N Engl J Med 2014;370(6):552–7.
41. Liaropoulos L, Goranitis I. Health care financing and the sustainability of health systems. Int J Equity Health 2015;14(1):80.
42. Salari P, Di Giorgio L, Ilinca S, et al. The catastrophic and impoverishing effects of out-of-pocket healthcare payments in Kenya, 2018. BMJ Glob Health 2019;4(6): e001809.

43. Kairu A, Orangi S, Mbuthia B, et al. Examining health facility financing in Kenya in the context of devolution. BMC Health Serv Res 2021;21(1):1086.
44. Barasa EW, Molyneux S, English M, et al. Setting healthcare priorities at the macro and meso levels: a framework for evaluation. Int J Health Policy Manag 2015;4(11):719–32.
45. Dzeng E, Curtis JR. Understanding ethical climate, moral distress, and burnout: a novel tool and a conceptual framework. BMJ Qual Saf 2018;27(10):766–770.
46. Dzeng E, Curtis JR. Understanding ethical climate, moral distress, and burnout: a novel tool and a conceptual framework. BMJ Publishing Group Ltd; 2018. p. 766–70.
47. Ramírez-Elvira S, Romero-Béjar JL, Suleiman-Martos N, et al. Prevalence, risk factors and burnout levels in intensive care unit nurses: a systematic review and meta-analysis. Int J Environ Res Public Health 2021;18(21):11432.
48.. Shapiro GK, Schulz-Quach C, Matthew A, et al. An institutional model for health care workers' mental health during Covid-19. NEJM Catalyst Innov Care Deliv 2021;2(2). https://catalyst.nejm.org/doi/full/10.1056/CAT.20.0684. [Accessed 20 July 2022].
49. Mabetha K, De Wet-Billings NC, Odimegwu CO. Healthcare beliefs and practices of kin caregivers in South Africa: implications for child survival. BMC Health Serv Res 2021;21(1):486.
50. Abubakar A, Van Baar A, Fischer R, et al. Socio-cultural determinants of health-seeking behaviour on the Kenyan coast: a qualitative study. PLoS One 2013; 8(11):e71998.

UNITED STATES POSTAL SERVICE® | **Statement of Ownership, Management, and Circulation (All Periodicals Publications Except Requester Publications)**

1. Publication Title
CRITICAL CARE CLINICS

2. Publication Number
000 – 708

3. Filing Date
9/18/2022

4. Issue Frequency
JAN, APR, JUL, OCT

5. Number of Issues Published Annually
4

6. Annual Subscription Price
$266.00

7. Complete Mailing Address of Known Office of Publication (Not printer) (Street, city, county, state, and ZIP+4®)
ELSEVIER INC.
230 Park Avenue, Suite 800
New York, NY 10169

Contact Person
Malathi Samayan

Telephone (Include area code)
91-44-4299-4507

8. Complete Mailing Address of Headquarters or General Business Office of Publisher (Not printer)
ELSEVIER INC.
230 Park Avenue, Suite 800
New York, NY 10169

9. Full Names and Complete Mailing Addresses of Publisher, Editor, and Managing Editor (Do not leave blank)

Publisher (Name and complete mailing address)
DOLORES MELONI, ELSEVIER INC.
1600 JOHN F KENNEDY BLVD. SUITE 1800
PHILADELPHIA, PA 19103-2899

Editor (Name and complete mailing address)
JOANNA COLLETT, ELSEVIER INC.
1600 JOHN F KENNEDY BLVD. SUITE 1800
PHILADELPHIA, PA 19103-2899

Managing Editor (Name and complete mailing address)
PATRICK MANLEY, ELSEVIER INC.
1600 JOHN F KENNEDY BLVD. SUITE 1800
PHILADELPHIA, PA 19103-2899

10. Owner (Do not leave blank. If the publication is owned by a corporation, give the name and address of the corporation immediately followed by the names and addresses of all stockholders owning or holding 1 percent or more of the total amount of stock. If not owned by a corporation, give the names and addresses of the individual owners. If owned by a partnership or other unincorporated firm, give its name and address as well as those of each individual owner. If the publication is published by a nonprofit organization, give its name and address.)

Full Name	Complete Mailing Address
WHOLLY OWNED SUBSIDIARY OF REED/ELSEVIER, US HOLDINGS	1600 JOHN F KENNEDY BLVD. SUITE 1800 PHILADELPHIA, PA 19103-2899

11. Known Bondholders, Mortgagees, and Other Security Holders Owning or Holding 1 Percent or More of Total Amount of Bonds, Mortgages, or Other Securities. If none, check box ► ☐ None

Full Name	Complete Mailing Address
N/A	

12. Tax Status (For completion by nonprofit organizations authorized to mail at nonprofit rates) (Check one)
The purpose, function, and nonprofit status of this organization and the exempt status for federal income tax purposes:
☒ Has Not Changed During Preceding 12 Months
☐ Has Changed During Preceding 12 Months (Publisher must submit explanation of change with this statement)

PS Form **3526**, July 2014 [Page 1 of 4 (see instructions page 4)] PSN: 7530-01-000-9931   PRIVACY NOTICE: See our privacy policy on www.usps.com.

---

13. Publication Title
CRITICAL CARE CLINICS

14. Issue Date for Circulation Data Below
JULY 2022

15. Extent and Nature of Circulation

			Average No. Copies Each Issue During Preceding 12 Months	No. Copies of Single Issue Published Nearest to Filing Date
a. Total Number of Copies (Net press run)			286	262
b. Paid Circulation (By Mail and Outside the Mail)	(1)	Mailed Outside-County Paid Subscriptions Stated on PS Form 3541 (Include paid distribution above nominal rate, advertiser's proof copies, and exchange copies)	171	162
	(2)	Mailed In-County Paid Subscriptions Stated on PS Form 3541 (Include paid distribution above nominal rate, advertiser's proof copies, and exchange copies)	0	0
	(3)	Paid Distribution Outside the Mails Including Sales Through Dealers and Carriers, Street Vendors, Counter Sales, and Other Paid Distribution Outside USPS®	69	63
	(4)	Paid Distribution by Other Classes of Mail Through the USPS (e.g., First-Class Mail®)	0	0
c. Total Paid Distribution (Sum of 15b (1), (2), (3), and (4))		►	240	225
d. Free or Nominal Rate Distribution (By Mail and Outside the Mail)	(1)	Free or Nominal Rate Outside-County Copies included on PS Form 3541	30	21
	(2)	Free or Nominal Rate In-County Copies Included on PS Form 3541	0	0
	(3)	Free or Nominal Rate Copies Mailed at Other Classes Through the USPS (e.g., First-Class Mail)	0	0
	(4)	Free or Nominal Rate Distribution Outside the Mail (Carriers or other means)	0	0
e. Total Free or Nominal Rate Distribution (Sum of 15d (1), (2), (3) and (4))		►	30	21
f. Total Distribution (Sum of 15c and 15e)		►	270	246
g. Copies not Distributed (See Instructions to Publishers #4 (page #3))		►	16	16
h. Total (Sum of 15f and g)		►	286	262
i. Percent Paid (15c divided by 15f times 100)		►	88.88%	91.46%

* If you are claiming electronic copies, go to line 16 on page 3. If you are not claiming electronic copies, skip to line 17 on page 3.

PS Form **3526**, July 2014 (Page 2 of 4)

16. Electronic Copy Circulation

		Average No. Copies Each Issue During Preceding 12 Months	No. Copies of Single Issue Published Nearest to Filing Date
a. Paid Electronic Copies	►		
b. Total Paid Print Copies (Line 15c) + Paid Electronic Copies (Line 16a)	►		
c. Total Print Distribution (Line 15f) + Paid Electronic Copies (Line 16a)	►		
d. Percent Paid (Both Print & Electronic Copies) (16b divided by 16c × 100)	►		

☒ I certify that 60% of all my distributed copies (electronic and print) are paid above a nominal price.

17. Publication of Statement of Ownership
☒ If the publication is a general publication, publication of this statement is required. Will be printed in the OCTOBER 2022 issue of this publication.   ☐ Publication not required.

18. Signature and Title of Editor, Publisher, Business Manager, or Owner

Malathi Samayan

Malathi Samayan - Distribution Controller

Date
9/18/2022

I certify that all information furnished on this form is true and complete. I understand that anyone who furnishes false or misleading information on this form or who omits material or information requested on the form may be subject to criminal sanctions (including fines and imprisonment) and/or civil sanctions (including civil penalties).

PS Form **3526**, July 2014 (Page 3 of 4)   PRIVACY NOTICE: See our privacy policy on www.usps.com.

Moving?

Make sure your subscription moves with you!

To notify us of your new address, find your **Clinics Account Number** (located on your mailing label above your name), and contact customer service at:

Email: journalscustomerservice-usa@elsevier.com

800-654-2452 (subscribers in the U.S. & Canada)
314-447-8871 (subscribers outside of the U.S. & Canada)

Fax number: 314-447-8029

Elsevier Health Sciences Division
Subscription Customer Service
3251 Riverport Lane
Maryland Heights, MO 63043

*To ensure uninterrupted delivery of your subscription, please notify us at least 4 weeks in advance of move.

ELSEVIER